CONTENTS

To the memory of Dr R.M. Gibson, OBE,
and to his original team,
Miss Dorothy Daley
Miss Marie Finlay
Miss Betty McIntyre
and
Miss Grace Parbery

FOREWORD

If a person becomes ill he will either succumb or survive.

If he survives, recovery might be complete or incomplete. When recovery is incomplete he suffers from residual disability.

The pathological diagnosis does not describe the degree of disability nor does it necessarily lead to appropriate management. The significance of disability in any one person must be viewed both objectively and subjectively and relates to many other factors such as an individual's personality and resources. Moreover any person may be affected by more than one pathological condition each of which may contribute in various ways to his overall state.

The physiological changes of ageing adversely affect our capacity to adapt to illness. For some people, progress through life may be punctuated by illness which may result in an accumulation of disabilities. Nevertheless, we know from experience (and this is supported by scientific evidence) that aged people can benefit from mental and physical activity and that much of what society sees as the inevitable accompaniments of ageing are in fact the result of social attitudes rather than the inevitable effects of the ageing process.

People admitted to geriatric units characteristically are those unfortunate enough to have developed disabling illness and as a result have multiple problems which must be solved if they are to be able to manage outside of hospitals and institutions. While in some disease states we can expect complete recovery, in others expectations cannot be placed so high. Indeed it is true to say that it is impossible to predict the outcome of any illness in a particular person. This is especially apparent in certain conditions such as strokes, arthritis and Parkinson's Disease which, as everyone knows, commonly result in physical and mental disability.

If we accept this philosophy that the outcome of illness cannot be predicted for any one person, then we can understand why the management of disability in ageing people must be based on problem solving and why it is important to set realistic goals.

Through problem solving we seek to provide remedies which will improve health, prevent complications and help compensate for disability by making the greatest use of residual abilities. At the same time, we build on gains as they occur. Thus there is the need for

1

continual reappraisal and reassessment which are not an end in themselves but means towards an end.

Problems such as body image disturbance associated with strokes, impaired special senses, confusion, anxiety and depression commonly occur in patients referred to geriatric units. Such problems are frequently associated with heart and lung disease. Further, if due to the nature of the illness itself a person is disinclined to, or afraid of, physical activity, this very inactivity can result in increasing weakness. Thus disability tends to beget more disability.

If people thus affected are to achieve their main aim (and that is to live at home) they will need to build up their physical strength and to compensate for disability by acquiring new skills which make the best use of residual abilities.

Problems for disabled people do not cease at 'knock off' time. Therefore the techniques of enablement and training must be practised in the practical context and continue 'around the clock'. This applies particularly to people who have difficulties with comprehension and who, therefore, will learn these new skills through repetition of patterns of movement. Those people who have the greatest disabilities also have the greatest needs.

Again unless techniques are consistent for each patient under all circumstances, progress will be impeded, dangerous situations will result and the chance to teach relatives to use and gain from methods of management will be lost. It is therefore necessary that the techniques of enablement and retraining be incorporated into the nursing process. The nurse then becomes the teacher of both the patient and carer, and is able to assess the value of techniques in all practical situations before they are handed on to relatives and carers.

Ideally geriatric units should have staff trained in various disciplines who understand the principles of geriatrics and who work together to solve problems. Through sharing knowledge everyone can enhance their own contributions and those with specialised training can use their time in teaching and in testing standards.

In writing this book Margaret Mort is sharing her knowledge and experience gained over many years. Miss Mort first trained as an artist and teacher. As well as this she has an innate flair for design. When she trained as an occupational therapist she brought these skills with her. In 1960 she joined the William Lyne Unit of the Royal Newcastle Hospital, New South Wales. She brought with her the experience she gained in Oxford working with Lionel Cosin in the management of confused elderly people.

As early as 1957 the William Lyne Unit of the Royal Newcastle Hospital had laid the foundations of the 'multidisciplinary team' approach under the guidance of the late Dr Richard Gibson, Miss Grace Parbery (social worker), Miss Betty McIntyre (occupational therapist) and an enlightened nursing staff. Using nursing staff in the processes of enabling, rehabilitating and retraining was at first seen as a logical way of overcoming shortages of other specialised staff. However, it soon became apparent that this approach was a necessity if such activities were to achieve the greatest effectiveness.

Further, if severely disabled people were to be managed at home it became obvious that relatives must be taught techniques which took advantage of the patients' strengths and used balancing to avoid lifting. In carrying through these principles it was necessary to take a functional and simplified approach which in the long run proved to be not only expedient but also the most rational one. By standardising techniques and equipment, Miss Mort developed this approach which is described in this book.

Most people contributing to the care of ageing and disabled people have not had special training. For this reason it is necessary to keep a text such as this as simple as possible if it is to reach and help the people most in need and the majority who provide the care for them. Thus this book avoids, where possible, the use of confusing terminology and describes principles which can be applied to situations. For instance, the term 'reality orientation' does not appear as a separate chapter. However, much care and space is given to teaching the importance of first attending to basic needs, and to instruction in the techniques of orientation.

This book does not discuss or offer training in specialised techniques such as those specifically directed to management of spasticity or incontinence. Such information, though important, is beyond the practical scope of this book. That is not to imply that all manner of special techniques cannot be used along with those described. However, the benefits derived in achieving independence include the alleviation of incontinence and being able to stand without fear is surely a most practical way of treating spasticity and preventing contractures in the lower limbs. As well, that is a simple treatment which can be done easily at home.

This book is a practical guide for dealing with disability in ageing people. It should prove valuable to a wide variety of people such as nurses, doctors, families and carers, volunteers and paramedical specialists.

Kevin Grant
Director of the Department of Geriatrics
Royal Newcastle Hospital

PREFACE

The programme described in this book has developed over a period of more than 25 years at the Royal Newcastle Hospital in New South Wales. It grew in response to the practical needs of patients who, having been treated by conventional means, were left with residual disabilities to a degree that their successful return to the community was jeopardised. When such people return home without help in overcoming their disabilities, and when relatives are not advised in management techniques, a breakdown in family relationships is likely to occur. Nursing home or other institutional care may be seen as the only answer.

The retraining programme presented here is a problem-solving process, designed to serve in such situations. One of its main strengths is its coordination of many services under one director, combined with close team-work between the staff, the patient and his relatives.

Most of the problems encountered can be grouped in one of three categories — psychological, physical and social — but it should be remembered that varying combinations and degrees of all three may be found in any particular case. Where these aspects are separated in the text it is for the purpose of simplifying the discussion. They should never be treated in isolation in the individual patient.

Physical retraining methods are designed to help those with learning or emotional problems as well as those who are better motivated and more mentally alert. They are based upon the repetition of routine movements, used by all who work with the patient. They should be started as soon as possible in his treatment programme. Involvement of the patient is an essential element.

The movements used to retrain the patients are known as 'drills'. This word has been questioned because of its military connotation, but despite searches through dictionary and thesaurus, and discussions with many interested people, no other word has been found which includes the basic idea of learning a movement by accurate repetition of its components. To those who have negative feelings about the term it should be emphasised that the 'drills' are adjusted for the individual patient as necessary. His own special pattern of movement is then used by those who work with him.

In this book, as in the retraining programme, everyday words have been used rather than technical terms or jargon. Words which may cause difficulties have been listed in the glossary. It is hoped that non-technical language will make the book accessible to a wide range of readers, just as the programme itself is available to doctors, administrators, nurses, assistant nurses, therapists and their aides, wardsmen, relatives and patients. The chapters have grown out of lectures to people in all these categories and from their requests for a text book on the subject.

For clarity, and because of the clumsiness of combined forms such as 'he/she' and others of its kind, 'he' has been used for the patient and 'she' for the helper throughout the book. Anyone who sees this as discriminatory is at liberty to transpose the pronouns to suit his/her own preferences. Patients and helpers may be either male or female in any situation described.

It remains for me to thank all those who have played a part in the production of this book; the relatives, patients and fellow members of the retraining team out of whose experience it grew, the students whose interest and questions helped to integrate the material, and the original team members, led by the late Dr R.M. Gibson, OBE, by whom the foundations of the programme were laid. Particular acknowledgement should be made to the following: Dr L.Z. Cosin of Oxford who introduced me to the discipline of Geriatrics in 1950; Dr Kevin Grant and Miss Betty McIntyre for kindly looking over the chapters as they were written and giving me advice and encouragement; Mrs Lee Hughes for taking more than her share of lecturing to free me for writing, and for her faith in the project; Mrs Margaret Henry and Mrs Margaret O'Leary for reading the manuscript and for helpful suggestions; Gloria Gerrish for clerical help and Cheryl grant for the drawings.

Finally, I would like to thank the Administration of the Royal Newcastle Hospital for their approval and support for the production of this book.

PART ONE
Philosophy and Administration

This section discusses the background
to Retraining for the Elderly Disabled and shows
how this discipline is part of the larger
Geriatrics Service.

1 CONCEPTS AND PRINCIPLES

A general picture of the Newcastle method of retraining, defining a few major terms and introducing basic concepts.

Definitions

Geriatric Retraining is the method by which the many forms of treatment and the many services which are needed by the elderly sick can be brought together in an integrated framework of medical and social care. The dictionary defines 'geriatric' as: 'relating to the branch of medical science dealing with old age and its diseases', and 'retraining' as: 'bringing a person again to a desired state or standard of efficiency by instruction and practice'. The two definitions combined give a clear statement of the subject of this book, so long as the term 'old age' is extended to include people, not yet chronologically old, who need the help of such a service. The onset of old age varies with the individual, his situation, and the customs of his community. Stanley Matthews was 'The Old Man of Football' at forty, while Stanley Bruce was considered rather young for a Prime Minister at the same age. Some of the diseases which are clearly best treated in a Geriatric unit can develop much earlier than the statutory age of sixty five, while every illness in a person over that age will, just as clearly, not automatically require its services. It is the need of the individual and not his chronological age which determines his suitability for retraining.

The question has sometimes been asked, 'is it physiotherapy, occupational therapy, nursing, or what?' It is none of them, but incorporates something from all of them. It is a separate discipline, and like the patients for whom it is designed, it is better not divided into compartments.

Formal training in any one of the paramedical services is usually not enough to ensure that the graduate will understand and carry out retraining techniques as an integrated member of the team, but any interested and intelligent member of any one of them can become adept at retraining with a little further investigation, study and practice.

Development

In its developed form, Geriatric Retraining is a multidisciplinary service, which forms part of an even more complex Geriatrics service. It is complementary to the acute and maintenance phases of the service, and is integrated with them by team organisation under the leadership of a Geriatrician. In the beginning, however, it developed in response to growing community needs, under the leadership of a few isolated people with vision, who saw the problem of the increasing number of elderly people in the community. Changing social conditions made many of the problems too difficult for family and neighbours to manage unaided, but the old solutions of almshouse, nursing home, or workhouse, were satisfactory on neither economic nor humanitarian grounds. The pioneers had enough practical concern to seek an acceptable alternative, and the geriatrics service, with special emphasis on retraining and on home care was the result. They involved others, and gradually the teams developed, as needs were identified and specific skills were required to meet them. In many places the needs which led to the development of the original teams are only now being recognised and similar small bands of people are trying to provide a service. Geriatric Retraining, having developed in such a situation, can still find its place in small units as well as large. Its practical nature, and the simple equipment required to institute it, make it possible in almost any place where elderly folk are treated or accommodated.

Primary Aim

The primary aim of retraining is to fit the patient for return to his own home, with as great a degree of independence as he can achieve, and if necessary, with support in those areas in which he is deficient. The problems which make a return home difficult vary in kind and magnitude with each individual. These variations must be taken into account by any scheme for dealing with them and so an early report from the social worker on his home conditions is essential if the main goal of the retraining programme is to be achieved.

Multiple Problems — Multiple Solutions

In an early article in *The Practitioner*, Dr L.Z. Cosin discussed his method of identifying his patients' problems, and it is still very relevant:

> In the organisation of geriatric units I have advocated the replacement of the medical approach by what I have called the 'dynamic quadruple assessment'; dynamic, because any longitudinal study and solution of more than one problem with which the elderly sick are so often faced must be varied to suit not only the medical problems facing the patient, but also others. The dynamic quadruple assessment can be subdivided into the primary three; the pathological, the psychological, and the sociological, which must obviously be repeated as occasion demands and the circumstances facing the patient alter. As a result of the altered clinical condition, circumstances and status following the first three assessments, the fourth and most important of the 'residual disability' provides for courses of physical rehabilitation where necessary, and for compensation of that disability.
>
> The dynamic quadruple assessment then, provides solutions for the total problems of a sick old person, and the more solutions that are available, the more successful will the geriatric unit be in preventing prolonged ill health in the elderly.

Programme Planning

This multiple assessment, or a variation of it, is useful in treating the individual, and it also helps in planning for the group as a whole. Generalisations, averages, and stereotypes, are dangerous when applied to a specific person, but in planning for a group they are helpful in setting the guidelines and explaining the reason for choosing one option in preference to another. Planning for a group would be very difficult without some concept of common needs.

The Patients' Needs

An assessment of the needs of the majority is an acceptable basis for planning, so long as there is enough flexibility to allow for individual variations. The use of the dynamic quadruple assessment does make provision for this, and for change and growth. Geriatric Retraining programmes based on this concept provide for physical, psychological and sociological assessments and treatment, followed by a final assessment which in turn leads to the provision of the necessary equipment and on-going care for their return to the community. The patients' needs in this context are measures to combat those problems which prevent them from making a satisfactory return home, so planning must begin with knowledge of the homes.

The Needs of the Family

The needs of the family may well be different from those of the patient, and superficially at least, 'placement' in an institution may seem to be the answer to them. However, this does not take into consideration the emotional needs of relatives which are no less real than the material ones.

The distress of an old man who is separated from an ailing life partner by his inability to manage, or the guilt feelings of a daughter who can no longer care for a loved parent, can create their own problems. Retraining of the patient, and training of the relative in easier methods of looking after him, with the provision of the necessary equipment and services, can change an unhappy situation into an acceptable one, with benefit to all concerned. If, after a good try, and in consultation with the geriatrician and social worker, 'placement' is found to be necessary, it is arranged without guilt, if not without regret.

There are some factors which present great problems to the family, and these must be considered in planning a retraining programme. The main problems are incontinence, the need for lifting, night calls and wandering. Routine retraining methods must be designed to help with management of these difficulties. The need for a 'day off' may be evident, or even a longer break for a holiday, sickness, or a family emergency. Such occasions may be used for readmission of the patient, and a 'refresher course', so that when the family are ready to receive him again he will return with increased ability, and a holiday of his own to talk about. Thus there is a sharing of responsibility with the family, help being supplied at points where the family cannot help themselves. If no such provision is made for family needs, the patient may well have to go to an institution for permanent care, despite excellent treatment of his main illness. The very simplicity of retraining methods is in part due to the fact that the family must be able to carry them on after the patient has been returned to its care.

Hospital and Community Needs

The needs of the hospital are different again. They usually grow out of economic considerations, and include shortages of beds, space, staff, and equipment.

The tendency of older patients to have long-term problems, and a slower response to traditional methods of treatment, has led some acute hospitals to close their doors to them except in emergencies, or to transfer them as soon as possible to less high-powered institutions. While this solves the problem for the hospital concerned, it leaves untouched the problems of the patient and his family. Other programmes select those patients who are responding well and seem to have good potential and refer them for treatment in a 'rehabilitation unit'. While solving the needs of the stronger patients, this still leaves the slower and more disabled ones little alternative to custodial care in an institution. Smaller hospitals, and particularly those in the country, frequently have nowhere else to send the patients who fail to achieve independence, and so continue custodial care in their own 'Geriatrics Ward'. Even with the great kindness which usually prevails, this is not the ideal way to end one's life, and the lack of turnover of beds leads to a static situation where hope is lost. These solutions, while helping individual large hospitals to clear their beds, do little for smaller hospitals or the community at large. The problem has been transferred, but in most cases it has not been solved. Planning, then, must be for a reasonable turnover of beds and economical use of staff, together with the solving of the problems of the patient and his family.

Shared Responsibility

By sharing the responsibility with the family the geriatrics unit takes a middle path between leaving it to battle on unaided and taking all the responsibility from it by the provision of more and more custodial care. Geriatric Retraining, combined with domiciliary care, gives the seriously disabled patient, as well as the reasonably competent one, a chance to return home, and it also helps frail or fearful relatives to look after their own. This is its very purpose and planning should lead to this end.

The Initial Programme

There is a tendency to think that a new building, a full team, and settled plans are the ideal way to begin a new project, but this supposition needs to be considered before being accepted at face value. Growth in response to need can only happen if everything is not settled in advance, and as no two hospitals, and no two towns, are the same no complete plan can be made successfully out of someone else's experience. The team itself is unlikely to have cohesion just because it contains one of everything, but it will do so if each new member is appointed because her skills have been proved necessary. A complete new building is even less likely to be a success unless the people who are to work in it have the experience behind them to be sure of what they want and of what they do not want. From major matters such as the allocation of space, to minor ones such as the choice of door handles, the people who are to use them should be consulted, and these people should have opinions born of experience. There is no better experience than having to function in a less than satisfactory building first.

The initial programme may have to begin in the ward with a team of two, but even at this level something can be done. If a ward sister teaches her nurses a lesson in movement instead of lifting automatically, and arranges to have a few beds cut down to domestic height, the programme has begun. Many things remain to be added to this small beginning, but some of them at least will be self generating, as the attitudes of patients and staff adjust to this new way of doing things.

Early Development

Once a patient is involved in doing simple things for himself, he gains in confidence and motivation, and this in turn stimulates staff and relatives to further effort. Eventually it will be seen that the patient could go home if ..., and that is when growth will come in response to need. It may be a service or a piece of equipment that is needed, or perhaps both, but if this need is provided for, domiciliary care has begun. In ways similar to this a practical service can be built, which will eventually be much closer to the needs of the community in which it grows, than a grand plan transferred in total from somewhere else.

This more *ad hoc* approach means that ideas come from the team, and this usually produces enthusiasm and a determination to make it work. Involvement of this kind is invaluable and gives the team the job satisfaction which is so important to staff at all levels. Mistakes, when they are made, are on a small scale, and changes in direction are easier as a result. The one factor which can lead to disappointment and apathy is a negative attitude on the part of the administration. If people are trying to start in a small way, they need small gains to maintain their momentum. History, and particularly medical history, is full of stories of those who made good despite official opposition, but everyone with a good idea is not made of such stuff, and positive attitudes are as necessary in the administrators and planners as they are in those who carry out the schemes.

Co-ordination

If the retraining programme does prove itself, and begin to grow, the team will grow too, and regular formal meetings will become necessary so that work may be co-ordinated. Team-work becomes essential, to set a standardised way of teaching the patient so that he will not be upset by differing directions from different people. Team-work must be provided for in any programme which hopes to reach its maximum value to the hospital, the relative and the patient.

Attitudes

Attitudes are perhaps the most important single factor in a successful retraining programme. This statement applies to everyone concerned: administrators, doctors and the treatment team, relatives, the maintenance team, and the patient. The most important attitude is one of 'having a go'. To say something can't be done is to be defeated before one tries, and one will never know whether it was true or not. Small advances added together can produce results which looked impossible from the beginning. Nowhere is this more true than in Geriatric Retraining. One of the most rewarding aspects of retraining is to see the patient change his attitude from one of despondency or apathy to one of hope and active participation. This change is brought about almost entirely by the positive attitudes of the staff.

Routine Retraining

Routine retraining is a method, developed at the William Lyne Unit of the Royal Newcastle Hospital, whereby the daily routine is used as a therapeutic instrument. Rising, toileting, bathing, dressing, and moving about are all essential activities for the patient's return home. For this reason nurses are asked to teach the patient how to manage such tasks instead of doing them for him in the quickest possible way. Patients learn quickly in the real situation and the regular practice is built in, with no need to remember to do exercises. Patients with difficulties receive extra lessons from professional staff, while the routine drills go on day by day for every patient. This method is particularly valuable in helping with the specific learning problems of the sick elderly person.

Teaching

Teaching and teaching methods permeate the whole process of retraining, and function both vertically and laterally. Team members teach each other skills so that the patient will be taught the same method by any member of the team who is working with him. Senior members also pass on skills to professional and technical assistants, and in-service lectures are attended by all grades of staff to whom they apply. The continuous training programme helps to maintain staff interest as well as improving standards and interpersonal understanding. Many ideas and modifications come from the experience of the non-professional staff, and are as valid as the theory of the experts.

The teaching of the patient by staff members requires special skills which can be learned. This applies particularly to patients with some degree of dementia and, as these patients need to learn physical skills just as do those with intact mental powers, simple teaching techniques are included in the staff education programme.

Relatives of the patient often require to be taught the most practical method of handling a patient with residual disabilities and this task devolves upon the staff member most closely associated with the problem. The activities sister, activities nurse, dietician, occupational therapist and physiotherapist, are all involved from time to time in this aspect and, where multiple problems occur, more than one of them may work with the relatives.

The subject of teaching cannot be left without referring to the wider community. Lectures and seminars are arranged for teams from other hospitals, nursing homes and community organisations. The growing demand for these was one of the factors which stimulated the writing of this book.

Equipment

The choice, design, adaptation and provision of equipment is one of the most important functions of the geriatrics service, and it is in the retraining phase that this takes place. There are innumerable pieces of equipment on the market which are claimed to be of special value to the disabled patient. Even such a simple item as a walking cane is available in bewildering variety if one looks up the catalogues. As in retraining as a whole, so it is with equipment: the simpler the answer the better. The main consideration is that the patient should be trained in the use of his equipment while he is in the hospital, and that identical equipment should go home with him if he still needs it. If it cannot do so, whether size, complication, or expense is the inhibiting cause, the training he has undergone with it will be rendered a waste of effort. Insecurity and even falls are frequent results of a change in equipment without a properly supervised transition period. Many patients need specially adapted equipment, and this too should return with him to his home.

Extension to the Community

The hospital exists to serve the community and, in geriatrics at least, this can best be done by reaching out into that community. The patients are referred for the most part by their general practitioner, and after treatment, retraining, and final assessment, they return to him for continued medical care. The maintenance of the skills the patient has learnt, and the supervision of his equipment and services, however, are usually outside the sphere of the family doctor, and even if he would like to manage them himself, they are very time consuming if provided without some organisational backing. Originally the follow-up team was an extension of the hospital service, and that close co-ordination has much to recommend it.

If, as is now happening, a separate community service is to be provided, there should also be provision for very close consultation with those who are responsible for the early treatment and retraining. Unless this is so, there is a grave risk of overlapping, incompatible treatment methods, and misunderstanding, to the frustration of both teams, and consequent harm to the patient.

Retraining was designed with the primary aim of facilitating the patient's return to his home, but there are always some for whom this proves impossible and nursing home care is necessary. The time spent in retraining will not have been wasted if it has made care lighter, or if it has widened the choice among available nursing homes. If, in addition, the home both knows and uses the retraining methods as taught in the hospital, these patients should maintain their gains, or even continue to improve, instead of reverting to apathy and dependence, as so often happens.

A close relationship between on-going care and the hospital also makes possible the return of the patient to one of the earlier phases of the service, with minimal delay, if his condition should deteriorate or his cirumstances change, so that the resettlement plan needs revision. Should this happen, a request for consultation from the family doctor to the geriatrician will bring the necessary action, at the appropriate level for the individual patient. This may well mean that he will be brought again to a desired standard of efficiency by further instruction and practice.

2 THE PLACE OF RETRAINING IN A GERIATRICS PROGRAMME

The links between the Retraining programme and the Acute and Maintenance phases of the Geriatrics Service.

Retraining is the name given to one of the phases in the overall management of the many problems of the elderly sick. It is not itself a treatment, but a framework which incorporates and integrates the treatments and services which are needed to help bridge the gap between dependence in hospital on one hand, and managing at home on the other. For convenience in discussion a complete geriatrics service may be divided into three main phases, but the divisions between them are a merging of one into another rather than a definite line. The three phases are 'Acute', 'Retraining', and 'Maintenance', and because of the inter-relationship between them it seems necessary to outline the functions of all three and so to place the retraining phase in its proper context.

The Acute Phase

The acute phase usually begins with a crisis of some kind. Illness, injury, or a change in the patient's social condition will lead to a request for admission to hospital, and his immediate needs will be met by the usual hospital routine. In those patients for whom the admission is an isolated incident, examinations, investigations, and treatment related to the presenting illness may be all that is needed for a return to complete independence. In geriatrics (including some younger patients with chronic disability and/or multiple pathology) the situation is rather different. The presenting illness is often only the last of a series of problems which the patient has acquired over a period of time, and all have a part in his present difficulties.

These problems may be physical, psychological or social in nature, and are likely to be a combination of all three.

While they remain operative the successful treatment of the

presenting illness will not necessarily make the patient fit to return to his life in the community. In fact to return him to the unsatisfactory situation from which he came, without doing something to change it, is usually an invitation to early readmission. For these and other reasons, thorough medical and social investigations are necessary in the acute phase, and are the basis for realistic planning of treatment and management in the other two. Both treatment and management are more diverse and far reaching than they would be for the presenting illness alone, and the management should be considered early and not as an afterthought associated with discharge.

An example of this is the case of an elderly woman who was admitted with a fractured femur after a fall at home. She had fallen during a dizzy spell, was slightly confused, and found to be anaemic. The social worker's report gave a picture of a frail old person, living alone, with no close relatives and few visitors. The house showed signs of her failing ability to keep it clean, and the main items in the refrigerator were a loaf of bread, margarine, and jam. Tea was also in good supply.

The need for more than treatment of the fracture is obvious, as the fracture is only a symptom of her deeper problem. Thorough medical and social diagnosis in the acute phase led to appropriate surgical and medical treatment, followed by retraining, which in its turn led to realistic assessment of her residual needs. On this assessment a plan was made for maintenance at home with support from domiciliary services. These included visits from the community nurse to give injections for anaemia, a housekeeper to do her heavier work, Meals on Wheels to provide a better nutritional standard, and a weekly visit to the Day Centre to supply motivation and social contacts. Thus the unsatisfactory chain of events which led to her admission was broken, and she herself told a member of the staff that one of her luckiest days was the one on which she broke her leg.

It is the presence of multiple, long-standing, and sometimes irreversible problems which most strongly demonstrate the need for the geriatrics service, and Geriatric Retraining is one of the tools available to the geriatrician in managing them.

The Retraining Phase

Procedures begun in the acute phase will obviously be continued in the retraining phase if they are still indicated by the patient's condition, but the emphasis will change progressively from being looked after to looking after himself. There may be a move from the acute ward to a retraining ward, or a journey to a retraining area, but the absence of such facilities does not preclude the opportunity for retraining. In fact, some of the most valuable lessons in this phase are given in the ward situation. However well appointed and staffed, activity rooms, gymnasiums and other special areas are in a sense artificial, and ward conditions are more like those of home. Many a patient who has been proud of his ability to move in bed during day-time instruction, has called for help from a nurse at night. This behaviour in the real situation in the ward is closer to what he will do at home than the special effort he makes in the stimulating conditions of a lesson. For this reason, those abilities which are necessary for living at home, or which lead to a less dependent state in an institution have been made the corner stone of retraining, and their application is a matter for the ward, whether or not extra training is available from staff in specialised departments.

This often requires a change of attitude on the part of ward staff, and an understanding of the patient's long-term needs as well as his more obvious immediate ones. Misplaced helpfulness can produce even greater degrees of dependency than a more offhand approach, and if it holds the patient back from regaining his independence it is not as kind as it looks. In retraining an attempt is made to assess the patient's real needs unemotionally, and to set realistic goals for him. It is the responsibility of all staff to help him achieve these goals.

Retraining is prescribed by the geriatrician for all those patients who have problems in resuming their previous way of life after admission, and for those who, though not yet independent, no longer need the special care of a sick ward. It is designed to provide stimulation, motivation, mobility training, and increased skill in activities of daily living such as dressing and cooking. It also involves the provision of suitable equipment, both for treatment and to help compensate for residual disability. When each patient reaches his own best level of performance it provides for a team assessment of his achievements and continuing needs. The final plan for his return to the community is built on this information, and interested relatives must be involved as well as members of the staff. If it is indicated, training in special aspects of care is given to supporting relatives to give them confidence, and to ensure continuity of methods for the patient. Help from the domiciliary services is arranged at this stage, and only when all is ready does the patient go home to enter the third or 'Maintenance Phase'.

The Maintenance Phase

The ailments of our later years tend to be chronic, and recurrent or progressive in nature. The maintenance phase is needed to deal with the problems associated with this circumstance. There are many frail people who can be maintained at home or in the home of a relative if adequate domiciliary services are available, and who would much prefer this to a move to a nursing home. The provision of this care can be justified on both humanitarian and economic grounds, as has been well documented elsewhere.

The acceptance of responsibility in this area by hospitals ensures that elderly people are not sent home to fend for themselves in the very situation which brought about their breakdown. Most communities have a number of fine services available, but these are sometimes used with less than their full potential because co-ordination is inadequate. Retraining helps to minimise the patient's needs for equipment and services, while the practical assessment which follows points up real needs at the time of discharge. Continuity at this stage, with feedback to the geriatrician if problems arise, gives the patient his best chance for a satisfactory resettlement.

While the geriatrics service continues to provide maintenance in this way, directed by the geriatrician, the regular medical care of the patient becomes once more the responsibility of his general practitioner.

Examples of the dangers of individual services without co-ordination are numerous, but one will suffice to illustrate the point. A patient who had spent some time learning to walk and to do efficient transfers so that his frail wife could look after him, but who was known to have poor motivation, asked for a wheelchair from a kindly local group, 'because the hospital wouldn't give me one'. At much expense to themselves the group provided the best they could buy, without consultation. A few weeks later a call came from the wife to say she could no longer manage. On investigation the patient was found to have lost his hard-won walking ability, and to have developed contractures of his hips and knees. All this was the result of not getting the regular weight bearing which was a considered part of his resettlement plan and which he could not avoid before the advent of his wheelchair.

This case has been outlined to demonstrate the importance of follow-up procedures, and co-ordination of the services. A regular meeting of representatives of the hospital team and of the main services, under the chairmanship of the geriatrician, has proved a satisfactory solution. Special needs of individual patients can be explained to those who will now be serving them, while difficulties encountered in the home can be reported, and appropriate measures taken before they have become insuperable.

Direct consultation between the geriatrician and the general practitioner is a key part of the maintenance phase. The latter makes the initial request for consultation and, if necessary, admission to the hospital. At discharge a letter from the geriatrician outlines what has been achieved and the plan for domiciliary care. Medical care reverts to the general practitioner but domiciliary services continue to be administered from the hospital.

Further consultation is encouraged, and if readmission becomes necessary it is arranged at the request, or with the approval, of the patient's own doctor.

The overall plan of an efficient geriatrics service is not complete without provision for new or recurring problems after resettlement has been achieved. This is not failure, but an inevitable feature of chronic and degenerative illness. In certain conditions (for example, Parkinsonism and multiple sclerosis), a regular 'refresher course' is part of the original plan. In others a new illness may create new problems, or a change in social status, such as the death of a supporting relative, may necessitate readmission. In the many contingencies of this nature which may occur there need to be as many solutions, and flexibility is essential. The patient may need reassessment and further treatment in any one of the three phases which have been described.

3 TEAM-WORK AND LEADERSHIP

The organisation and development of the team, communication, internal stresses, and the role of the leader.

In the preceding chapter geriatric retraining was placed in its context in a well-developed service attached to a large general hospital. The complicated structure would have little relevance to smaller units, or those just starting, if the developed services themselves had sprung, ready made, to life. They too, however, had small beginnings, and the earliest of them started without facilities, without the experience of others to draw on, and with minimal staff. In many cases they also had to face the opposition of those who held the purse strings. This is recorded to encourage those who are starting today, and who feel that the facilities available to them are insufficient for their needs.

The one essential is a team, however small, which has a vision, and the enthusiasm to say 'how can we?' instead of 'we can't because . . .'. Geriatric retraining is founded on team-work, and the interdependence of all who are involved in it.

Team-work

In some ways the word team-work is rather overworked, and almost every talk or article about a subject in which two or more people are involved either starts or finishes with a reference to it. Team-work is an accepted concept, and we all like to think we belong to a good team. Despite this, some aspects of team-work are not quite as obvious as the constant referral to it would lead one to expect.

The Concise Oxford Dictionary defines a team as 'a set of persons working together', and team-work as 'combined effort, organised co-operation'. Thus friendly relations with one's workmates, and an occasional bout of shop talk over morning tea, does not quite fit the definition. A good team is structured. It has a leader or captain, and members who contribute different skills

24

which can be aimed towards a common goal. It should also have the ability to 'back up' if one member is under stress or absent, and it must make provision for communication, combined policy making, changes in tactics, and the solution of disagreements and internal problems when they occur. In other words, it should produce 'combined effort and organised co-operation'.

The Composition of the Team

The original team was 'two or more beasts of burden harnessed together', and the human team may also consist of only two members. Many large projects began with no more, other members having been added as results proved the value of the work, and as the need for additional hands or additional skills was demonstrated. Retraining is no exception, and a start can be made if there is a doctor who will refer dependent patients and take an interest in their return to independence, and a ward sister who will ensure that her nurses encourage it.

The number and composition of the team depends upon the availability of personnel as well as the funds to pay for them, and so teams will vary widely between different hospitals and districts. The needs of the elderly sick, however, are much the same throughout the community, and the fact that there is no physiotherapist available, for instance, should not mean that a patient with Parkinson's disease gets no exercise. Retraining, being a less specialised discipline, and designed to be administered by all members of the team, allows for this 'back up' if one member is unavailable. The resettlement needs of the elderly sick have been shown to be physical, psychological and social in nature, and the team, however constituted, must cover all these factors.

As well as doctors and nurses, teams in larger units may include permanent full-time members of ancillary services such as dietitians, occupational therapists, physiotherapists, speech pathologists and social workers, with the availability as needed of podiatrists, hairdressers, limb and splint makers, and a variety of voluntary agencies. Many of these may also lead smaller teams of technical assistants (aides) in their particular disciplines.

When it is remembered that the retraining phase is part of a larger whole, it is obvious that it must be related backwards to the acute phase, and forwards to the maintenance phase. Good communication between all three teams is essential. The other two teams may be just as diverse as the retraining team. In the acute phase it may include doctors, nurses, social workers, physiotherapists, occupational therapists, speech pathologists and dietitians. In the maintenance phase the family doctor, community nurses, housekeepers, providers of 'Meals on Wheels', and the staffs of day centres, clubs, and other relevant services may also be involved.

There are usually four team members who are involved from the beginning to the end of each case. These are the doctor, the social worker, the patient and a responsible relative. The doctor, ideally a geriatrician, is responsible for all aspects of treatment, and for the role of director of the whole service. The medical social worker is the chief link between the patient's home background, his family, the community services, and the rest of the team. The patient and his family are the reason for the whole exercise, and must be actively involved in it. They should never be seen as merely passive recipients of service.

Co-ordination and Planning

The larger and more diverse the team becomes, the more necessary is the regular meeting of its members, so that all may work together towards agreed goals, and so that misunderstandings may be resolved and overlapping avoided. Ward rounds and case conferences are concerned with treatment and management of individual cases, while policy matters are usually best handled at a separate administrative meeting. These meetings do not take the place of more informal discussions between individual members of the team, but they do ensure that the whole team is aware of aims, policy, problems, significant changes and the agreed allocation of responsibilities. The function of the various meetings which have developed within the Royal Newcastle Hospital's retraining programme, and which have proved their value, may be of interest.

The Ward Round

The ward round is the occasion when the patients see the doctor routinely, in a less formal way than in their medical examinations, and in the company of representatives of the rest of the team. Their physical skills, and particularly any changes in ability, are demonstrated, and problems reported, and the patients have a chance to speak for themselves. Deeper discussion and particularly controversial matters are kept for the case conference, when the patients are not present. Similarly, only minor medical problems will be dealt with during the round and more serious or personal matters will receive individual attention at another time.

The weekly chance to show the doctor and the team just what progress he has made has great value in motivation and morale for the patient. It also ensures that the team has a clear and recent picture of him when he is discussed in the case conference which follows.

The Case Conference

In the retraining phase the case conference is the main co-ordinating medium. All members of the team attend and are expected to contribute. In relevant matters the observations of the nursing aide who toilets the patient may be as vital to understanding his needs, and her opinion as worthy of consideration, as those of the more senior members.

Although every patient is seen on the ward round which precedes it, not every patient is necessarily discussed at the case conference. Those who are progressing without problems are excluded so that more time can be spent where it is needed. Patients who are discussed are the new patients, those who have problems, or are to have a change in their management, and those who are considered to be ready for discharge. So that no patient will be left for too long without formal discussion, those who are not discussed are given a 'review' date, and even if there is little to report their cases will be brought up when that date arrives. A few of these review patients will also be considered, therefore, with the three more active groups which have been listed.

New Patients

A new patient's medical diagnosis and relevant features of his condition, including any precautions to be observed, are outlined by the doctor, and if not already instituted, treatment is prescribed. Social conditions, background and possible family support, as they affect his treatment, are outlined by the medical social worker. In this way problems and assets can both be considered in planning his programme. A person who lives alone, for instance, will need to achieve higher standards of independence than one who is returning to an over-protective relative who will insist on waiting on him whatever happens. Similarly, it is important to know the lay-out of the home, and whether the patient takes a shower or a bath. Much time can be wasted, and the patient may even be endangered if these details are not known from the beginning.

Changes and Problems

The initial plan for each patient is based on the information received during his first discussion in the case conference. Changes may be needed in the light of his response to treatment, or because there has been a change in the factors upon which the plan was based. These changes will be brought about by discussion and decisions at subsequent meetings and so the second group of patients discussed will include those with problems which need team consideration, and those whose status has changed in some way which will affect treatment.

Pre-discharge Arrangements

When a patient is deemed by the team to have reached the best level of performance of which he is capable (without a great deal of extra time for minor gains) an assessment of his abilities in the activities of daily living (known as an ADL) is prepared. This highlights not only his achievements, but more importantly, his areas of weakness. This is presented at the case conference, and plans and arrangements for discharge are made in the light of this knowledge. Arrangements for the delivery of equipment and the provision of domiciliary services are set in motion after further consultation with supporting relatives. A letter or phone call from the geriatrician to the family doctor advises him of the plans. Only when all is ready will the patient be discharged.

Relative Interviews

Interviews with interested relatives happen routinely at the beginning and end of each patient's time in hospital, and in between if requested by the relatives or if there are changes which need discussion.

The preliminary interview is used to gain a clear picture of the background of the case and to inform the relatives about the programmes and to involve them in it. The final one is used to return the main responsibility to the family, with the offer of such help as has been decided upon as explained previously.

The doctor and social worker conduct the relative interviews, and the Activity Sister (a key member of the retraining team) is present at the final one when discharge is arranged. This group is kept as small as possible because many relatives become anxious and upset in the presence of too many people when discussing their problems and concerns.

One of these concerns is the fear of not being able to manage the care of a disabled person, and relatives with this problem are asked to attend the hospital themselves to receive professional instruction in handling their own patient. Lessons will be continued until the patient and relative gain enough confidence in each other to work together as a new 'team', or until it is decided that they will not be able to manage. In this case, nursing home placement may have to be considered. The help available from the family is taken into consideration when services are allocated and family help is co-ordinated with domiciliary services so that the maximum benefit may be gained from both.

The Domiciliary Care Meeting

Because of the long-term, and sometimes degenerative nature of the diseases which are prevalent in geriatrics, and because of the residual disabilities which are often a feature of them, 'follow-up' is essential. Equipment and services are provided, and another meeting is held for efficient on-going care as well as for administrative purposes. At this meeting representatives of the various domiciliary services, and of the hospital, meet under the chairmanship of the geriatrician.

Information about the special needs of new referrals can be made known to the Domiciliary Team, and its members can report back any problems or changes encountered in the home. Such reports lead to reassessment of needs in response to change, either for better or worse. Readmission, refresher courses and changes in services or equipment may result. The discussion may also lead to a home visit by a selected member of the team. However careful the assessment and planning at the end of retraining, there can always be a difficulty which was not foreseen. Many of these can be dealt with early, and before they become intractable, as a result of a report to the Domiciliary Care Meeting by one of its members.

Communication with the family doctor is also effected through this meeting in appropriate cases.

Administrative Meeting

The complex organisation we have been considering must provide for changes and growth if it is to continue to adjust to changes in the community it is designed to serve. It must also make provision for teaching its philosophy to new members of staff, encouraging new methods and ideas where they apply, and solving the disagreements and internal stresses which appear from time to time in the best of teams.

A good idea is welcomed for discussion and possible implementation by the whole team, but unilateral changes and decisions are not acceptable. Such decisions can breed misunderstanding and the person making them is often unaware of their implications for other members of the team or to the service as a whole. Open discussion is the solution. All this and more is the function of the administrative meeting where the whole team is asked to enter into discussion, to help in decision making, and to abide by team decisions once they are made.

Leadership

To function efficiently, most teams need a leader whose task it is to represent it to outside agencies, and to give it cohesion within itself. The leader must be one to whom all team members can give support, and whose casting vote is acceptable when the members themselves are unable to reach a decision. Because the retraining team is dealing in the treatment of sick people, the geriatrician is *ex officio* its leader, though responsibilities in their own fields must obviously be delegated to members of the various disciplines. In larger units these delegates must themselves act as leaders of their smaller teams which unite to make the larger one.

Communication in the Smaller Unit

These various meetings have proved necessary and helpful in the

interlocking structure of a large unit. Team-work and communication are no less necessary in a smaller organisation. Fewer meetings may be needed, but the small team will still need to meet regularly to discuss business, both medical and administrative, if it is to
reach its potential. An opportunity should be given for discussion
of all the matters outlined in the larger programme, but a single
meeting may suffice to cover the whole range.

It must always be remembered that patients are individuals with
many needs, and that just as many solutions are needed whether
they present in small or large numbers. It is the number of calls for
service which grow with population, and not the variety and quality of the services required. Good team-work from the beginning,
even by a small group, will ensure that any growth is in response to
needs and not just 'empire building'.

Summary

Tea-break team-work, though pleasant, is usually not structured
enough for efficiency in any but the smallest teams. More formal
meetings are needed so that all members may understand the programme, and be aware of policy, problems, and solutions. The
larger the team the more necessary such meetings become. In
every case the doctor is the leader with final responsibility for the
decisions taken. The team members, having put their point of view
forward as forcefully as they please, should abide by the decisions
until the team as a whole agrees to change them.

4 SIMPLIFICATION

Simple, practical methods are recommended in goal setting, organisation, management, reporting and equipment.

Introduction

The Newcastle Method of Geriatric Retraining has been specifically designed to serve the needs of the elderly sick and their families. It involves 'management' as well as 'treatment', and in it the home and the community join the hospital in a shared responsibility. Careful planning is necessary at all levels to make such a service economically viable as well as socially useful. Three elements of design provide threads which run through the whole scheme, contributing to this end. These are: (a) the setting of goals and priorities; (b) the optimum use of existing assets; (c) simplification.

The word 'design' incorporates the concept of order. Things happen 'by accident or design', and in the process of designing something we put its components into some kind of order to serve a specific purpose. In most cases this involves the three processes listed above. The concept applies to overall planning of the service as well as to the more detailed plans for its component parts. It also applies to the specific design of new equipment and the actual activities presented to the patients. In each area 'good' or 'bad' design depends to a large extent upon how successfully we use these principles.

Goals and Priorities

The goals set should be realistic rather than idealistic, so that some degree of success can be achieved. If an idealistic and distant goal is set, at least there should be smaller, more readily achievable goals leading to it. If possible, these should be tackled individually providing a series of definite achievements. Passing another milestone gives encouragement, however long the journey.

The conscious setting of goals helps us immediately to simplify our plans without the loss of essential elements. Elements which do not contribute towards achieving the goal can be seen as 'optional extras'. These can be deferred until more important aspects are successfully launched. This applies, however attractive an idea may appear if considered independently. Priorities can usually be set with confidence if we compare the contributions made by different options to an established goal. This general statement applies at all stages, from individual articles to the whole retraining programme.

Optimum use of Existing Assets

Many people are deterred from starting a retraining programme because they are introduced to the concept by an organised inspection of a fully developed service. Some reject the whole idea as too complicated and expensive for their own limited resources, while others produce elaborate schemes which demand buildings, equipment and staff (in that order) before a start can be made at the patient level. Both reactions mean that existing patients, who need help immediately, will be denied it.

The principle of using present assets to their best advantage is the happy medium between these extremes. A cleared space at the end of an existing ward is more valuable than a $2,000,000 building which is not yet started. A folded newspaper stiffened with a ruler makes a better back slab for a patient who is ready for it than the latest design from Europe with a three-month delivery time. Similarly, active participation by patients in an informal sing song led by an interested nurse will be of much more value than mindless time spent watching the world's best entertainers on an expensive television set. It is the staff who motivate and retrain the patients, and if they themselves are motivated they can do so anywhere. 'Start where you are' is another general precept which applies throughout the retraining programme.

Simplification and the Elimination of Inessentials

Many factors in the field of Geriatrics emphasise the need for the simplification of techniques and the elimination of inessentials from the programme. Some of these factors are:

(a) The impaired learning capacity of many of the patients who enter the retraining programme.
(b) Pressure for beds, which means that extra time spent on one patient is usually time denied to another.
(c) The difficulty in obtaining qualified personnel in units outside metropolitan areas.
(d) The need to make the most of limited funding by putting first things first.
(e) The need to build staff morale in a field which is seen by many as 'depressing'. The strongest weapon against this negative attitude is to use staff skills to the full by involving them in retraining instead of custodial care.
(f) The need for a scheme which can be understood and carried on by relatives, whatever might be their previous experience or ability in patient care.

Some of the areas in which simplification is needed and has been attempted in the Newcastle Method are as follows.

Programme Content (see Chapter 5)

This can be simplified by taking the following steps at the planning stage:

(a) Study goals, defining the major one, and allotting priorities to minor ones.
(b) List requirements in order of urgency.
(c) List possible existing solutions.
(d) List possible new solutions.
(e) Give solutions priorities related to the major goal.
(f) Arrange the use of existing facilities so as to make a start.
(g) Introduce new activities and services in order of urgency and in response to proven needs.
(h) Be prepared to change or eliminate items which do not fulfil their purpose.

Team-work (see Chapter 3)

The retraining team will vary in size and composition between hospitals, and depending upon local conditions. One aspect of work which is common to all teams is the need for good communication. In larger teams this may be difficult to achieve unless an efficient framework is provided within which it is simplified. Regular mandatory meetings for the whole team provide an answer. Some of the ways in which regular meetings simplify communication and eliminate unnecessary work are as follows.

(a) Communication through all levels of responsibility is possible without complicated and time-consuming appointment systems.
(b) 'Ringing around' to elicit or give information becomes unnecessary.
(c) Unnecessary 'overlapping' and omissions are avoided in the team effort.
(d) Decisions are made after discussion, and are better accepted and understood than directives from a single authority.
(e) Difficulties and disagreements can be tackled as team problems instead of personal confrontations.
(f) Pooled knowledge of a situation will give a balanced view and make a wise decision more likely.
(g) Decisions can be taken more quickly, and jobs allocated with the immediate knowledge of the whole team.
(h) 'Nobody told me' becomes invalid, either as an excuse or a complaint.

Efficient simplification of communication procedures and the elimination of many unnecessary stresses can result from the provision of a single point of reference in the form of a regular meeting. This applies to matters of policy and administration as well as to decisions about the treatment needs of an individual patient.

The Time Table (see Appendix B)

Because the major aim of retraining is a satisfactory return of the patient to life at home, it is logical to use the activities he must perform there as a basis for his treatment. These are all present already in the daily running of the ward, so the ward time table can be made the starting point of his programme. Other activities are fitted into this framework as they are introduced, but routine retraining goes on all around the clock, and only patients with specific needs require individual attention from the ancillary staff.

Team meetings are given a fixed place in the programme after discussion, and individual team members arrange their own time tables around these fixed points. It has been found practical to provide individual activities in the morning session, so that patients can move freely between the ward, the activities room, and their specialised treatment areas. Group activities are provided in the afternoon so as not to be disrupted by too many comings and goings.

Individual time tables for both patients and staff are simplified by a rational major time table, related to a major goal.

Staff Training Programme

The philosophy and techniques of geriatric retraining as an entity are not taught in the training schools for ancillary staff, nor in the nursing profession. In fact, the courses mentioned may even tend to inhibit thinking along these lines. The institutions seem to concentrate upon demonstrations of safe lifting and quick, efficient ways of doing things for the patient, rather than teaching students to elicit the patient's active involvement. As a result it has been found necessary to provide 'on the job' training for all new staff members who work with the patients. This can prove too time consuming to be possible unless simple, direct methods are employed. Those employed in the Newcastle Method are:

(a) A discussion of aims and principles with the person in charge of the retraining programme as part of original orientation.
(b) Inclusion as appropriate in ward rounds and case discussions.
(c) Practical demonstrations with patients in the real situation by established team members.
(d) 'Mini lectures' by established team members when interesting or unusual problems are encountered in the programme.

Staff training in geriatric retraining methods is a continuous process, which is integrated as much as possible into the daily routine, and deals with the actual problems being encountered rather than a large range of possible contingencies. It is additional to the basic training received in their own specialities by all members of the team.

Equipment (see Chapter 18)

There is an enormous amount of commercial equipment available. all of which is claimed by its suppliers to be invaluable in training patients. Much of it is extremely complex, and if used correctly does all that is claimed for it, but in geriatric retraining simple basic equipment has many advantages over such items. Some of these are:

(a) Equipment is to be used by patients who find difficulty in coping with elaborate detail.
(b) Many patients are unable to look after their own belongings, including their equipment and its parts.
(c) Use of the equipment will be supervised by support staff as well as qualified ancillaries.
(d) Moving and detachable parts are prone to damage and loss.
(e) Equipment used in retraining is provided in the home if still needed. Relatives must be able to supervise it, and cost must also be considered.
(f) Simple basic equipment, adapted as necessary, simplifies ordering and storage procedures.

Simplification of equipment involves the three procedures discussed at the beginning of this chapter.

(1) Goals and priorities — if these are set the choice of good, adaptable basic equipment will be possible, rather than a general ordering of items because they are traditional, look impressive, or might 'come in handy'.
(2) Existing assets — for independence the patient must learn to get in and out of bed, up and down from a chair, on and off the toilet, and so on. To do this no equipment is needed other than beds, chairs and toilets, etc., which are already available. They will also be available at home, and should be used. If a patient needs a lower bed or a higher chair, a good basic item can be adjusted more accurately and more cheaply than a new one can be bought.
(3) Simplification — by going through these first two steps, some degree of simplification is achieved automatically. Individual items should also be simplified. This subject is discussed in detail on page 367. This involves the elimination of moving and removable parts whenever possible, and concentration on safety factors as well as basic function.

Teaching Methods (see Chapter 11)

In the Newcastle Method, teaching is carried out by many grades of staff, for patients with widely ranging ability to learn. This is made possible by incorporating simple, direct teaching in the design of the programme itself. Staff members are themselves taught 'drills' by a method appropriate to the patients. This involves a careful job breakdown, and step by step presentation. The movements are the basic ones needed for essential daily living transfers, and staff are required to give a lesson in their application every time they attend to the patient. Thus repetition is built into the system. The 'three Rs' which are taught to the staff are:

(1) *Relevance.* Patients learn more quickly and willingly if they understand the relevance of what they are being taught. There is little doubt about the relevance of the basic drills. Some of the other areas of instruction may be less relevant. It is a waste of retraining time to persevere with any skill a patient will not use after discharge. The volume of matter to be taught can be greatly reduced and simplified by ensuring that it is relevant to the needs of the individual case.

(2) *Repetition.* If the pupil has not learned, the teacher has not taught. It is the responsibility of the teacher to use a method which does ensure that the pupil can learn. In geriatric retraining the most universally successful method is that of repetition. It has been used with success for retarded and demented patients, but it by no means degrades the well preserved. It is, after all, the method used by skilled sportsmen to perfect their skill, and by most actors to learn their lines. Intellectual understanding can be added where the patient can function at a higher level, but learning by repetition is available to all. It is the most practical way to teach necessary basic skills.

(3) *Rewards.* Elderly patients are no exception to the rule that rewards bring better results than punishments. Praise for what has been done well gives the patient heart to try again those aspects he has not yet mastered. A rose pinned on the lapel of a patient who has negotiated steps down into the garden will give him pride in his achievement, just as concentration in a game will be improved by the provision of inexpensive prizes. Recognition of effort as well as accomplishment is asked of staff members as part of their simple teaching method.

Supervision (see Chapter 12)

The involvement of all grades of staff in the retraining programme makes supervision essential. This does not mean a supervisor sitting at a desk to watch what goes on. The professional staff should work with their patients in the presence of their junior co-workers. In this way standards are demonstrated, and at the same time the seniors will become aware of the work being done by the others. Where the patient and the support staff are managing well the routine methods will bring results. Where a problem is noticed it is the responsibility of the senior person to help find a solution. Keen observation is the best way for the specialist to decide which patients need attention outside the routine programme.

The patient who is almost independent is particularly in need of supervision. 'On the job' observation at this stage can demonstrate remaining weaknesses in safety or performance while there is still time for more practice. No problem should emerge for the first time in the final assessment.

Supervision is simplified if staff members are aware of things as they happen, and see their implications in the patient's treatment.

Retraining 'Drills' (see Chapter 15)

The retraining 'drills' of the Newcastle Method have been simplified by relating them to the principal movements required for independence in transfers. The four main movements which are needed can be combined in various ways to meet almost every situation. Body mechanics are the bases of the movements, which are designed for the patient as he is in his present state, and not as he might be if and when recovery takes place. For example, a patient with a lower limb amputation is taught to be independent in his drills and the one-legged use of the walking frame before any decision is made concerning his suitability for a prosthesis. This involves learning to place his remaining foot under the mid-line of his body to enable him to stand and balance on one limb. He will thus achieve a degree of independence whether or not he graduates to a prosthesis. Because the movements have been thus simplified, the patient can begin to learn from the first time he sits up in bed.

Walking, which has in some cases been made so complicated that weeks of preparatory exercises are involved, has been brought back as closely as possible to the natural way we all learnt the skill in the first place. Elderly patients respond very well to learning to walk by walking, with necessary support which is withdrawn as they improve in skill and confidence. The simple direct method means that the great majority of patients can be taught to walk, despite serious physical or mental disability.

Creative Activities (see Chapter 7)

The aim of providing creative activities in the programme is to stimulate the patient's interest in something outside his immediate problems, to encourage mental and physical skills, and to give him the satisfaction of accomplishment. Crafts and hobbies provide for all grades of skill, but in the special circumstances of the retraining programme a simple job, well done, is needed rather than a difficult one which will create problems of its own. The finished job should be useful, meaningful to the patient, and pleasant to look at. It should also show fairly quick results so as to give the patient the satisfaction of seeing it completed. Simplicity is the key to success. It applies in the following areas:

(1) The variety of choices offered — most elderly folk find it difficult to choose if too many ideas are put forward.
(2) The processes employed in the activity — fine work involving good eyesight and steady hands is usually unsuitable.
(3) The number of processes involved — simple repetitive processes bring the best response.
(4) The tools employed — work done directly by the hands on the material gives great satisfaction, and is more easily understood. If tools are used they should be as simple as possible.
(5) Design — simple lines in construction, and minimal decoration help the production of accurate work. Complicated design usually looks untidy and amateurish.
(6) Colour schemes — a simple colour scheme using dark and light tones of one or two colours usually looks cleaner and brighter than one using all the colours of the rainbow.
(7) Starting and finishing — crafts which involve a lot of staff time for starting and finishing should be avoided unless they have some special purpose for the patient concerned.

Simple crafts done well are satisfying to the patient. Patients should begin with small, simple items, and more difficult processes should only be added when they prove themselves ready to manage them.

Group Activities (see Chapter 6)

Group and social activities need to be simplified, partly to make them available to the wide range of abilities in the patients, and partly to save too much staff time being spent in preparation. The simplification must be done with tact, however, or some patients may find the activities childish or beneath their dignity. Activities which involve patient participation are preferable to entertainment of a passive nature. Actual activities may be simplified versions of a more complicated game, or something which is already simple by nature. It is necessary to present the activity slowly and with clear explanations of what is about to take place. For instance, in a sing song the songs should be simple ones, well known to the patients, they should be clearly announced before starting, and they should be sung at the patients' pace in a lower key than would apply in a younger group. Patient participation is quickly lost if the activity seems either too difficult or too childish.

Assessments (see Chapter 8)

Much valuable time can be saved if the reason for an assessment is considered before it is made. Long wordy assessments are time consuming for the person who makes them, and also for others who must read them. Simplification can be effected by using a scale instead of wordy sentences. Only those assessments which are relevant to the occasions should be made and the patient should be observed in real situations rather than judged by a battery of formal tests in an artificial one. In retraining, what the patient does and will do has more relevance than what he could do if he would only try.

The most useful assessment is done while working with the patient, so that it is a living progressive process. It can be supplemented by further, more formal testing in doubtful areas, but there is no substitute for knowledge of the patient as a person in planning his programme and assessing his needs. In the Newcastle Method three main assessments are required.

(1) For the individual staff member's own use in planning her particular part of the patient's programme. Each will assess the aspects which are relevant to her needs.
(2) For reports, as necessary, to the staff case conference. Each member should be ready to answer questions on various aspects of her work with the patient, but reporting should be limited to changes in status, problems for discussion, or matters of interest to the team as a whole. Repetition of things

already known and receiving attention should be avoided.

(3) The final assessment before discharge. Decisions concerning the patient's readiness for discharge, and the equipment and services he will need are based upon this assessment combined with those of the doctor, the social worker, and the responsible relative. The form used in the Newcastle Method has been simplified as to content by revisions over a number of years. A limit of two quarto pages has ensured the exclusion of unnecessary items, and the use, wherever possible, of a simple marking scale has helped to keep verbosity at bay. It has also made it possible for those studying it to identify deficiencies in the patient's performance at a glance. Simplification of the assessment form also helps in keeping the assessment itself simple but comprehensive.

Elimination of inessentials has already taken place in the design of the form, but it can be carried further when some section does not apply to an individual. For instance, only those patients who will have to prepare their own meals need to be tested formally in the kitchen. (See Appendix C.)

Reporting and Book Work (see Chapter 8)

It should always be remembered when instituting a new form or requiring an extra report, that time spent by treatment staff in completing these is time taken from the patients. The simpler and fewer the reports, the better the results they claim to record are likely to be. The three design principles should be applied.

(a) *The setting of goals and priorities* — does it help to achieve a useful goal? Should it take priority over treatment in the allocation of time?

(b) *Optimum use of existing assets* — does it ensure the best use of qualified personnel? Could it be done more economically by a clerk? Would a word of mouth report to an existing meeting suffice? Is the information already available elsewhere? Could an existing report be supplemented to cover the problem?

(c) *Simplification and elimination of inessentials* — is another report really necessary? If so, is it simple and well designed? Is it easy to fill in, and to interpret? Can eliminations be made in content, frequency of submission, or verbal elements? Can it be completed in one session, or will it mean breaking into other work on a number of occasions?

The havoc caused by 'work to rule' strikes demonstrates the need for this kind of thinking in procedural matters. It is easy to draw up an elaborate form. It takes understanding and skill to produce a simple, efficient one.

Conclusion

Complexity has no value in its own right unless all the components which produce it have a useful part to play. There are many instances of the rejection of geriatric retraining as 'too hard', in places where it is obviously needed. This has happened chiefly because the concept of simplification has not been understood. This chapter has attempted to show that by a series of simple steps a relatively complicated goal can be reached.

PART TWO
Programmes and Activities

This section deals with the choice of
programmes and discusses various
activities which may be included.

5 THE OVERALL PROGRAMME

The introduction of a retraining programme is discussed with some of the practical considerations involved. The need for a variety of activities is stressed.

Introduction

The overall programme for geriatric retraining, as described in earlier chapters of this book, may seem complicated and formidable at first sight, but it should be understood that it is presented here as a developed service in a large hospital. To attempt to reproduce such a service ready-made would be unrealistic and unlikely to produce the results most suitable to local conditions. The initial programme should provide for stages of development and consolidation rather than a large initial capital outlay with once and for all decisions about policy and method.

A simple, useful programme can be achieved in most existing institutions if entrusted to an enthusiastic and well-informed leader who is capable of developing a positive attitude in the rest of the staff. Given this basic asset, the programme will grow as the institution becomes able to absorb it.

The first consideration in planning such a programme is its integration with existing time tables and methods of work in the institution, and the less disruption it causes the more readily it will be accepted by existing staff. Some changes are inevitable, but the most important one is a change in attitudes. Resistance will be reinforced if the changes are too great or too early, but if the simple initial programme can prove its usefulness further developments are likely to be accepted. What that usefulness is will depend upon the type of institution involved, and so in planning the programme it is necessary to clarify one's aims in introducing it. For example, a hospital may want better treatment results and a quicker turnover; a nursing home may want maintenance of morale and a better quality of life for its permanent residents; and a day centre may want to play a preventive role as well as maintaining the gains a patient has made in hospital. Obviously three

47

separate programmes are necessary, with different emphases, although all three may well use similar basic activities.

The overall programme is thus a framework for development upon which individual programme sections can be built in response to the special needs of the institution concerned. In the early stages, human assets are the only indispensable ones.

Initial Survey

Whether the programme is a new venture in a new setting, or a development in an established institution, it is equally necessary to conduct a survey to discover how best to introduce it. This does not mean an expensive exercise by a firm of consultants, but a good look over the ground by the person who will be doing the work. The person responsible for introducing the programme will need to be very clear in her own mind about her aims and aspirations, and have positive suggestions about how they can be achieved if she is to gain administrative support in their implementation. She will also need to see the problems of those who will be affected by the scheme, and be ready to discuss them in a positive way if she is to gain acceptance from the existing staff. One way to achieve this is to ask all the questions of herself before they are posed by others.

Most of the relevant questions will come to mind if prompted by the 'Who? What? Which? When? Why? Where? and How?' method. These basic questions, listed systematically, help to produce positive ideas in many areas, and demonstrate the need for further investigation or discussion if no immediate answer presents itself. For example, the word 'Who?' may suggest such questions as:

Who will benefit from the programme?
Who will decide which patients should attend?
Who will transport the patients from the ward?
Who will decide on the day to day programme?
Who will provide meals?
Who will take the patients to the toilet if they need help?
Who will be responsible for ordering, storage and accounting?
Who will attend administrative meetings?
Who will attend medical case conferences?

Who will approach outside agencies for support?
Who should be called if a patient is ill?
Who is enthusiastic already, and likely to help?
Who seems antagonistic and will need tactful handling?
Who should be kept informed of problems and progress?
Who should be invited to the 'Official Opening'?

All of these questions, and many more posed by local conditions, will be suggested by the simple word 'Who?'. Similarly, the
other 'trigger words' in the list will produce their own questions to
which an answer must be sought. From these a practical plan will
begin to emerge. A plan for a recreational programme which was
prepared for a medium-sized country hospital in this way, is given
in Appendix B.

Assets and Liabilities

During the survey period a list of assets and liabilities can also be
compiled, and this will help the planners to make the most of one
and to avoid the other. When the programme is to be introduced
to an established institution, such a survey of the existing situation
is imperative. The nurses who take pride in their patients' appearance, the people from the church who sing hymns on a Sunday, the
relatives who bring in Mum's knitting, or take her for a drive, and
the cleaners who tell the patients the news or put on the bets, are
all in their own way pre-empting the programme, and should be
looked upon as assets, even if some of their activities need to be
channelled a little differently. An over-polished floor, high beds,
over-rigid ward routines, disgruntled members of staff, apathy
from those in high places, and too generous visiting hours, may all
be seen as examples of liabilities. Such things will need tact and
patience if they are to be overcome. The plan which incorporates
existing strengths, and minimises known liabilities, is the one most
likely to succeed.

Programme Content

In choosing the content of a Geriatric Retraining Programme, two
sometimes conflicting subjects must be considered. The first is the

ideal of a complete and efficient service, and the second is the availability of resources. No set list of activities can be provided which will suit every situation, but there are some principles which provide a frame of reference to help even the most deprived unit to make a start. Some of the most important can be listed as follows.

Begin With What is Already Available

Geriatric retraining is more a matter of attitudes than activities, and things which we all do every day are the only activities which are essential to the programme. The dependent patient who is dressed, fed, put in a chair and left snoozing in front of a television set will withdraw further and further into himself as time goes by unnoticed. On the other hand, the patient who is encouraged to put his own arm into his sleeves, to take at least a few mouthfuls from a spoon in his own hand, and is spoken to as a person whenever he is receiving attention, will respond as far as he is able, and at least have an opportunity for progress. If the deadly TV session can be exchanged for something more active, such as winding bandages, folding linen, giving out teas, collecting cups, tidying a locker, and so on, and if the staff can give adequate encouragement and praise for such activities, a retraining programme has started.

There is Little Difference in Value Between Different Activities

In an experiment in which activities were tested for their value in stimulating a group of geriatric patients to greater spontaneous activity, all the activities employed were shown to do so, but no activity could be shown to be more effective than the others. The average age of the patients was 82 years, and there were 24 patients in the group. The experiment was set up so that the group was given a month of an activity, and then a fortnight with no specific stimulation. They were tested at the beginning and end of each session for social interaction and self help in getting themselves up and dressed in the morning, during the evening meal, and while undressing and going to bed in the evening. The activities tested were domestic, craft, social, combined craft and social, and group activities. The report on this research states that 'no significant differences in terms of power to increase behaviour scores of the group were found among the different social and occupational therapies employed; but they all had in common the ability to interest and stimulate the confused patient. The response varied very much with the individual. What suited and amused one did not interest another'.

This finding has been quoted at length, to give confidence to those who must begin with less than a full range of activities for their patients.

Any Activity which is Introduced should have a Definite Purpose

There are many reasons for introducing activities, but the most valid reasons fall into one or more of the following categories.

Motivation. Helping the elderly people to feel that life still holds something for them, and that it is worth being involved in what is going on around them.

Mobilisation. Helping those with physical problems in moving about and doing things for themselves to function more easily or more independently.

Development of Independence. Encouraging the elderly to do everything that they can for themselves and teaching nurses, relatives and others to resist the temptation to be over-protective.

Socialisation. Encouraging the elderly to behave appropriately in social situations, to interact with other people, and to regain or maintain an interest in people and events.

Reorientation. Helping those who have become confused or dis-orientated to come back to reality, or to adjust to new and threatening situations.

Improved Quality of Life. Adding interest and satisfaction to an otherwise dreary and monotonous or pointless existence.

Maintenance of Physical and Mental Skills. Ensuring that function is not lost through inactivity, apathy, or lack of opportunity to practise existing skills.

The Programme Should Start with Simple Activities Done Well

It is a truism that 'Nothing Succeeds Like Success', and small early successes will lead on to better things, while initial failure at something more difficult is not easy to live down. In each section of the overall programme, therefore, it is wise to choose initial activities in which the person introducing them is confident, and which are well within the capacities of the people for whom they are being organised.

Major Equipment Should Not be Ordered too Soon

The equipment needed for geriatric retraining is essentially simple, and there can be considerable waste if expensive equipment is ordered before a need for it is demonstrated. Unfortunately some institutions insist on a complete initial order, with little provision for subsequent orders in response to need. This leads to over-ordering 'just in case', and makes it difficult to vary the programme or introduce new ideas. A smaller outlay and better use of equipment result from a less rigid system of supply, and this is strongly recommended wherever it is possible.

The Time Table Should be Widely Distributed

A formal time table should be worked out, fitting as closely as possible into the existing hospital or institutional routine. Copies should go in advance to the administration, as well as all whose work impinges upon the new programme. This will include those who deal with food, and those who clean the wards, as well as the nurses and treatment personnel. Time should be given for objections and suggestions before the programme is actually started, and every attempt should be made to allow for these if they are in any way reasonable. Remarks should also be asked for after a fair trial. In this way objections, which are bound to occur, will be out in the open, and not persisting as a destructive undercurrent. Those who are satisfied in this way will be your allies against the incorrigible negative thinker.

Administration

Provision in the programme of time for administration and preparation is essential. How much time is needed will vary greatly with the size of the undertaking, and the type of activities which are to be used, but even the simplest programme will not continue to function well if no-one has time to think. Depending upon the individual programme time will be needed for such diverse duties as medical rounds, case conferences, home visits, the training of relatives, the design and adaptation of equipment, staff meetings, staff education, ordering and storage of equipment, record keeping, reporting, and the preparation of crafts and activities. Any of these which apply should be planned for, so that full attention can be given to patients during treatment sessions, and full attention to administrative duties when the patients are absent. Except in special circumstances it should not be necessary for staff to work through their lunch hour and tea-breaks, or to take work home.

Choice of Activities

The choice of activities will depend upon the aims of the programme, the facilities of the institution, the type of patient involved, and the skills and interests of the staff. The staff should be willing and able to acquire new skills when needed, but those they have should never be wasted. Ability to sing, dance, tell a good story, collect stamps, grow pot plants, make pikelets, or demonstrate beauty culture, can be made the basis of a section in the programme, and are likely to produce enthusiasm in the group because they are of real interest to the person offering them.

Activities will be discussed in detail in a subsequent chapter, but for programme purposes they may be classed as follows.

Routine Retraining. Drills in mobility to improve independence in using chair, bed, toilet, bath, car, etc., and in walking ability (Chapters 15 and 16).

Activities of Daily Living. Training in dressing, eating, cooking, household tasks, shopping, writing, etc. (Chapter 7).

Orientation Retraining. Should permeate other activities, but also includes news readings, discussions, reminders of time and place, and programmes for the blind (Chapter 6).

Social Activities. Also known as 'non-specific social stimulation'. These include music, parties, community singing, outings, and entertainments (Chapter 6).

Group Activities. Patients work together on a common project.

Christmas decorations, a mural, sale of work, group exercises, making a fruit cake, are examples (Chapter 6).

Sport and Games. These are usually played in a modified form. They may include table games, blackboard games, group and team games, and outdoor games (Chapter 6).

Individual Creative Activities. Crafts and hobbies, depending upon local conditions, available teaching skills, and supply of materials (Chapter 5).

Outings and Special Occasions. Bus drives, barbecues, Cup Day, National Days, Christmas, Easter, and so on (Chapter 6).

Entertainments. Visiting groups, mannequin parades, concert parties, staff revues, television (Chapter 6).

Provision for as many of these groups as possible should be the eventual aim in a complete retraining programme in order to serve a wide and varied list of needs and to allow for change so that the programme will not become repetitive and dull. The purpose of the individual programme will determine the order in which activities are introduced and their relative importance in the scheme. Four different time tables designed for four very different situations are given in Appendix B.

Rotation of Programmes

In providing an activity programme for elderly patients, their need for a feeling of security must be balanced against the risk of boredom. There is a wide variation in the ability of people to cope with change at every age, and this is so in the population of the usual geriatric unit. A really adventurous programme might well appeal to some of the clients, but these would tend to be the better preserved, and those best able to manage their problems independently. The patients least able to accept change, exuberance, and over-stimulation, are the sick, the withdrawn, and the timid, and these are the patients who most need help if they are to return to a more active way of life. For this reason it is helpful to have a structured programme which remains unchanged, while individual activities are rotated to provide variety. For instance, games might be played daily from 3 p.m. to 3.45 p.m. but a different game could be chosen every day for eight days before the cycle starts again. Thus the security of knowing that games would be played is balanced by the interest of wondering which one it might be today. This rotation of programmes within a framework is particularly important for patients who attend a day centre on the same day each week. To have the same meal, the same songs and the same game week after week can negate much of the value of the visit.

Homework Problems

In the part of the programme devoted to creative activities, many patients become extremely enthusiastic about their work, and this gives great satisfaction to the teacher, but also has its problems. Requests to continue the work in the ward at night or at weekends, or if a day patient, to take it home, are frequent, and on the surface reasonable, but homework should not be included in the programme unless there is a staff member available to supervise it, or voluntary help provided for starting, finishing, and the correction of mistakes. Enthusiastic homework by patients usually results in less than voluntary homework by the staff. Occasionally, there will be a patient who can work successfully without help, but it creates difficulties if one patient has his request granted and others must be refused.

Preparing, Fixing and Finishing

If craft work is to be provided, there needs to be planned time for preparing, fixing and finishing. There are few crafts which sick and disabled folk can manage alone, and if the tasks mentioned are carried out while they are working, the supervision becomes inadequate and standards fall. The value of the whole project can be lost if the patient is discouraged by mistakes, or distressed by having them fixed in full view of the group.

Preparation time is also necessary for social activities, games and discussions, though perhaps less urgently than for crafts. Nevertheless, the acceptance or otherwise of a new activity is frequently dependent upon adequate preparation.

The Multiple Time Table

Because geriatric retraining is carried out around the clock, it is necessary to have separate time tables for the patients and the various staff members who attend them. The patients' time table is obviously the key to the others, but the planning of the latter is of equal importance. Thus the occupational therapy staff may be preparing the afternoon activities while the nurses are serving the patients' lunch, and the nurses may read their reports while the occupational therapists conduct a song session. Such co-ordination is essential to harmony and the smooth running of the programme. The larger and more complex the unit, the more need there is for consideration of such matters. In clubs and day centres it may be simpler, but even there it should be arranged that the staff members are available when the patients are present, and that meetings, preparation and accounting take place as far as possible in their absence. This is stressed because to the majority of geriatric patients their contact with understanding members of the staff is the most meaningful part of their day.

Recurring Events

Certain recurring events need to be allowed for in the time tables of both the patients and staff. The weekly medical round and case conference are examples of these, and for the patients, the visiting hours have special significance. The administrative programme will necessitate annual events (stock taking, a 'spring clean' and a report), monthly events (statistics and administrative meeting), and weekly events (accounts, orders and stores). In the activity programme special days, festivals, the local show, and possibly a sale of work are spread through the year, recurring annually, and giving opportunities for variations in the programme which can be built up in advance and enjoyed in retrospect. All such events and duties must be considered as part of the overall plan.

The Final Result

However careful the planning, in a subject with so many variables as geriatric retraining, and particularly in one where the human element is so important, there will be some things which succeed and some which do not. There is no lack of alternatives to a less than satisfactory activity, so if, after good preparation and a fair trial, something has not proved its value we should have the humility and courage to lay it aside and try something else. It may well be that at a future date, with a different group, it will be a tremendous success. If the overall plan is good, and we are prepared to adjust those aspects which do not fulfil our expectations, a successful and rewarding programme is sure to result.

6 GROUP ACTIVITIES

The value of group activities is discussed. Some useful activities are listed with suggestions concerning their introduction.

Introduction

Each patient is an individual, and his programme should fill his individual needs, but this does not mean that all his activities must be carried out in isolation. In fact, apart from a few life-long 'loners', most patients respond best to activities they can perform in company, and often in co-operation with others. A new patient who is introduced to an active group will usually become involved himself in a very short time, but the same patient offered an activity in a ward where no-one else is occupied is likely to reject it fearing to be the odd man out. The success of a group of elderly patients attempting some co-ordinated effort depends to a large extent upon the skill of the leader of the group in allocating suitable tasks for the individuals in the group, and in her ability to transmit her own enthusiasm to its members.

Group activities, while not as directly related to independence as the retraining drills, have a distinct part to play in stimulating the patient to find a new interest in his surroundings. They help him to see that he can still enjoy social occasions, can relate to other people, and is needed to play his part in whatever is going on. All the work put into retraining and walking practice can become too intense if there are no lighter moments. Group activities provide these. Whatever Jack's age, 'all work and no play' can still lead to dullness. The activities discussed in this chapter have been called 'non-specific social stimulation'. They are often the starting point along the way back for patients who have apparently decided that they have come to the end of the road. They also provide recreation and a break from concentration on their disabilities for those who are already well motivated.

The Value of Group Work

To the Patient

Working in a group towards a common goal gives satisfaction to most human beings, both at work and at play. If it were not so there would be little point in clubs, teams and the multitude of co-operative ventures available in almost any community. The patient entering the hospital community as a stranger can feel some such satisfaction if introduced early to a suitable group. If the place he is asked to take suits his abilities and his needs, the group can play an important part in building morale and self esteem, but it must always be remembered that a poor choice of activity can have the opposite effect.

To the Staff

By treating patients in a group rather than completely individually, more patients can receive attention. This is particularly helpful when there are numbers of patients with the same disability, or in times of staff shortage. For instance, exercises common to a number of patients can be given in a group, and the time saved can be used to give more individual attention to patients with specific individual needs.

Group activities can provide a number of tasks of differing complexity and for differing aptitudes. These can be used by the staff to involve a patient who is not yet able to manage more than one simple process as well as the more able patient who can be involved as a leader or supervisor. The group also provides a medium for encouraging withdrawn and lonely patients to react again with other people, and to make friends with their fellow patients. The sensitive staff member can make good use of introductions, careful placement of patients and patient-to-patient help as therapeutic tools.

Leaders and Helpers

Modern writings on group dynamics usually insist that leadership should come from the group itself, and should not be imposed by a figure with authority. This can work well in a group of motivated people with intact mental and physical capacity. It has been tried and found wanting among the elderly disabled. Anyone who has

worked with this type of group will know that the person who has
the ideas, the energy, the organising ability and the enthusiasm to
emerge as a leader is ready to go home. Rooms full of disinterested
people, sleeping or vaguely watching television in some hospitals
or nursing homes where no leader is present demonstrates this
point. Even when a person has been employed for this purpose the
level of activity decreases markedly when she leaves the room.
This does not mean that the group as a whole has not enjoyed the
activity, but rather that they are sick and disabled, and need
encouragement and leadership if they are to be involved.

The statement above may seem heresy to the modern school of
thought but it should be remembered that the people with whom
we are dealing have grown up in earlier days when overt leadership
was the norm. Reliable leadership provides security for such
people and frees them to enter into the spirit of the current activity.

If spontaneous activity or leadership should appear in the group
it should naturally be encouraged and the staff leader should stay
in the background. She should not, however, cease to observe, but
should always be ready to come to the rescue if things should begin
to go wrong. An example could be a patient who offered to lead
the singing or call the housey numbers, but who forgot the words,
or whose voice proved too weak for the task. The appointed leader
has the dual responsibility of seeing that the would-be helper is not
upset and that the group as a whole can continue to enjoy the
activity.   If the group is a large one and extra helpers are available, these helpers should be informed of the kind of activity to be
undertaken and the reason for introducing it. They should help
those patients who are obviously having difficulty with the activity,
but should do so as unobtrusively as possible.

In some cases they may take a small group away from the main
one and provide an alternative activity more suited to the needs or
inclinations of the selected group. This may be something more
simple for those who can't keep up, or just as legitimately, something more taxing for those who find the main activity too simple.

What the helpers should not do is stand on the sidelines and
look bored, or carry on a private conversation in competition with
the main activity. Most people do not enjoy being watched by an
outsider, and the presence of someone who is not involved in the
activity almost invariably leads to self-consciousness and loss of
involvement by the group.

Group Exercises (see Appendix C)

Exercises lend themselves very well to group work. In the Newcastle programme three main exercise groups are used.

General Exercises

General exercises are given daily in the activity rooms. They
usually take place after the mid-day break, and before the time set
apart for group recreation and social activities. All patients who
are fit enough are involved, and all staff members who are available take part as leaders or helpers. The exercises proceed for a
maximum of 30 minutes. They are designed to ensure that each
joint is put through its range of movement, and to provide practice
in listening, concentrating and following directions. Staff members
stand with those who cannot manage unaided, and relay the mes-
sages or give physical help as needed.

The exercises are presented with a light touch, and patients are
asked to do their best even if they cannot perform the complete
movement. Paralysed limbs are aided by the patients' own strong
ones when this is possible, or by a member of staff when it is not. If
help is needed it is given in such a way that the patient is involved,
if only mentally. Passive movements without the patient knowing
or caring have no place in group exercises where involvement is
part of the goal. These group exercises are non-specific and
patients and staff are instructed not to proceed beyond the point of
pain. More specific exercises are the province of the physiotherapist. Staff members are instructed to watch the patient's face,
when moving any limb passively, and to stop whenever there are
signs of distress.

Note. If a physiotherapist is available she should be responsible
for this activity, but being non-specific, it can be delegated to
another team member.

The Mat Class

The mat class is provided for a small group of selected patients. It
is usually conducted by the physiotherapist or by an aide who has
received instructions from her and is responsible to her.

A padded mat and a pillow are placed on the floor for each
patient, and chairs are provided for those who need them. A set of
wheelchair steps is also at hand. The patients learn to go down
onto the floor, to perform a set of exercises, and to get up again
onto a chair. The going down and arising are important to patients

who are subject to falls as well as to those who wish to return to gardening or to other activities where this ability is needed.

The exercises themselves are closely related to 'bed drill', using the same movements for moving up, down and across the mat, for turning over, and for sitting up. Moving in this way on the mat reinforces the bed drill, allowing the movements to be performed more freely because the fear of falling has been removed. Other exercises are given for strengthening and loosening the patient's movements and for developing balance and confidence.

Patients who seem to benefit most from the mat class include those with Parkinson's Disease, balance problems or a tendency to fall, multiple sclerosis, and strokes in the later stages of retraining. Some old stroke patients who have stiffened because they have not remained active at home also do well when given a 'refresher course'.

A list of mat class exercises is given in Appendix C.

The Hand Class

The hand class is usually presented by aides, directed and supervised by the occupational therapist. In the Newcastle programme it is not introduced during the in-patient period, but is reserved for the Day Centre. If it is thought to be valuable for an individual in-patient he can be referred to the out-patient group at the appropriate time.

Each patient in the group is given a small box containing some simple equipment, and the contents of the boxes are used in a series of exercises. The equipment can be varied from time to time to prevent boredom through over-familiarity with the contents. Some examples of the exercises and equipment are:

(a) A baton which is passed around the circle from left to right and then from right to left. This is about 1.5 in (4 cm) in diameter to give a comfortable grip.
(b) A box of a set number of matches which are tipped out onto the table and then returned to the box one at a time.
(c) A bean bag which is bounced on the back of the hand, or passed from patient to patient by tipping it from the back of one hand to the back of the next.

Many simple devices of this kind can be used. A fuller list is given in Appendix C.

As with the general exercises, the hand class should not be given too seriously, but should be made fun. Gentle competition between patients may be encouraged from time to time, and inter-patient exchanges should be used. Ideas which come from a patient should be included if possible. For instance, one patient suggested pegging a piece of cloth onto a length of line held by two other patients. This caused a good deal of hilarity, and involved many patients with each other.

Group Activities of Daily Living (ADL)

The activities of daily living can be conducted in groups, although these will usually be smaller than the groups which can exercise or enjoy games or parties together. Some examples are as follows.

Dressing Classes

Patients who are having trouble dressing and undressing can work together at taking off and putting on their shoes, pulling a cardigan off over their heads, or at doing up and undoing buttons. The main practice in dressing and undressing is given at the time when this is the normal activity of the day, but these 'real' sessions can be reinforced by a dressing class which gives practice in details and demonstrates the easy way.

Cooking

Too many cooks may spoil the broth, but a few patients working together employing division of labour may produce something which would be impossible to one of them working alone. A plum pudding is a good example. The group can discuss the recipe, fit patients can be asked to help fetch the materials, patients with varied disabilities can prepare the different fruits, and all can be asked to stir. Any patient with special skill in cooking may be asked to keep an eye on things, and one or all can be asked to remember when to take it out of the oven. No Christmas party is more appreciated than one in which the patients have all taken a hand in baking the cake.

On a smaller scale, two or three patients may work together to produce afternoon tea, to serve it, and wash it up, or a husband and wife team can cook their own mid-day meal in preparation for combined efforts at home.

Group Recreation

Group recreation is provided for daily in the Newcastle programme. It takes place in the afternoon when the patients have completed their various treatments and retraining activities and need some lighter activity. The programme covers at least a fortnight before an activity is repeated, except in unusual circumstances. The activities chosen are those which demand the patient's participation. Entertainment of the passive kind is used sparingly, and usually takes the form of concerts provided by voluntary groups from the community.

Because of the varying abilities and backgrounds of the patients the activities should be of general interest. Even so there may be some to whom the activities do not appeal. If possible, these patients should be given a chance to take part in the preparations or help a patient less able than themselves. Without a much higher patient/staff ratio than is usually available it is not possible to provide activities to suit each individual on every occasion. Patients reject group activities for a number of reasons, but most join in willingly if they realise that they can help others by doing so, and that tomorrow the programme may be more to their taste. For some ideas on motivating and involving patients see Chapters 12 and 13.

Some examples of group work are as follows.

Group Crafts

Patients can work together on large craft projects such as a mural, or decorations for a special occasion such as Christmas, Easter, or Cup Day. They may each do part of the whole scheme with the individual parts being assembled together, or they may work on the same material. They may become involved in producing shared articles for a sale of work in a common cause, or join together in a simple task such as untangling and sorting the materials. Individual crafts may tend to isolate patients as they become interested and concentrate more deeply on what they are doing, but group crafts can be a shared event over which they hold discussions or even arguments. Group potting of indoor plants has much the same socialising effect, and has more appeal for some male patients. An extension of group crafts is the simple puppet show where the craft group can produce the puppets and the setting, while the show is produced by others who can work the puppets and provide the voices. If a tape recorder is available the problems of stage fright and missed lines can be overcome by taping the voices (and music, if any) in advance.

Group Games

Group games are almost limitless in number, and can be varied to suit the abilities of the patients who are to play them. They can be simplified forms of adult games such as indoor bowls, or adapted versions of games most of us remember from childhood. To be accepted the latter must be presented in the spirit of 'let's have fun' and if this is done, fun is usually the result. Some of the games which have been successful are as follows.

Blackboard Games. These can take the form of quizzes or discussions, and are often made competitive by playing one side of the room against the other, men against women, or grandmothers against the rest. Noughts and crosses, spelling games, travel and memory games can all be played with the help of a blackboard.

Table Games. These include boxed games such as dominoes, checkers, scrabble, and group games such as beetle, housey and hoy. If there is an element of skill care should be taken in matching opponents, or unobtrusive help should be given to the weaker players. A patient who is allowed to lose consistently or to feel inferior may well reject not only the game in question, but other more important aspects of his programme. It must always be remembered that the player is more important than the game.

Floor Games. Indoor bowls, 'Ninepins', and both deck and peg quoits can be used successfully. If there are patients in the group who must remain seated for their throw, then all competitors are asked to do the same. The walking into position and sitting and rising can provide useful exercise for the patients who need to practise these skills. The rules of all such games can be simplified to suit the group, and distances can be adjusted to the strength of the players.

Less formal floor games can be provided by marking out a 'court' on a large sheet of cardboard, or if conditions are suitable, on the floor. An example is a game with rules very like darts, but with a large numbered circle on the floor, and bean bags to throw into the divisions. The variety is limited only by the imaginations of the people concerned.

Outdoor Games. Many of the games already discussed can be played out of doors if a suitably equipped area is available. Modified forms of croquet and 'putting' can be arranged with minimal equipment, as can 'invented' games in great variety. The weather is usually the deciding factor in such activities. It must be remembered that elderly people do not stand up well to extremes of either heat or cold.

Some games which have been found useful are listed in Appendix D.

Group Discussions

Group discussions are useful for helping patients to get to know each other, for reminding them of current events, and for providing an opportunity for self expression. The factors which affect the success or otherwise of group discussions are the composition of the group itself, the choice of suitable subjects, and the skill of the leader in 'keeping the ball rolling' unobtrusively.

Relatively small groups are usually more responsive and lively than larger ones and more likely to gain the participation of reserved and hesitant members. For instance, a group of 20 will probably enjoy the activity more if divided into two groups of ten. This should be done if the group contains withdrawn, aphasic, deaf or confused people who need help to be able to take part and benefit from the activity.

The group leader needs to be knowledgeable about the subject for discussion, or at least to be interested in it. She also needs tact in giving each patient a share of the floor, and the ability to keep the discussions from becoming boring, one sided, hurtful, or too controversial.

Discussions can vary in structure and subject matter. Some examples are:

(a) Set subjects such as gardening, recipes, hobbies, holidays, weddings, work, and numerous other general topics.
(b) Free-ranging sessions where one topic leads to another in a group 'chat'.
(c) Quizzes where selected questions lead to discussions.
(d) Newspaper readings followed by discussion.

(e) Discussion of current topics of interest to the group.
(f) Local history — stories of how things were. Out-patients may be asked to bring in old photographs or treasures.
(g) Orientation sessions focused on the present — the date, the place, current events and modern changes.
(h) Music played and then discussed.

The person leading the group should always be aware of the response of the members and should change the subject or the whole activity if interest is not maintained. A discussion can often be led quite naturally into a singing session or a game if the patients' attention has begun to wander.

Music and Singing

Music and singing have a valuable part to play among the group activities, and should not be neglected because the leaders of the group are not musicians. If any member of staff has musical skills these should of course be used, but the most valuable asset in the leader is to be able to involve the patients. This can be done without a trained voice or the ability to play an instrument.

As with other activities, the best results are obtained by starting at a simple level, and working up to whatever standard the group can reach. Some simple starting points are as follows:

(a) Ask the group to sing 'Happy Birthday' and 'For He's a Jolly Good Fellow' on all appropriate occasions.
(b) Discover whether any group member has a good voice or can play an instrument and if so, encourage their use. Mouth organs, concertinas, recorders and other simple instruments can entertain the group and give status to the performer.
(c) If a patient mentions that his daughter plays the violin, sings in a choir, or has some other musical skill, send her an invitation to play for the group.
(d) Ask the patients to sing well-known marching songs such as 'Pack up your Troubles' and 'Tipperary' at appropriate times during exercises. The soldiers sang them unaccompanied too.
(e) Make use of rhythm. Home-made percussion instruments played to a rousing tune on the record player can be fun if the session does not go on for too long. Quick steps and marches have proved the easiest rhythm for beginners. Pipe and brass bands provide music of suitable volume. A patient or member

of staff can emphasise the rhythm by standing in front and wielding a baton or playing one of the louder instruments.

(f) Discuss music. Play an interesting band on a record and ask members of the group for comment. Ask patients to discuss their favourite tune. Tell the story of a composer, and play something he wrote. Have an Irish or Scottish afternoon, and play appropriate music. Ask patients of other ethnic groups if they can tell about their music, and perhaps bring examples from home. Many more variations will come to mind to suit local interests.

(g) Have a sing-song. This may start spontaneously as a patient who enjoys music sings as he works. If this can be picked up by the staff or other patients it is usually well received by the group. Even a more formally programmed session can be kept simple and still provide enjoyment for the group, if not for the listener. More details of the programmed sing-song will be given in the following paragraphs.

The Singing Session

Value. Singing together is enjoyed by many people, whatever the quality of their voices. Soldiers on the march pick up their feet more briskly, people in buses find the journey goes more quickly, and people in church find more involvement in the service if they can join with others in a song. Among the older generation are many to whom 'community singing' was a recognised form of entertainment, and sing-songs around the piano were a feature of family life. Others have sung the songs of two world wars, or sung bush ballads around the camp fire. These past experiences provide a wide range of songs available to the group, and most patients enjoy hearing and singing them again. Some patients with speech problems find particular release in singing because they find that the words come back in song even though they are unable to produce voluntary speech.

Choice of Songs. The really well-known community songs are usually the most satisfactory for 'warming up', as they do not demand too much of the singers, and give them confidence to go on. If any patient knows the verse it may be good practice for him to be asked to sing it while others join in the chorus. Requests from the patients should be encouraged, and sung if possible.

It usually helps patients to remember songs they would like to sing if types of songs are introduced in groups. Such groups include songs from the first and second World Wars, Irish, Scottish or plantation songs, songs using somebody's name, or songs of Australia. Occasionally, younger staff members like to sing some of their own popular songs, or do a 'hokey pokey' or a conga. If some such staff involvement can be introduced during the session it is appreciated by the patients and gives them a little break in their own efforts.

Action songs and rounds can also be used to make a change and add some physical activity or humour to the programme.

Accompaniment. Whether or not an accompaniment is a help depends upon the understanding of the accompanist. If the accompanist can play softly and at the patients' speed the patients will sing along and enjoy doing so. Unfortunately, there is a tendency for some pianists to feel that by playing loudly and strongly they will make up for the weaknesses of the voices and carry the group along with them. Among the elderly disabled this is not usually so. Loud or fast playing results in the withdrawal of the singers who find the opposition too strong. On the other hand, they will nearly always respond to the leader who can ask for help, saying 'I'm not much of a singer, but I think singing is fun. Let's have some fun together.'

Whether or not there is an accompanist, the person conducting the singing should take time to announce each song, and remind the group of the opening words. If the accompanist plays one song after another without a break, most of the songs will be half over before the majority of patients join in. This too can lead to withdrawal from the effort.

How Important are Words? Songs are made up of words and music, but many people remember a tune long after the words have gone. This can be an embarrassment if it is not provided for in advance. The conductor can explain before starting that if those who have forgotten the words will hum the tune or sing 'la la la' to it they will help those who do remember the words to keep going. Large print books of words may be helpful, but they encourage the singers to look down to read rather than to look up to sing. In doing this they reduce the rapport between singers and the leader. The leader should certainly face the group and give encouragement rather than burying her head in a book. She too can sing 'la la la' if it becomes necessary.

Variations and Solos. Singing sessions can become flat and lifeless if there is no variation from old songs sung in unison by the group. If a patient or a helper can provide a solo, a welcome change can be made. What the solo can be will depend upon the ability of the singer, but recitations, comic songs, and solos on an instrument are helpful as well as the usual ballads. Action songs and rounds can break the monotony or the singing can be divided into two sections by a period of percussion playing to a record, or a musical quiz.

As in all activities, the leader should be aware if the group is tiring or losing interest, and should have a change of activity ready if this is so. The participants should leave their song period feeling happy and wanting more.

The Problem of Tears. Singing can have a strongly emotional effect upon some people, and the old and sick are not immune. Some patient will cry even during happy songs if those songs touch a chord of memory. There are also some songs which ask for tears. 'Home Sweet Home' is a prime example. If there are tears a simple change to another group of songs may suffice, but if any patient is obviously deeply affected it may be necessary for a helper to ask him quietly if he would like to go outside. The patient should be given the choice in this matter because in many cases they prefer to stay. They usually explain that they are 'not unhappy', but that the singing made them feel a little 'full up'. On many occasions such patients have said later that they felt better for their 'little cry'. Tears of this kind should not be ignored, but neither should too much fuss be made.

Patients who have had a stroke are particularly liable to tears of this nature. For further comment see Chapter 17.

Visiting entertainers often have difficulty in accepting weeping by some of the people they have come to 'cheer up'. It is both wise and kind to warn them that this may happen, and explain that the emotional release is not necessarily a bad thing. A staff member should, of course, attend to any patient who is excessively moved by the entertainment.

Special Occasions

On a few occasions each year there are opportunities to take

advantage of a special day to add interest and variety to the programme. All the public holidays can be used, and national days of
other countries. The local show, Cup Day, and other national or
local events can provide the theme for a celebration. An annual
event such as an 'Open Day' or Sale of Work might also be considered. These big days should not be confined to the retraining
staff and patients, but as many of the rest of the staff as possible
should be asked to take part. The patients can work as a group for
days, or even weeks in advance for the occasion. The craft groups
can prepare suitable hats for the day, for example, glengarries for
St Andrew's Day, easter bonnets, jockey caps for Cup Day, and
so on. Patients who like to cook can make cakes or sweets which
pick up the theme, other staff members can be asked to lend suitable recordings or tapes, and a small display of pictures, posters
made by the patients, relevant objects and ornaments can be set
up. On the day activities are organised around the theme, with as
many things as possible being related to it. This may include
games, quizzes, singing, dinner music, items on the menu, the
wearing of favours and hats, and anything else that the occasion
may suggest. Dancing by staff members is usually well received.

Special occasions are not difficult to organise because they just
mean giving everyday activities a special slant. They do stimulate
both the staff and the patients, and make for interest in the unit,
good will, and a heightened level of co-operation and communication.

Group Entertainment

In the retraining programme entertainments have limited value
because the audience is made up of relatively passive recipients
rather than active participants. The most successful entertainments
are those in which some audience participation is demanded. An
occasional concert is stimulating and adds variety. Colour slides
are useful if followed by discussion and reminiscences by the
patients. A fashion parade will be more valuable if patients can be
included among the models. Most 'live' entertainments can be
adjusted to include active patient involvement, and this effort
should be made.

Background music and television are rarely helpful. If the
patients are being activated it is not helpful to have competition

from obtrusive sounds unconnected with the business in hand. In a busy activity room there is plenty of sound made by the people themselves. Many patients in the retraining situation have difficulties in concentration and in coping with multiple stimuli. Noise which is unrelated to the main activity can only add to their problems. Confused patients, and particularly those who tend towards restlessness and wandering, are usually adversely affected by too high a level of sound, and irritation usually results. The provision of background noise is usually considered by those who supply it to be preferable to the quiet which is so noticeable a feature of groups of unstimulated elderly folk. It does not in fact stimulate them, but makes it harder than ever for them to chat amongst themselves. The stimulus should come from real people to whom they can relate.

Television which is used actively is a different matter. Some patients have their favourite programme and feel deprived if they have to miss it. A small group which is really watching and can discuss the programme later is a very different thing from the group of disinterested patients nodding in a circle around the room while a flow of sound is used to disguise the lack of activity and human exchanges.

When there are important current events or special entertainments the television can be used with effect as part of a group programme. The Melbourne Cup should be watched as part of a Cup Party, groups of interested people can watch a test match, Royal visits and Anzac Day can be celebrated and other special programmes can be used in stimulating patients. Passive viewing without involvement, on the other hand, acts as a soporific, and works against the retraining programme as a whole.

The Individual Within the Group

Group activities have value administratively, and in some aspects of patient care, but it should never be forgotten that a group is made up of individuals, and is valuable only when it is meeting their needs. In the retraining situation the group leader should be aware of the response of the frailer members, and ensure that they are not being over-extended. She must see that the quiet patient has his turn as well as the extrovert, and that no-one is allowed to look silly in front of the rest. Individual physical needs should be seen to as they arise, but the wise leader prepares for them in advance. For instance, access to the toilets should be kept clear, and suitable passages left so that patients can be reached by the staff. Knee rugs should be available for any patient who complains of the cold, and patients who are known to like fresh air should be seated if possible near windows or doors. Some care should also be taken that patients in higher chairs should be placed behind the shorter patients and those in low chairs. No group can be expected to function well if half the people are unable to see what is being done. Care for individual comfort in such ways helps the group as a whole as well as the individual whose needs have been met.

7 INDIVIDUAL ACTIVITIES

The value of individual activities is discussed and some problems are noted. The satisfaction engendered by 'making things' is related to the degree of success and a plea is made for simple forms.

Introduction

Group activities have much to offer in geriatric retraining as described in the previous chapter. It is often necessary, however, to give people more individual attention than is possible in the group situation in order to discover their full potential. This applies to both physical and psychological treatment. Individual activities include gardening, cooking and writing, as well as the many crafts and hobbies which are available. If a patient already has an interest, it is usually helpful to encourage that, rather than to introduce something new which he is likely to drop as soon as he resumes his life at home. If the activity is new to the helper, it is an opportunity to learn enough of it to add one more subject to the programme.

Individual activities can encourage the individual patient, and make possible a closer knowledge of him as a person. They can also provide a background to treatment and so eliminate the long hours which are spent waiting for treatment by doctor, nurse, or therapist, or for bath, transport, or routine retraining procedures. Individual activities are not disrupted by the removal of patients for reasons such as these, whereas a group activity can be completely destroyed.

Choice of Activities

Almost any activity can be used therapeutically for some patient at some time, and the more activities the helper can offer the more success she is likely to achieve with her patients. If she herself is enthusiastic about some hobby or interest, it is more than likely that she will be able to enthuse her patients with it, so long as she offers it at a level at which they can succeed. Some activities have a wider appeal than others, and it is obviously better to use these as basic features of the programme, but other, possibly less obvious activities should be introduced from time to time if the programme is not to stagnate. Some of the more basic activities are the following.

Crafts

Crafts have a wide appeal to most people once they overcome the initial feeling that they may not be able to manage. Many people are already interested in using their hands creatively and many others have wished to do so without taking the necessary steps. Even those who have no such feelings usually enjoy producing something once they tackle a job and bring it to a successful conclusion.

As well as being readily accepted by most patients, crafts have characteristics which make them a useful tool for the staff. They offer great variety, so that they can be graded for the individual, they produce useful end results, they create interest in other staff and relatives, and they can be adapted for treatment or recreation depending upon the need of the patient.

Domestic Activities

Domestic activities should be used for specific patients as part of their retraining. This applies particularly to those who live alone, or who will be alone by day while a relative is at work. They are also of value to patients whose interests and skills are to be found in this area. Electric fry pans and small electric cookers can overcome the problem of segregation of the 'cooks' from the main group when staff shortages make supervision difficult in divided areas.

Hobbies and Interests

The patient's own existing hobby should be considered when his programme is being planned. It is likely that he will already be motivated towards it, and will also be likely to continue with it when he leaves the hospital. Music, gardening, and art can all be used in the retraining programme, as well as stamps, coins, shells and other collections. Care should be taken in suggesting an established hobby if the patient's disability will prevent him from reaching a standard to satisfy himself, but in most cases it is a good starting point for gaining his interest.

Past Employment

Past employment often provides clues as to the best choice of activity for a patient. This applies particularly to the former craftsman. Woodwork, metal work, bootmaking, dressmaking, and so on, all have processes which can be put to use. Patients with such skills can often help with the making of adaptations to equipment, building up a shoe, or supervising the work of a fellow patient who is learning a process which was involved in his trade. The use of existing skills in this way, even if it amounts only to giving advice, has great value in showing the patient that he still has something to offer.

We should think out our reasons for providing activities for the elderly person before deciding on the form these activities should take. The provision of crafts just because it has become traditional to use them can mean that the programme is not fulfilling the needs of the group concerned. Demented patients, for instance, may respond better to simple group projects, intellectuals to crossword puzzles or chess, and dedicated housewives to serving the morning and afternoon teas. If crafts are decided upon, they should be presented at a level well within the patient's competence to succeed.

Creative Activities

The oldest description of creative activity is 'in the beginning' — the story of Creation as told in the Old Testament. Today's craftsmen can see parallels with their own actions and satisfactions in their work. There is light by which to work and show off the end product, there is the collecting together and sorting of materials, there is the start with simple articles and working up to the masterpiece, and there is checking as each process is finished to 'see that it is good'. Finally, there is the satisfaction of standing back and observing the finished article — 'and God saw everything that He had made, and behold it was very good'.

The feeling of satisfaction and the rest after a successful effort are the craftsman's reward, and provide the main reason for introducing crafts in a retraining programme.

Creativity and the development of tools to extend his own powers are two areas in which man has progressed far beyond all other members of the animal kingdom. Both these advanced skills are combined in the field of crafts, and most people find great satisfaction in applying them. The bird with her nest, and the spider with her web, are both creating something, but the design and the method of building are dictated by instinct, and not by creative thought. Their efforts are far removed from the limitless ways man can devise to produce an egg basket or a fishing net. It is his involvement with decisions about such things as shape, size, colour, texture, and so on, which leads each person to see an article as his own, and his satisfaction will depend to a large extent upon how much of himself has gone into its production.

Reasons for Using Crafts

Our reasons for introducing crafts in the overall programme, and our reasons for presenting them to the individual patients both need to be considered. The former are matters of policy, and the latter are based on individual needs. The advantages and disadvantages of crafts in these two areas are as follows.

Crafts in the Overall Programme

Advantages.
  Most patients enjoy them.
  They can be varied to suit individual needs.
  They can be taught in groups so that supervision is localised.
  Something is there to show for the work.
  They can be used for specific physical and mental treatment.
  They can be increased in difficulty as the patients progress.
  They satisfy many of the basic human needs, particularly the final three (page 118).

Disadvantages. Unless carefully controlled they can be abused. Pressure by relatives or staff to produce more, attempts to make money for the institution rather than to satisfy the patient, and staff who want to make 'foreign orders', are examples.
  Some crafts demand excessive preparation time from the staff.
  Poor choice of activities can lead to waste of materials, purchase of expensive equipment, and disappointing results.

People who do not understand the treatment aspects of the whole programme tend to associate it with the tangible crafts instead of the intangible benefits to the patients. This is particularly important when applied to lay administrators, and those who are responsible for funding.

Crafts in the Treatment of the Individual

Advantages.

They give a wide choice, so that it is usually possible to find a suitable activity for each patient.

They give a good opportunity for assessing the patient's ability and motivation.

They give great satisfaction if well chosen.

They can be increased in difficulty to help the patient to progress, or decreased to help a deteriorating patient to continue doing his best.

They give patients something to discuss besides pain and illness.

They make a good starting point for a relaxed interview with the patient.

They give opportunity for self expression in colour, form, etc.

They give saleable articles if the patients are working together for a common cause.

They impress relatives and friends whose praise reinforces the patient's positive feelings about himself.

They can provide a measure of improvement.

Disadvantages.

They can disappoint a patient if he makes a mistake.

Some people are not interested in them, but are expected to conform if the helper forgets why they are being offered.

Pressure to produce too much or too quickly can cause distress.

Patients may not be able to afford the finished product, yet feel compelled to buy it.

There can be danger in the use of some tools.

Crafts can encourage withdrawal from social contacts if taken too seriously.

Selfish and greedy patients tend to demand more than their share of attention, while the quiet, timid patient may be forgotten.

The Patient's Reason for Working at a Craft

Whatever the helper's object in offering an individual a certain craft, she must also have a reason which has meaning for the patient in order to gain his interest. His reason for attempting it may well be different from hers in wanting him to do so. Some of the more useful reasons to use in motivating the patient include the following.

Treatment.

To provide a specific movement in a natural way.

To increase dexterity, particularly if the non-dominant hand must be used.

To strengthen existing movements.

To encourage better posture.

To increase the range of movement in stiffened joints, and such other physical benefits as may be applied to the patient in question.

To help improve concentration.

To provide an interest and help the time to be well spent.

To provide a counter-irritant to worry or sadness, and other such reasons as may be appropriate.

These reasons will be suitable for the better preserved of intellect, but are usually meaningless to the confused, demented or really resistant patient. More personal reasons are usually preferable for such people.

Personal Reasons.

Gifts for relatives or friends. A baby basket for a new grand-child, a cheese board for a son, or a coat hanger for a helpful neighbour.

Something to use himself. A pottery ash tray, a tray for his pylon stick.

Work for a 'cause'. His Church Fete, a local children's home, a raffle for his club.

Help to another patient. Doing one simple process while the other patient produces the article. Sorting materials, winding wool or stuffing a cushion. Also, if proficient, doing a part which is too hard for the other patient.

Starting or finishing a basket, preparing bases, machining a cushion.

Economic Reasons.
   Items to sell at a small profit to augment finances.
   Learning a craft to continue at home as a 'cottage industry'.
   'Mend and Make Do' activities.

The reason which will motivate one patient may have the opposite effect on another, and so it is necessary for the helper to choose her presentation of the task to suit the one person she wishes to enthuse.

Fashion in Crafts

There is usually an ebb and flow of interest in different crafts at different times, and the wise group leader is aware of these and uses them to advantage. Sometimes it is widespread and general like the recent renewal of interest in cord knotting, and sometimes it is purely local, because someone in the group had a particular skill and their ideas took flight. If the fashion is general, the patient's involvement will be a link with what is happening in the community, and pictures in magazines, exhibitions and talks on the subject can all be used to encourage the interest. If it is local, it can provide a talking point for the group.

The main problem with fashions is that there is a tendency to overstock materials or buy expensive equipment for a craze which is likely to wane as fast as it waxed. The leader should also discourage slavish copying of an article by the patients. The value of crafts lies partly in their individuality, and variations in size, colour, texture, and so on, should be encouraged. Machines are better than people at producing identical articles. The craftsman's skill lies in not doing so.

Simplification of Crafts

In encouraging the patients to tackle craftwork we must always remember that the important thing is the effect of the craft on the patient, and not the effect of the patient on the craft. This concept leads a few people to say that standards do not matter, so long as the patients enjoy doing it. The problem here is that most people do not enjoy doing something they are unable to do well, and most of the results we hope to get from providing crafts depend upon a successful end product. It is the teacher's responsibility to present something at the level at which her pupils can learn, and to help them to grow from there. If we wish to do this with a group of adults with a wide range of ability, experience, and disability, we must develop our own skill in assessment (see Chapter 8), and adjust the work to the patient.

Many helpers, who are good at crafts themselves, have some difficulty in finding simple starting places for their patients. The major crafts, many of which can be used in activity programmes, involve the craftsman in an apprenticeship of five or more years. Basketry, carpentry, metalwork, needlework, pottery, tiling and weaving are all crafts of wide potential, providing opportunities for the development of great skill and invention. What is more to our purpose in retraining, they include some processes which are simple and direct, and can bring satisfying results even to a complete beginner. In using crafts in the treatment or motivation of elderly patients, it is our task to search out these simple processes, and make sure that what we offer is within the workers' powers. If the reasons for providing crafts are studied it will be apparent that success in the chosen activity is necessary to achieve the purpose of that activity. The patient who is tackling a craft for the first time must start with something at which he will not fail. Much of his satisfaction will come from being told that he has done so well that he is ready to move on to the next step.

Important Factors in Simplification

Minimal Use of Tools. One of the major advances in the development of man was his invention of tools, but we still find great satisfaction in using our hands directly on some materials, and in some processes where no tool comes between us and our work. Pottery, weaving, basketry, and tiling all provide such processes, which can in themselves produce completed articles. Plaiting, lacing, beadwork, sanding, polishing, and folding are also possible with very simple direct tools, or none at all. Such processes come easily to most people, as they demand neither great manipulative skill, nor complicated thought processes.

Single Repetitive Processes. The single, repetitive process such as weaving cane in and out to build up the wall of a basket, is easier to learn and do well than a task which requires a series of different moves, such as framing a picture or plaiting the border of the same basket. Such processes are the basis of simplification and should be used to good advantage. It is sometimes better to ask a patient to help another patient by doing one of these simple repetitive jobs for him than to give him the full responsibility for a job on his own. Such processes include sanding, polishing, cutting stakes for basketry, winding wool, randing (simple weaving) in basketry, finger weaving on a frame, tearing paper (papier mâché), and bead threading. Single repetitive processes are the basis of mass production methods, and can be used to advantage in retraining, so long as the person in charge makes sure that patients move on to the next step as soon as they are ready. Boredom with the task will nullify its value.

Anticipation of Difficulties. When preparing a job for a patient it is important to be aware of his limitations, such as poor eyesight, coordination, or mental capacity, and to allow for them in what you ask him to do. For instance, a formal pattern in beadwork may be beyond a patient with poor concentration, but a haphazard mixture of blending colours will be possible. In this way he will produce an acceptable article which is not meant to be accurate rather than a poor one which is. A patient with a tremor which would make it very difficult for him to stick tiles down accurately could manage if the person preparing his work could stick down those around the edge, and let him do a haphazard, or 'crazy' pattern in the centre. Again, a good article will result, because it is intended to be 'crazy', and is not that way as a result of the patient's disability. Elimination of a problem by forethought is an essential form of simplifying the job for the individual if he is not to be distressed rather than pleased by his work.

Supervision and Progress Checks. When a job involves a number of different processes, these can be simplified for the patient by being taught one at a time. The simple processes can be given first, the helper doing the harder ones until the patient is ready to tackle them. When the patient begins a new process the helper should supervise closely and, if it proves too difficult, should be ready to help before the patient loses heart. Once the process has been mastered the patient should be left to do it alone, but the helper should check the work for mistakes at salient points. There is no joy for the patient in a mistake which is found only when the article is finished, and no remedy is possible. The salient points for checking are places where changes occur, for instance, changes in shape, material, colour, pattern, tool or process. This is the equivalent of quality control at each stage on a production line.

It is also wise to check each patient's work at the end of each session, and to rectify any mistakes at once. If this is done routinely, the patients will not build on mistakes the next time they tackle their work, or start their session by seeing their mistake corrected. It is a good rule never to put a mistake in the cupboard.

Simplification of Choice

Many elderly patients, and particularly the mildly demented, find difficulty in decision making. When faced with too many alternatives they tend to become flustered, and solve the problem by rejecting them all. As in other areas of treatment it is necessary to start at the patient's level, and to increase the difficulty of the task as he improves.

There are many ways of offering a choice of crafts to a patient, and his response to that choice depends upon the helper choosing the one which suits him best. Discussion of a few typical ways of offering work to a patient who is about to start a new piece of work will illustrate this point.

Method 1. What Would You Like to Do?

This question may suit an established patient who knows what is available, and who is well motivated and confident. It is too vague and places too much responsibility on a new and hesitant one. It gives him too wide a choice, and too little information upon which to base his decision. The answer is likely to be 'nothing today, thank you'.

Method 2. Would You Like to Make a … ?

Here the choice being offered is between doing something and doing nothing, rather than a choice between different activities. The patient may say 'yes' just to please you, or 'no', because it seems safer. This question almost suggests a negative or at best neutral response, and not a positive choice which is needed to involve the patient in what he is about to do.

Method 3. Which of These Would You Like to Try?

(Show the patient samples of as many alternatives as you think he is ready to consider.) This is a positive and encouraging question. Most patients can choose between two alternatives, and the act of choosing involves the patient with the activity. Seeing a finished article lets him see what he is attempting, and so provides a definite goal, while the word 'try' gives him a face-saving way out if the task proves too hard. His ability to choose will develop with confidence, and should be matched by increases in the number of alternatives offered.

Method 4. I've Brought You This ... to Try. Have a Go, and If It's No Good We'll Try Something Else.

This method is a trial and error one which gives both the helper and the patient room to manoeuvre. Particularly in the early stages, some patients say 'no' to any activity, and a question which can be answered negatively is useless. The patient who is not ready to make a positive decision will often respond to this approach, as he can accept the task without promising anything, and without responsibility. The task offered should itself be simple, and praise for a good try is an essential part of the exercise. Once the patient has set his hand to the task it is unusual for him to withdraw it. A successful conclusion is the best base for a more involved choice for his next job.

Craftwork and Motivation

Crafts are naturally interesting to some people, who are already aware of the satisfaction of creating something, but to others they are a new experience, and one they are afraid to tackle in case it is beyond them. Some people feel that crafts are unsuitable for the latter, and an alternative activity should be offered. This may be so in a few cases, but it has been found that careful selection of the right craft with the right degree of difficulty leads in most cases to great satisfaction and pride when the article is brought to a successful conclusion. In fact, the less a patient expects to succeed, the greater his pleasure is likely to be when he does so. As this feeling of accomplishment is a major reason for providing creative activities it would be a pity to deny it to patients just because of an initial show of reluctance. For more detailed discussion of motivation see Chapter 12.

Programme Problems

Much has been written about simplifying activities for the patient, but it is also necessary to keep the programme simple for the staff. If crafts are part of a comprehensive programme it is hardly practical to provide alternative programmes for a few, and thus create the need for two or more types of preparation, and double supervision. The programme should cater for many different needs and interests, but not all at the same time unless the staffing and space available are more generous than is usually the case. It is usually better to spend time in involving the patient in the programmed activity than in providing an alternative which will divide the group, and necessitate separate supervision.

Some Easy Starting Points

The easy processes of major crafts which were mentioned earlier can be used as starting points and some of the more useful ones are listed here.

Basketry

Randing — this involves weaving a single fine cane in and out around a series of heavier upright canes to build up the wall of a basket. It is simple repetitive movement, and can be learnt by most patients with the exception of the grossly demented, and stroke patients with constructional dyspraxia. The helper at this stage will have to do the two borders for the patient, but as the wall is the part one sees the patient can still feel that it is his own work.

Carpentry

Despite modern ideas about 'unisex', the majority of male patients like a job that they can think of as being 'male'. Anything to do with the working of wood is usually acceptable. Some examples are:
(a) *Sanding and Polishing* — wood blocks on masonite to make cheese boards, bread boards, or occasional table tops. Cigar boxes to make trinket boxes. Fruit boxes for storage boxes and so on.

(b) *Gluing* — parquetry offcuts, small timber offcuts, or used matches to make articles as above, and tray bases, wall pictures (murals), etc.

Metalwork

(a) *Modelling* — copper sheeting for pictures, letter racks, fire screens.
(b) *Impressing* — silver foil, aluminium foil, to cover many items from jewel boxes to lamp stands.

Needlework

(a) Coarse wool embroidery and tapestry cushions, aprons.
(b) Simple toys — cut wool, stuffed, knitted.
(c) Cross stitch on gingham or dobby check.

Pottery

(a) Pinch pots, modelling, rolling.
(b) Plaster carved pots for succulents.

Tiling

Gluing and grouting tiles on tea pot stands, plates, bowls, lamp stands, occasional tables.

Weaving

(a) Finger weaving on picture frame, bath mats, tea cosies.
(b) Plaiting — pull up ropes, binding a lamp stand, place mats and coasters.

Paper Craft

Greeting and Christmas cards, labels, sweet boxes, note books, collage.

This chapter is not included as a treatise on crafts, but to provide some simple but practical ideas so that a start can be made. There are many good books on the subject available in libraries and shops if any particular craft needs to be developed.

Some Useful Minor Crafts

Some minor crafts have proved their value in activity programmes.

The most successful of these have the following features in common:

The materials are reasonably cheap.
Processes can be graded from simple to moderately difficult.
Tools, if needed, are simple and safe to use.
Mistakes are easily rectified.
Designs are simple but effective.
Colours can be varied to suit individual tastes.
Results are produced quickly.
Useful or interesting products are the result.

Some examples which involve some or all of these criteria are as follows.

Plastic Beadwork

Many articles can be made from beads cut from 4 mm tubular plastic threaded on to strings of 1 mm gauge of the same material. Strings of glass beads can also be rethreaded to make new necklaces.

Shellwork

The mounting of shells on flower pots, trinket boxes, etc., or the making of shell 'animals' by gluing different-sized shells together to form body, head and limbs.

Pressed Flowers

These can be gathered, pressed, and mounted to form designs on cards, calendars, trinket boxes, lampshades, etc. The design is covered with transparent plastic film for protection.

Rug Making

Scraps of material, thrums, or any available thread can be hooked, woven, or sewn. The base can be hessian, canvas, or a warp stretched on a frame.

Stool Seating

Seagrass, cord, or twisted or plaited reed-like material can be used. Tapestry or pieces of upholstery material can be placed over a padded wooden box, or a hassock can be sewn and stuffed.

Added to activities such as these are the 'fashion' crafts which come and go from time to time. Some examples are stuffed clowns, woolly toys, plastic waste paper baskets, draught stoppers for doors, and similar items. While they are in fashion the demand for them from the patients is high, but such interest is likely to fade after a time. Fashions can be used to advantage while they last, but materials for such activities should be ordered in moderation to avoid waste when the demand slackens.

Other Individual Activities

When a craft session is in progress most of the patients will be happy and interested, but a few would be better employed at some other pursuit, and should be encouraged if this can be managed. Doing 'homework' for the speech pathologist, writing letters, reading the morning paper, polishing shoes and working on a jigsaw puzzle are all legitimate alternatives which are not difficult to provide within the craft session setting.

If a patient has an interest like tinkering with broken clocks, polishing silverware, soaking off and sorting stamps, or looking down a microscope, the activity will be just as valuable as crafts in his particular case. He should be encouraged to follow his own interests when this is possible because he will be better served by those when he goes home than by some new activity imposed by others. His interest and involvement are the important factors. No single form of activity has been proved to be 'better' than the others.

Conclusion

Individual activities have an important place in the retraining programme if they are used with a purpose and not merely because they are expected. The actual activity has little intrinsic merit, but any activity which interests the patient will have value in helping to develop and maintain motivation. Activities which are introduced into the retraining programme, but which are not directly related to activities of daily living have this motivational purpose. How they are offered and accepted is more important than which activities are actually chosen.

8 ASSESSMENT

Introduction

Assessment is a word which has expanded its meaning so much in recent years, that a current edition of most dictionaries is needed to find a satisfactory definition. Webster probably comes nearest to its usage in retraining, 'assess': 'to analyse critically and judge definitively the nature, significance, status, or merit of.' Heinemann's Australian Dictionary puts it more succinctly: 'to estimate or judge.' Both have come a long way from the Concise Oxford (1962), which is concerned exclusively with its application in fixing and imposing taxes.

Sophisticated modern treatment techniques have been matched by sophisticated systems of assessment, to a point where there has appeared a tendency to see assessment as valuable in its own right. In geriatric retraining assessment has two functions, and unless it fulfils one or both of these, it is of little value to the patient. These functions are to assist in the realistic planning of treatment, and to measure progress. Assessment should lead to decisions and action, and not to the production of one more lengthy report. In this chapter assessment will be discussed in its relationship to the patient and his retraining programme. It will be seen as the critical analysis of the patient's condition — those assets, disabilities, and needs, upon which his retraining programme is based. It is a dynamic process which continues throughout that programme, with more specific emphasis at crucial times along the way. These assessments are not made for their own sakes, but to be used as guides to treatment and measures of progress.

Specific Assessments

Every time we work with a patient we must assess the level at which to approach him, his ability to cope with what we are offering, his needs for equipment, and how he is responding to the activity. Our own adjustment to these continuous minor assessments determines to some extent the results we obtain from the patient. At certain times in the course of retraining there is need for a more specific and formal assessment which may need to be communicated to the team. This communication may be either verbal or written. Specific assessments are made as follows.

Selection of Patients for Retraining

The selection of patients for retraining is the responsibility of the doctor, but where a full team is operating the social worker's findings will have a strong bearing on his decision. Upon the combined social and medical assessment of the patient will depend the aims and intensity of treatments applied by the rest of the team. Case selection depends upon the practical needs of the patient and his family rather than an illness-based assessment of suitability for retraining. He will not be excluded by the severity of his disability, learning difficulties, or emotional problems if any aspect of the retraining programme can help the whole situation. 'Treatment' of the limbs, muscles or joints may be a lost cause, but the elimination of lifting, the choice and supply of suitable equipment, the training of relatives in effective management, and the provision of domiciliary services may provide a solution other than nursing home admission.

The method of selection which assesses a patient as 'doing well, and suitable for rehabilitation' does not necessarily apply in the selection for retraining. The patient who is not doing well, and who may not get home unless something is done is the one who needs retraining most. Initially the combined assessment of the doctor and social worker delineate such needs.

The Initial Group Assessment

Assessment should begin with our initial approach to the patient. All members of the team will make such assessments in their own way, and with their own emphases. At the first case conference the main points of these preliminary observations will be brought forward and a composite team assessment will emerge. This is unlikely to be unanimous and should certainly not be taken as definitive. It will give a many-sided view of the problems to be faced, and point up areas in which further investigations are necessary. Treatment will begin at this point and as the patient responds the assessment must be reviewed and refined. Medical and social assessments are the primary ones at this stage, showing as they do the present capacity of the patient for activity and the future prospects for his resettlement. Factors which are included in the initial group assessment are:

(a) Medical

Diagnosis — Information is needed concerning relevant signs and symptoms, and the presence of other pathology besides that of the presenting illness.

Relevant treatment — The team needs to be aware of current investigations, drugs, diet, radiotherapy or other treatments which may affect aspects of their own work.

Complicating factors — Does the patient suffer from other conditions such as hypertension, a cardiac condition, a skin problem or dementia as well as the presenting illness?

Pain — The team needs to know whether pain is an unavoidable part of mobilisation, whether the painful part should be used or rested, and whether the patient may be given analgesics.

Psychiatric history — Does the patient experience depression, hallucinations, feelings of aggression, or a tendency to wander away?

Prognosis — Is retraining expected to bring improvement, maintain current levels of independence, or discover easier ways to manage the problem?

Precautions — Are there any contra-indications for specific activities?

Stamina — How much can and should the patient be expected to do?

(b) Social

Family support — Is the family willing and able to offer help? Are family relationships close? Are the relatives disinterested or over-protective?

Family unit — Does the patient live with a spouse, a son or a daughter, or in lodgings? Does he live alone or is he alone for part of the day?

Quality of available help — What is the strength, health and mental capacity of the main supporter? Can the helpers provide physical support or supervision?

Community help — Has the patient good neighbours? Does he receive support from a church or club? Is he already receiving domiciliary services?

Housing — What is the condition of the house? Are there any hazards such as difficult access, stairs, or an outside toilet? Is the home cluttered with furniture or small rugs?

Furniture — Is the furniture well placed and of a suitable height? Does the patient take a bath or a shower?

Resettlement — What are the possibilities, problems, and essential factors in resettlement? What are the patient's feelings and wishes about the future?

Individual factors — What is known of the patient's previous personality and his past employment? Are there any relevant economic factors, 'touchy subjects', or individual needs?

(c) *Early Observations by Other Team Members*

Initial attitudes — When first interviewed did the patient seem resentful, frightened, unresponsive, plaintive, hopeful, enthusiastic, determined or unrealistic?

Problems — Did the patient express any complaints or worries? Did he bring suitable clothing and equipment? Have there been any misunderstandings?

Abilities — Has the patient shown any skills or deficits in learning, understanding, following directions, making friends, motivation, self-organisation or orientation?

Initial Assessment for Routine Retraining Procedures

The helper should know as much of the foregoing information as is available in the patient's notes and at the case conference before retraining goes any further than essential transfers. Armed with this information the helper can approach the patient with confidence and begin to make her own assessment of those factors which relate to her part in the treatment.

There is no need for academic assessments with batteries of tests, sophisticated equipment, and complicated forms. This is a practical assessment of what the patient can and cannot do, and it provides the base on which his retraining will be built. It has three main sections.

(a) Investigation by the Helper. The reading of any referral forms and the patient's case notes, and the noting of relevant information at case conferences or in conversation with other team members should be attended to before any action is taken.

(b) Informal Talk with the Patient. The helper should ask the patient about himself, explain what is going to be done, answer questions, and try to build up the patient's confidence. This talk need not be long, but it should never be omitted. The patient should be given the opportunity to express his fears, to mention his symptoms, and to make his excuses (see Chapters 11 and 12). During this talk the following points should be assessed. They should be brought out in conversation rather than in a series of questions.

Motivation — Is the patient resistive, accepting or enthusiastic about his retraining programme?

Orientation — Does he know where he is, where his home is, and how long he has been ill?

Understanding — Does he know why he has come, what has happened to him, and what you are saying to him? Is he in touch with reality?

Confidence — Is he afraid of the whole programme, or of certain aspects of it? Does he feel that it is too much for him, or is he over-confident and likely to take risks?

Manner — Is he withdrawn, diffident, responsive or self assertive?

Self organisation — Is he able to make his own decisions, and manage his own affairs, or is he dependent upon others to make sure he does the right thing at the right time?

Memory — Can he remember what has happened, and what you have said, or does he forget most of it before the conversation is over? Does he remember personal data such as age, address, and where he is?

Responsiveness — Is he withdrawn and unresponsive, does he respond but not initiate conversation, or does he sometimes take the lead?

Communication difficulties — (The speech pathologist's report should be consulted if available.) Can he express himself? Does he understand what you say to him? Is he deaf? Do hand signals mean more than verbal instructions? Is he distressed and frustrated by inability to speak?

Physical problems — Does the patient suffer from obesity, oedema, an unhealed wound, tremor, deformity or paresis? Is he excessively short or tall, and are there any other physical conditions which should be observed?

Note. Information of the kind listed should come from a conversation which takes the form of a friendly chat. The natural flow of information is usually inhibited by the appearance of a note book and pencil. While the helper is assessing the patient she is also being assessed. By the end of the conversation a friendly understanding should have been reached so that the patient feels confident enough in the helper to try the next stage of retraining.

(c) Wall Bar Assessment. The basic wall bar exercise (see Chapter 15), combined with the information provided by sections (a) and (b) above, demonstrates the level at which retraining should begin. It provides a practical medium for assessing the patient's physical abilities. The patient is seated on a sturdy chair, facing the bar, and the standing exercise is taught step by step using the method designed for his particular disability.

The patient should be told that this is being done to find out what his difficulties are so that he can be helped overcome them. If the patient has complained of pain he should be asked to tell us as soon as he feels the pain. Due regard should be paid to any problem he has mentioned himself, whether or not it is seemingly valid. His confidence in the helper will be greater if he feels that she has listened to him.

The appropriate standing drill should be carried out, with the help of two people if necessary. The patient should be involved as much as possible, and close observations should be made. Points to be noted include the following:

Is he trying to do what he is asked? Is he resisting passively or actively? Can he follow directions? If not, do any of these reasons apply?
Is he deaf? Does he not understand you? Does he lack concentration?
Is he afraid? Does he talk over you about a different subject?
Is he unaware of his own limbs? Has he an old injury or disability which has not been recorded? Has he forgotten the necessary movement pattern? Is he playing up?
Are any of his limbs flaccid or spastic?
Has he significant stiffness in any major joint?
Does he complain of pain on attempting the movement?
Has he any significant deformity?
Is he strong or frail?

Is he breathless on exertion?

Does he tire quickly?

Does he suffer from stress incontinence?

Can he take his own weight?

Can he balance without being held? Without holding on?

Can he transfer his weight from one foot to the other?

Can he rise from a normal height chair?

Does he need a built up chair? Temporarily or permanently?

Can he see out the window? (If the wall bar is not at the window, can he see across the room?)

Can he tell you what he can see on his left side? His right side?

Can he understand directions given on one side but not the other?

Does he look away if spoken to by the person on his weak side?

Does he ignore anything that happens on his weak side?

Can he sit down again, slowly, and without flopping?

Is he pleased with his effort, indifferent, or depressed by it?

If the patient does a good standing drill, and seems ready for it, an attempt at walking should follow. In any case a suitable walking aid should be chosen, and the patient encouraged to stand with it as he stood at the bar. Reactions to this should be noted as above.

The information gained in this way is primarily for the helper's own use, and whether or not it is recorded will depend upon her own needs. Unless the information is to be passed on to others, short notes should suffice. Time spent in elaborate reporting is time which is usually better spent with the patient.

Initial Assessment for Non-specific Activities

Non-specific activities, such as crafts, hobbies, games and social activities, are included in the programme to stimulate and interest the patient, and give him the opportunity for the satisfactions of achievement. If they are to fulfil this purpose it is essential that the patient should not fail when he attempts them. Maintaining the patient's dignity is also part of his treatment, and so he should not be asked to do anything he perceives as childish or a waste of time. For these reasons the helper should assess her patient's abilities and difficulties very carefully so that she can offer activities to suit the individual. These should be neither too complicated nor too easy. In assessing the level at which to start the patient, she should consider these factors:

(a) *Intellectual capacity* — previous standards (job, interests, education) modified by the results of his illness (concentration, learning capacity, confusional state, anxiety, etc.).

(b) *Physical status* — strength, stamina, mobility, manual dexterity, vision, hearing, balance, paralysis, wounds, etc.

(c) *Signs and symptoms* — breathlessness, dizziness, tremor, pain, stiffness, deformity, posture, patient's own complaints.

Most of these factors can be seen overtly, or will emerge from a short conversation. Others may become obvious when the patient actually starts the activity. For this reason the original assessment should not be considered as complete, but should be altered in the light of experience with the patient. Such alterations should not be allowed to upset the patient or make him feel that he has failed. The activity should be offered in the first place on the understanding that it will be changed if it is unsuitable, and the helper should accept the blame if it proves to be so. This will give the patient heart to try again, and it is indeed partly true, in that her assessment has been at fault.

Progress Assessments for Case Conferences

When a patient is to be discussed at a case conference, each member of the team should be ready to contribute her assessment of the patient as demonstrated in her own area. These reports should come from observation of the patient, and should be short and to the point. They should refer to his real problems, and should never be vague or emotional in content. What is relevant will depend upon the reason for discussing the patient at all. From his response to routine retraining, individual and group activities, the helper should be able to assess his progress at psychological and physical levels, his degree of independence in many situations, his ability to communicate, and his adjustment to his present condition. She should also have noted his problems and weaknesses, so as to bring them to the attention of the team for discussion if necessary.

When the team reaches a consensus of opinion that the patient is approaching his own best level of performance, a request will be made for a final assessment, with ADL (Activities of Daily Living) assessment.

Final Assessment

All team members should be involved in the final assessment, and

if they have doubt about any aspect of the patient's performance
they should make it known at the meeting so that a strong effort
can be made to overcome the difficulty before the ADL assessment is required. In the week before the presentation of the final
assessment the patient should be given as much responsibility for
his own care as possible, and his actual performance in real situations should be carefully observed. An ADL done as a test can be
very misleading, as the patient may do especially well because he is
trying to impress, or especially badly because he is nervous of his
'exam'. The person who knows her patients well, and is observant
in day-to-day situations, can complete much of the ADL form
without formal testing. Formal testing can be used in areas where
there is doubt. 'On the job' assessing is a skill which needs practice
and experience, but once it is mastered it becomes almost automatic. It depends upon accurate observation of what is happening
not only in the group but with other individuals at all times, and
not just in the patient's formal treatment session. It is worth the
effort because of its greater accuracy in forecasting the patient's
actual performance when he goes home.

The final assessment should give a picture of the patient's
strengths and weaknesses in the activities of daily life. A copy of
the Newcastle ADL form may be seen in Appendix B. Medical
and social assessments combined with his test form the composite
assessment which is the basis of the interview with the patient's
relatives before discharge. Plans for the patient's discharge are
finalised at this interview, and so the ADL test plays a major part
in determining the patient's need for domiciliary services, and support. It is also of value when a decision concerning nursing home
placement is necessary.

The Activities of Daily Living Assessment Form

The form used in the Newcastle Geriatrics Service was designed
specifically for that service, with reference to the form used at the
Bellevue Hospital, New York. It has been revised a number of
times over the years, in response to new needs as demonstrated in
practical use. These changes have been of a minor nature, and
have referred to details and not principles. Some points worth noting in the present form are as follows.

The Format (see Appendix B)

(a) The form is printed on thick paper to make it durable and easy to handle.
(b) The form is on quarto sheets, punched to fit the hospital's case charts.
(c) The report is limited to two pages to ensure concise recording and for easy reference.
(d) Headings on the first page conform to those of other records kept by the hospital.
(e) The key is included in the heading to help standardise marking judgement.
(f) Headings and subheadings have been used so that areas of difficulty may be discerned at a glance.
(g) The first page deals with items which are best observed in the ward.
(h) The second page deals with items of more general application.
(i) Verbal reporting has been kept to a minimum.
(j) Space has been provided for extra comment on problems of an individual nature not covered by the general questions on the form. If this is insufficient the blank side of the sheets can be used for extra comment.

Content

(a) Headings cover the main areas of activities of daily living as related to the home.
(b) Subheadings break these areas down into the most important components.
(c) Less important components have been eliminated. If one of these is important in an individual case it can be referred to at the end of the report.

The Main Headings

Feeding. Feeding difficulties gain more significance in replacement at home as the degree of family support lessens. Use of utensils may be overcome by adapting handles, serving cut-up foods, or even using fingers instead of forks. In a few cases actual feeding of the patient may be necessary. Cleanliness of eating is recorded so that relatives can make suitable arrangements for the patient's meals before the return home. Inappropriate behaviour at the family table is managed with less embarrassment and risk of hurt feelings if provided for from the beginning.

Food intake is affected by many factors in the elderly, and if known, these should be recorded. Lack of interest, forgetfulness, dental deficiencies, difficulty in swallowing, habit, medical conditions, ignorance of the principles of diet, loneliness, and attempts to manipulate other people are some of the most common causes, and should be mentioned if still unsolved.

Management of medication is recorded here as most elderly patients find this easier if tablet taking is associated with meal times. This can be a vital factor in ability to live alone, and should not be left to chance.

Bed. The two main problems in bed drill are the need for lifting, and the need for even light attention at regular intervals during the night. These aspects should be borne in mind while marking this section. Ability to manage bed drill can be crucial to successful resettlement. Relatives need to understand the problem before the patient returns to them, and training of the relative is often indicated.

Dressing. Ability in self-dressing may be vital to patients who live alone, but of less importance where there is good family support. Suitable clothing and adaptations are often more practical than a long series of sessions in practising the skill. If these are used, their main features and value should be explained to the helping relative. Simple dressing tricks and short cuts should also be discussed.

The importance of suitable footwear should be stressed, as a return to slippers or fashion shoes may so easily lead to falls or deterioration in walking ability.

Prostheses and supportive equipment should be listed, and the ability of the patient to apply them to himself noted. Any known difficulties or special features should be explained to the relative.

Hygiene. Fear of falls in the bathroom is common among both patients and their relatives. If this is apparent, or if the patient is actually in danger of falling, this should be noted so that the relative may receive the necessary instructions, or the services of the community nurse may be provided. The method of bathing tested should be the one the patient will use at home, and any special circumstances, including the need for adaptations to equipment, should be recorded.

Independence in using the toilet has important implications for management at home. Mobility, transfers, and dressing may cause as much difficulty in this area as frequency, urgency, and other problems related to the illness. Incontinence and night calls are important factors in the failure of resettlement. They must be accurately observed and recorded so that relatives may be made aware of the problems in advance. Extra training time for the patient, advice in management to the relative, the provision of special equipment, and the linen service should be suggested as necessary.

Mobility. Walking ability is so variable, and problems so individual, that short explanatory remarks are usually needed in the assessment. These should cover any aspects of danger, accepted variations from normal gait, and relevant recommendations for management by the relative.

It is usually possible to mark the other subheadings in this section with reference to the key. Their importance in each case will depend upon the home situation, the patient's projected life style, and the amount and quality of family support.

Communication. Problems in communication can be extremely frustrating to patient and relative alike. If a speech therapist is available, her advice to relatives may be invaluable to both. The aspects of communication listed here are the less specific ones which appear in everyday contacts, and which may have a bearing on the patient's ability to manage at home. It should be completed after consultation with the speech therapist if one is available.

Domestic. It is neither possible nor necessary to complete this section for every patient. It should be kept for those patients who live alone, and those who will be alone for extended periods during the day. Time saved by sensible selection can best be spent in extra training in this area for those who really need it. When marking cooking abilities it is essential to consider safety, motivation, and organisation as well as simple physical ability, because nutrition will depend upon what the patient does when left alone rather than upon what he can do in a test situation.

Provision of housekeeping services, Meals on Wheels, and day centre may be indicated by problems demonstrated by this section of the assessment. Simple aids and equipment may be indicated and supervision may be required.

General. This heading covers those aspects of the patient's mental capacity which have been found to have a strong influence upon his independence. They qualify the physical skills which have been tested in other sections. It is not possible to give a thorough psychological profile in so short a space, but major areas of concern should be indicated. Difficulties in this area usually show the need for discussion with a relative, and careful follow-up arrangements by an appropriate member of the team. When the problems mean that the patient is endangered, they may indicate a change in domestic arrangements, such as a move to live with relatives, or to a nursing home.

Because this area is more subjective than the physical ones, the opinions of the team as a whole should be sought if major changes for the patient depend upon the assessment.

Difficulties not Noted, and General Remarks. Relevant facts which are important to the individual patient are entered here. Some typical examples are:

'Tends to forget his walking aid, but is unsafe without it.'
'Responds best to a light touch. Enjoys a joke.'
'Daughter has learnt bathing techniques, but would benefit from nursing help until she gains confidence.'
'Patient tends to withdraw if left to herself. ?Day Centre for continued social stimulation.'

Any helper who really knows her patients will have observed some aspect of the patient's problems which needs further comment after the rest of the form is completed, and this section provides the space for such observations. If there is any safety factor still causing concern, it should be noted here.

Equipment Suggested. Any equipment which is necessary for the patient's safety or independence, and any adaptations needed in the home should be listed. If they differ from the basic equipment supplied, or have been adapted in any way, such variations should be noted. Specific details as to size and modifications should be stated accurately so that the patient takes home equipment which is the same as that on which he has been retrained. This section has a particularly important part to play in continuity between the retraining period and resettlement at home.

The Key to Marking

The key to marking, as seen in the upper right hand section of the form has been designed to be as factual as possible and to minimise variations in marking standards between individual observers. Points are given on a scale which delineates actual ability to perform a task. The scale is related to the amount of help needed. Qualitative statements such as 'good', 'fair' and 'poor' have been avoided as being too subjective, and leaving too much room for individual variations in interpretation.

A series of crosses has been chosen in preference to verbal or numerical reporting. This gives an instant visual picture of the patient's status, making it possible to determine problem areas at a glance. Where the crosses give an inadequate picture, it is always possible to add an explanatory note, but lengthy reporting is usually unnecessary.

Marking Standards

Some people find it hard to overcome the idea that an assessment is an examination to be passed. They feel that it is kind to give a high rather than a low rating where there is any doubt. In fact such a rating may send a patient home with an unresolved problem, or deny him a service which he really needs. Because of the factual nature of the key, marking is reasonably well standardised, but in cases where there is any doubt the staff are required to mark hard.

This is particularly important in areas such as mobility, bed drill, and management of medication, where safety is involved. Any doubt should be noted, as care in such matters is the best insurance against an 'accident' when the patient goes home.

The Value of the ADL Assessment in Planning Domiciliary Care

The content of the ADL assessment should be in the minds of all who work in the retraining team throughout the patient's stay, and high ratings in as many areas as possible should be their aim. The final, formal assessment is a definitive statement of the degree to which these aims have been achieved. It reports what has been accomplished in the retraining phase, and combines with medical and social assessments to form the basis of planning the maintenance phase.

Information from the assessment is used in the pre-discharge interview with relatives, and relatives are given the opportunity to learn suitable methods of managing the patient in areas where help is needed. In cases where it is relevant the information is also passed on to the community nurse and others who are to provide supportive services. In these ways the final ADL assessment is an important link between the hospital and the home, and helps to provide continuity of care for the patient.

Conclusion

Assessments have a very important part to play in geriatric retraining, as guides to planning, bases for action, and measures of progress. They may be formal or informal in character, but in all cases should be accurate, practical, and related to the needs of the patient concerned. Reassessments are necessary as the patient progresses, and at times when decisions are being made. Because of their influence on the future of the patient, they should not be taken lightly by those whose task it is to prepare them.

9 DISCHARGE PROCEDURES

A discussion of the retraining preliminaries to discharge, the post-discharge services, and the provision of continuity of management in the Maintenance Phase.

Introduction

The aim of retraining has been to fit the patient for a successful return home, and to enable him to play as large a role as possible in his own resettlement. It has been a problem-solving process in which training of the patient, the provision of practical equipment, and contact with the relatives have all played a part. When the time comes for discharge, a comprehensive assessment of strengths and weaknesses is matched with the patient's other assets such as a supportive family, a suitable home, and the available services. If problems are apparent these will be fully discussed, and steps taken to deal with them before the discharge is effected.

Assessment

Assessment plays such an important role in retraining that a separate chapter has been devoted to it. A detailed description of the pre-discharge assessment is given in Chapter 8, and should be understood. This assessment is carried out when the team as a whole decides that the patient appears to have reached his maximum, or that further improvement is likely to be of a long-term nature and could be achieved satisfactorily as an out-patient.

The function of the assessment is to show up any areas where some extra effort is needed or where domiciliary care may be required. It is used in planning discharge with the family, and deciding what level of help they will need. It is not an exam which the patient must pass, but a guide to future action. Marking must be accurate, and integrity and consistency are required of the assessor.

Pre-discharge Planning

The assessment form may be filled in by any selected member of the team, but the whole team is involved in assessing the patient's needs and in discussing ways to meet them. The final plan is then made between the caring relative and the doctor, supported by the social worker and the retraining sister as representatives of the team as a whole.

Working with the Relatives

Most people have had little experience in caring for a disabled person, and those who have, will usually have solved their problems with straight out lifting. This is as uncomfortable for the patient as it is burdensome to the lifter. The retraining programme will have taught the patient patterns which minimise lifting, and so it is logical to teach the relative to use the same method. Even if the relative is strong, and has little trouble with lifting it is better for the patient, both physically and mentally, to help himself as well as he can. The best way to use equipment is not always obvious to the layman, and advice on this, and some practice is often valuable. It is also helpful to discuss attitudes and expectations, and any special problems the relative may foresee.

Much of this can be accomplished if a team member who has worked closely with the patient can conduct a demonstration, discussion and practice session with the relative and the patient. Most relatives are grateful for such support and relieved to find that the help they must give is less taxing than they expected. When that help is beyond them the fact is demonstrated on neutral ground, and the knowledge gained helps them to make realistic decisions about placement without the emotional stress of having failed at home.

The following segments are usually part of the relative training session.

Discussion

The relative is seen without the patient and encouraged to express any fears and problems related to his management. Any previous difficulties that have been encountered are brought into the open. These problems should be taken into account when the patient's 'drills' are demonstrated later in the session. At this stage the relative often refers to personality problems between herself and the patient — 'he'll do anything for the nurses, but it's different with us'. Faced with this, the helper should listen, but not take sides either for or against. She should explain that this is one reason for the training session, so that the patient can demonstrate his abilities in front of staff and family and so avoid misunderstandings. During this part of the session the staff member should be a listener rather than a speaker.

Demonstration

Still without the patient, the helper should explain the principles of balance and movement involved in the drills, and demonstrate them herself by using the relative as a model if this is acceptable to the person concerned. For the principles see Chapters 15 to 17. The relative will need much the same lesson as a new member of staff, except that her lesson need only cover those aspects with direct application to the condition of the patient concerned.

Involvement of the Patient

When the relative has some knowledge of what is involved the patient is brought into the session. The staff member and the patient demonstrate each drill first, and then the relative is asked to take the part of the helper. She performs the same drill with instruction and help if necessary. Any difficulties are noted so that some adjustments can be made. If it proves necessary the patient may be given more practice.

The patient's use of any necessary equipment is demonstrated, and a lesson is given in the application of dressings, bandages or splints as required. In all these areas the part the patient can play should be stressed as well as the method to be adopted by his helper. The value to the patient of self help, and the dangers of slipping back if the effort is not made should be stressed in the presence of both the patient and his relative.

Specialised Problems

If the patient has more specialised problems, these should be referred to the person concerned. This may involve the registered nurse, the social worker, the physiotherapist or the speech pathologist if the problem is outside the scope of the team member involved in teaching the relative.

Final Discussion

When the patient and the relative have worked together to a point where either shows signs of fatigue, or when it is obvious that they do not need further practice, an opportunity should be given to the relative for further discussion with the helper. No pressure should be placed on the relative to undertake care of the patient. If the relative is satisfied that she can manage and seems competent to do so, the discharge procedures should continue through the social worker and the doctor. If further training sessions are needed these should be arranged.

In cases where the relative, despite retraining of the patient and instruction for herself, finds that she will be unable to manage, the matter must also be referred back to the doctor and the social worker for appropriate action. It is the responsibility of the person teaching the relative to show the facts as they are, but not to influence the relative's decision by her own attitude. Before a final decision is made they may decide to try at home with a promise of readmission if they are unable to manage.

Domiciliary Services

When the final ADL assessment is presented, and the case is discussed for discharge it should be obvious which of the various available services will be needed, and in what quantity. The whole plan of support will be discussed with the relatives to make sure that the help is appropriate and acceptable. The following services may be offered.

The Nursing Service

In the Newcastle programme this may be provided by the hospital's own domiciliary nurses or by community nurses working with the Department of Health or a voluntary agency. In each case the nurses receive training in the 'drills', and use them in their dealings with the patients. The nurse may be needed indefinitely to give physical help, or to supervise a patient whose ability to manage is in doubt. They may also visit as a temporary measure to give support and further training to an apprehensive relative until skill and confidence have been gained.

The Home Help Service

In Newcastle home help is provided on the recommendation of the geriatrician, by the Home Help Service of New South Wales. Liaison is maintained by the presence of a senior member of that service at the weekly domiciliary care meeting where difficulties can be reported and new instructions given. The Royal Newcastle Hospital subsidises the cost of housekeeping when necessary.

The home helps assist with normal household duties such as cleaning and washing, but must report social or health problems for investigation. They have particular value to patients who live alone, or those whose spouse is also frail and unable to do the work.

The Provision of Equipment

The domiciliary care services keeps a store of equipment which matches that supplied for use in the hospital. This equipment is provided on loan to the patient who still needs it on discharge. Patients are not encouraged to buy their own equipment because this is often different from the pattern used in his retraining, and can lead to unforeseen difficulties and falls. If hospital equipment is being used, the patient is also more likely to come back if he needs further help, and the social worker has a good reason for paying a visit if his ability to manage is in doubt.

If any item has needed adjustment or adaptation in the hospital that same piece of equipment will be sent home with the patient. For further information on equipment see Chapter 18.

Supervision by the Social Worker

If the home-going patient is thought to be at risk, and particularly if he lives alone, arrangements may be made for the social worker to see him regularly at a follow-up clinic, or on a home visit. In this way a developing problem may be recognised in time for help to be effective, and for preventive measures to be taken.

Meals on Wheels

Hot meals are delivered to the home by local voluntary agencies on the written request of the geriatrician, social worker or family doctor. The service is of particular value to patients who neglect to feed themselves properly through loneliness or lack of interest as well as to those who are physically unable to do their own cooking. The fact that someone comes to the door and says a friendly word may provide the high point of the day for the frail person who lives alone.

The fact that Meals on Wheels are available should not lead us to neglect retraining in cooking for those patients who are able to benefit from it, because the service is not limitless, and must be available to those with the greatest need.

Day Hospital, Day Centre and Club

Another book could be written on this subject but it is mentioned here merely as a service which can aid in the care of the frail patient who has returned home. Like the other services it is requested by the geriatrician after discussion with the retraining team and the relative. To be used to best advantage, it should be seen as part of the plan for maintenance at home, and not merely as an outing for the patient.

No limit is placed upon the patient's period of attendance at the day centre or out-patients' club. He may continue as a member so long as there is a need. If a change in his condition warrants it, a change may be made from one service to another. Increased independence may bring about a move from the day centre to the out-patients' club, or from either of these to a community group, social club or sports club. If possible, patients are encouraged to return to these clubs or interests they enjoyed before their illness. A decrease in competence may lead to a return to the more supportive group, or even to readmission for a 'refresher course'.

Some of the indications for attendance at clubs and day centres are listed:

(a) A frail elderly patient living alone and in need of supervision or social stimulation.

(b) Confused or 'difficult' patients whose relatives need a regular break if they are to continue to provide care.

(c) Patients who cannot be left while the relative is at work or out shopping.

(d) Patients who can continue retraining at a reduced level on an out-patient basis in the day centre.

(e) Patients who are at risk of slipping back if not regularly reminded of their 'drills', or stimulated to use them.

(f) Depressed or withdrawn patients who need social contacts but are unable or unwilling to seek them on their own initiative.

(g) Patients who attend for out-patient treatment such as the mat class or speech pathology, and who can benefit further from the day centre programme.

Help to the caring relative, or maintenance of physical ability and morale are the primary purpose of the day centre programme.

A Trial Home Visit

The ADL assessment as carried out in the hospital setting gives satisfactory and unequivocal results in most cases, but when there are unusual circumstances at home, or the patient needs familiarity with his surroundings (as in blindness), a visit may be paid to the home by the patient and a team member for an assessment of the patient's abilities on his home ground. Relatives may also gain confidence by trying out what they have been taught about managing the patient in familiar surroundings and with help available.

The visit is sometimes made on the understanding that it is only a trial run, and that the patient will return to the hospital while adjustments are made, and sometimes on the understanding that he may remain at home if no unexpected problems are encountered. In either case the plan should be stated very clearly to avoid any risk of disappointment or difficulty when the time comes for the return.

Occasionally it is helpful for the patient to have weekend leave so that he and his relatives can adjust to the new situation before the whole responsibility becomes theirs. This should never be encouraged too soon, or while the patient is still making good progress because difficulties which may later be overcome will give the relative and the patient a false impression of the problems they will have to face on discharge. This can lead to unnecessary apprehension, and even to a premature decision that the task will be too great.

Planned Readmissions

Planned readmissions are provided for patients with long-term or permanent disabilities who may be expected to deteriorate without regular 'refresher courses', and those whose relatives are likely to need occasional relief from constant or heavy care. In these cases the relatives are advised to take the opportunity for a holiday while the patient is receiving further retraining as an in-patient. If the need for readmission is foreseen, it is suggested at the time of discharge, giving the relative confidence that help will be available again when it is needed.

If the patient is unlikely to benefit from a further admission, the relatives are advised to contact local nursing homes for a bed. Patients who are likely to benefit include those with Parkinson's Disease, multiple sclerosis, rheumatoid disease, and those who have slipped back through inactivity, whether mental or physical.

Medical Care After Discharge

Part of the Newcastle discharge procedure is to return the patient to the care of his family doctor. A letter is written to the general practitioner from the geriatrician, giving an outline of what has been done for the patient and asking the practitioner to resume responsibility for medical care. The geriatrician remains available for consultation, and the various domiciliary services are under his prescription and control.

Subject to the approval of the general practitioner the patient's attendance at various specialist clinics may be arranged, and continued treatment may be provided through departments such as those of occupational therapy, physiotherapy, and speech pathology.

Retraining in the Maintenance Phase

Because many of the diseases of the elderly are of a progressive and/or fluctuating nature, and because many of the patients have difficulty in maintaining morale and motivation, there is often need for continued retraining during the maintenance period. This may be provided in a number of ways, the most common of which are as follows.

Supervision from a Relative

Relatives who have themselves received instruction in the various drills to be used by the patient are asked to see that these are carried out accurately, and to report back if they notice any marked deterioration in the patient's performance. The relative is in an excellent position to give instructions if the patient forgets and so to help maintain standards or even to improve them by further practice.

Instructions from the Community Nurse

Community nurses working with the retraining team are expected to use retraining methods in their dealings with the patient. They may also continue instructions in retraining procedures and management to relatives who are unsure and lacking in confidence. When the nurse is satisfied that the patient and the relatives can manage safely without her, she can reduce or even withdraw her services. When this is not possible, her regular visits and use of the drills will help the patient to maintain any gains he made in hospital, and even to add to them.

Out-Patient Attendance

Patients who have been able to return home and function adequately before reaching their full level of recovery may benefit from out-patient treatment in one of the ancillary departments. There, finer points of recovery or skill in self care may be encouraged. Discharge from the hospital bed does not necessarily mean that all treatment must cease. Care should be taken, however, that the patient does not become dependent upon his visits to treatment clinics for social stimulation when a day centre or club would better serve the purpose.

Day Centre and Club

The Day Centre and Out-Patients' Club provide social and psychological support for patients and their relatives. They should also play their part in the checking and maintenance of physical skills. Like other members, the day centre staff should know and use the retraining drills in their dealings with the patients. They should also be aware of the patient's performance, and report difficulties and signs of deterioration so that they can receive attention before they progress too far.

Discharge to a Nursing Home

Although the majority of patients who receive retraining are able to go home, there are a few for whom it is not possible. It may be that the patient has not achieved the required degree of independence, or it may be the result of social factors or family relationships. Whatever the case, some alternative accommodation is necessary, and a nursing home is the usual choice. Such patients should not be maintained indefinitely in the retraining unit, because they form a group of permanent residents which tends to grow if allowed to do so, and finally denies retraining to other patients who could benefit from it. The needs of the permanent patient, the type of activity required, and the staffing levels needed are all different from those of the person undergoing the dynamic retraining process. It is very difficult to do justice to both groups if they are housed in the same area. This does not mean that retraining should cease for patients who cannot go home, but that it should be carried on in the nursing home just as the home-going patient continues his with the relative and the domiciliary services.

Some difficulties have been experienced in this ideal situation for many reasons. These include lack of understanding on the part of some administrators and matrons, tight budgets, minimal staffing, and lack of training in the basic attitudes and skills required. For many years the Royal Newcastle Hospital geriatrics team has given help and advice when requested to do so, and a service is now provided by the Department of Health. Follow-up is provided between the hospital and the nursing home, and the patient's abilities can be demonstrated to the staff of the latter as they would be demonstrated to the caring relative in other circumstances.

Deterioration in morale and ability takes place very quickly in patients who leave the retraining unit only to have everything done for them without encouragement to do what they can for themselves. This applies to those who return home as well as to those who go to a nursing home.

Conclusion

The aim of retraining is to help the elderly patient bridge the gap between the dependence imposed by his illness or disability and the degree of independence necessary for a satisfactory return to the community. The problems vary from patient to patient, and are seen in many combinations, so there must be many solutions available to deal with them. This means that many different skills will be called into action, and the people who provide them must be welded into a team by good communication.

An attempt has been made to show how the Newcastle Method for Retraining the Elderly Disabled contributes towards and is integrated into the Geriatrics Service of the Royal Newcastle Hospital. Some guidance has been given as to how this method can be adapted for use elsewhere.

PART THREE
The Psychological Element

This section discusses the need for a
psychological basis to physical retraining
methods and proposes some practical
ways of involving the elderly in their
own treatment.

10 THE PSYCHOLOGICAL BASIS OF RETRAINING

The need for a psychological approach in retraining with a discussion of human needs and some suggestions for teaching methods which are appropriate for the elderly patient.

Introduction

The skills taught through routine retraining methods are mainly of a physical nature, but they need to be applied with psychological understanding if the fullest value is to be gained from their use. In order that this may be so, they are ideally associated with a programme of social and creative activities, and the drills themselves are presented to the patient with due regard for his mental as well as his physical condition. They were designed to serve the psychological needs of the elderly just as much as the physical needs. The attitudes of the person teaching them are just as important as her knowledge of the physical details of the drills. Both are part of the Newcastle Method, and both contribute to the patient's progress towards independence. Fortunately, most people can learn the necessary psychological skills which are not, as is sometimes thought, purely a matter of individual personality. The will to communicate well with the patient, and the humility to look for deficiencies in oneself if this does not come about are the main attributes necessary to attain these skills.

The Psychological Element in Retraining

The psychological element in the design and application of the Newcastle Method is intrinsic to the overall programme and is essential even at the physical level of retraining. Staff members are taught psychologically based methods of presenting the retraining programme as well as the physical processes involved in it. The two mainsprings of the psychological content are basic human needs (see pp. 118-22), and teaching methods which are suitable for the elderly (see pp. 122-7).

117

Basic Human Needs

Although not designed originally with Maslow's Theory in mind, the routine drills and the way they are taught come very close to putting that theory into practice. Maslow has grouped human needs under five headings, and has arranged these groups in the order known as his 'hierarchy of need'. He postulates that needs in his first group will take precedence over the second, and so on, when there is conflict between them. See Chapter 11 for a more detailed account. The groups as arranged by Maslow are:

(1) Basic psychological needs.
(2) Safety needs.
(3) Needs for affection.
(4) Needs for esteem.
(5) Self realisation.

They can be applied to retraining in the following ways.

Basic Psychological Needs. The routine drills are actually designed around basic psychological needs so that the patient is immediately aware of their relevance to himself. He must sleep, eat, eliminate and be sheltered to survive. Thus the areas of bed, feeding, toilet and dressing are appropriate areas in which to begin his retraining. At a more immediate level the helpers are taught that these most primitive needs should receive attention before those activities which fall into Maslow's later categories of need. The first priority is to make the patient physically comfortable, and only then to expect his undivided attention on whatever activity is envisaged. The helper's awareness and willingness to cope with these needs usually leads to a good relationship with the patient. This is invaluable when the time comes for the next step.

The psychological needs provide very strong motivation to action, whether acceptable or otherwise, and should be used positively for good. Any activity which helps the patient to achieve his goal while the need is actually being felt is usually readily accepted. For this reason, feeding is best taught at a meal, dressing and bathing in the real situation in the ward, and walking when a patient wants to get somewhere. Common sense, however, is important in applying this idea, for if the physiological need is too great it will take precedence over the need for the helper's approval, and even the need for safety. In such situations panic can be the result.

The very names of the drills show how close most of them are to basic physiological needs — bed, chair, commode, toilet, bath, dressing, feeding, walking, steps, and car drills. Their consequent value and acceptability as retraining media can hardly be denied.

Safety Needs. Safety factors are built into the retraining drills as part of their design, and are stressed in the methods recommended for their teaching. They are designed in harmony with body mechanics, making allowances for changes in those of the disabled person as a result of malfunction of limbs. Problems posed by such factors as sensory loss, retarded response, poor concentration and impaired balance are also relevant. The helper is taught to be aware of the patient's difficulties, and to help with these while encouraging him to use his strengths. Thus each move is a team effort between helper and patient and has been designed with this in mind. It is still necessary for the nurse to understand kinetic methods of lifting, and to use them in her own movements, but as the patient is also involved in the combined motion, the placement of his limbs, and the thrust of his effort must also be considered. The movements involve taking the patient's weight to earth through his own limbs or body, and if those limbs have unequal capacity the movement is adjusted accordingly. The drills are thus fitted to the patient as he is, and his returning strength is incorporated into them as he progresses. In this way he has the satisfaction of helping himself to the best of his ability at each stage of retraining, with the security of help in those things which are beyond him. The weaker limbs are not asked to function beyond their capacity, and so the danger of the weak member 'letting him down' is lessened for the patient and his confidence is increased.

Balance is essential to safety, and particularly so in the practice of geriatrics where fractures are so easily sustained, and so damaging in their results. For this reason SAFE POSTURE is preferred to so-called 'GOOD' POSTURE whenever a choice must be made. For example, a slight lean to the strong side is encouraged for the hemiplegic patient so long as his reactions remain slower or his strength defective on the hemiplegic side. Similarly, a patient who has a history of falls is actively encouraged to lean forward on to a low walking frame, rather than to 'stand up straight'. In this way he takes weight to the ground through his upper limbs as well as his lower ones, and so is safer if not more elegant. This gives confidence and allows independence to be achieved more quickly than a more traditional attitude to posture would do. It also provides another example of links with Maslow, in that good balance, a safety factor, takes precedence over good looks, a factor in esteem.

Confidence is a major factor in retraining, and it is produced by physical safety in the drills themselves, and also by a process of transfer from the helper. A light hold, a calm voice, and accurate directions all help in this, and demonstrate the helper's own confidence in what she is doing. Well-designed and well-kept equipment, with special emphasis on safety factors such as stability, brakes, and suitable adjustment for the individual also add to the confidence. The neglect of these factors can break confidence quite dramatically.

Affection Needs. The need for affection is one that is felt very strongly by many people who enter hospital. They may leave behind them the security of home, a loving family circle, a kindly neighbour, or even a pet. The efficiency of admission procedures, the endless questions, and the unfamiliar surroundings can seem anything but friendly, and the new patient can feel very much alone. Thus from the start the retraining staff should try to make the patient feel welcome as a person, and should ensure that physical comfort is attended to (group 1) and that fears are allayed (group 2). The fact that someone has bothered about these more personal matters will in itself demonstrate that the hospital staff is human and that affection is possible there.

When retraining starts, the team-work which is necessary between the helper and the patient is an ideal ground for building a friendly relationship. The willingness of the patient to tackle some of the more difficult procedures at a later date depends in many cases upon the trust and good will that have been generated in the beginning. The giving of praise for a good effort, and the obvious pleasure of the helper in each new achievement, both help the patient to feel that at least some of his need for friendship and affection is being met. They will also act as a motivating force as he tries to please those he has come to see as friends.

The presence of other patients is an asset not to be neglected in this connection. By introducing patients to each other with as much care for compatibility as a good hostess would use, the early feelings of loneliness can be alleviated. Long-standing friendships have developed from the caring interest of an established patient for a new and insecure one. The group activities of the programme can also be used to encourage inter-patient reactions and co-operation.

Needs for Esteem. The patient who was being cared for in the previous paragraph was having his need for affection met by staff members or other patients. Those other patients were also having a need met by these exchanges at the next level of the scale. The fact that a member of staff asks a patient to help, demonstrates esteem and gives satisfaction to that patient. Subsequent relation of the incident to admiring visitors can bring more esteem into the situation and help the patient to move further towards the goal of self realisation. Provided that they are capable of doing so, it is good therapy to ask patients to help each other in non-medical matters, to help the staff, or to be models for demonstrations to visitors. Performing a task at which they have some skill is in itself satisfying, but it is also important that the patient should receive adequate recognition and thanks from others. Retraining gives many opportunities for showing esteem, and these opportunities should always be taken. This is not just politeness, or even kindness, but part of the teaching method. The more disabled the patient and the more difficulty he is having in performing a task, the more necessary it is to note every small triumph and to show appreciation of it. The patient who, having stopped caring for her appearance, makes the effort to use her lipstick, the withdrawn patient who is seen to tap a foot in time to some music, and the disgruntled one who packs up the plates spontaneously at the end of a meal have all taken a step forward, and should all have the step noted and applauded in a manner appropriate to themselves. The satisfactory achievement of one goal is the best base from which to set out to achieve the next. The design of the drills, with progress by stages as a major feature, and effective job breakdown as the recommended basis for teaching, is well suited to the achievement of small goals, with appropriate recognition. It must be pointed out, however, that praise without sincerity can be counter-productive. Lack of sincerity is quickly sensed, and usually resented, so that insincere praise, far from showing esteem, tends to show a distinct lack of it, and so defeats its purpose.

Self Realisation. The appreciation by others of each goal achieved during retraining, whether physical or psychological, helps the patient to build confidence in himself, and to feel pride in his accomplishment. What he will be able to do eventually will be relative to his physical and mental status and so it is important that his goal should have been kept within his range. The patient who has been encouraged to aim too high is unlikely to reach the goal of self acceptance, although this is usually more important to his happiness and quality of life than purely physical success. For example, the double lower limb amputee, who has been encouraged in the early stages by tales of how good modern prostheses are, will feel failure and frustration at a later date if, for any one of many reasons, he has to be told that he will not be able to wear one. His chance for self realisation will suffer because he is unable, through no fault of his own, to live up to his own or someone else's unrealistic expectations. If on the other hand he is reminded that he, as a person, consists of his capacity for thinking, feeling, and expressing himself, and that these are unimpaired, he can begin to accept himself. At the same time he should be offered the immediate goal of progressive physical independence despite his disability. In accomplishing this he can once again feel proud of his achievements. Later, if improvement in his condition permits success with a prostheses, he has lost nothing. If it does not, he is spared the distress of failure in his main goal, because of the achievement of other goals at a more realistic level.

Because residual disability is inevitable in so many geriatric patients, the acceptance of what cannot be changed combined with an all out attempt to deal with what can, is the true basis of self realisation for the patient. The building of false hopes is unjustified, just as much as the taking away of hope in such time-worn phrases as 'you'll never walk again'. As in most things, the middle way has much to recommend it. 'Let us try, and see how far you can go!'

Teaching Methods for the Drills

The learning capacities of the elderly, and the teaching methods best suited to them have indicated certain requirements in the drills to fit them specifically for the group for which they were designed. The more important of these requirements are as follows.

Repetition. Soldiers are drilled 'by numbers' to perform complicated tasks step by step, so that when those tasks must be performed in a tense situation they will come accurately, safely, and efficiently without any need to think how they should be done. This is the principle behind the teaching of 'drills' in the Newcastle Method. The movements are learnt by the patients at a physical rather than an intellectual level, making retraining available to those with dementia or sensory loss related to parietal lobe injury, as well as to the well preserved. Obviously the latter will learn more quickly, and probably more thoroughly than the former, but the former are by no means excluded.

Start Where the Patient Is. Before his first lesson, and as often as necessary thereafter, explanations are given to the patient about what is being done. Even if he does not understand, the fact that the explanation has been given will help him to feel confident in his teacher. Physically he will be given as much help as he needs with what he cannot do, while being encouraged to do for himself the things he can. He should not be asked to attempt anything far beyond him, but small new goals should be offered and small new achievements added to the old. Good foundations are thus established for further progress. The drills have been designed with this form of progress in view, so that even if a patient has to be helped through every part of the movement, the movement itself will be the same as the one he will eventually perform independently. Withdrawal of help as it becomes unnecessary is the responsibility of the helper.

The Patient Sets the Pace. The variation of ability, both mental and physical, in any group of elderly patients is very wide, and the pace must be varied to suit their different capacities. Unlike the situation in a school there is no selection according to ability in a retraining unit, and yet the programme must offer suitable treatment for everyone. The physical aspects of the drills are similar for all, so long as they are offered at the correct level and in a manner suitable to each individual. Each patient will need to learn at his own speed, and for this reason classes in the usual sense have only limited application. The more able person can quickly lose interest if the pace is too slow, while the more disabled one will lose confidence and give up if it is too fast. For this reason progress should be linked to the achievement of each individual, and not to a class time table.

Set Attainable Goals. The design of the drills incorporates a line of progress which is followed systematically, thus providing a series of goals to be reached one by one. Success in achieving the nearest goal is the stimulus to move on to the next, without making the patient too sharply aware of a distant goal which may very well be beyond him. This is an important factor in the maintenance of morale and the will to keep trying.

No Need for Change. Retraining is based upon habit building, and the fewer ingrained habits the patient has which do not blend with the moves he is trying to learn, the easier it will be for him to acquire the new skills. It is important, therefore, that the method itself should not produce habits in the early stages which must be discarded later. The movements have been designed so that there is no need for change. For instance, the movements used by the nurse to sit a patient up in bed for the first time are the same as those he will use himself when he is independent. Much time can be wasted if a habit must be broken before retraining can begin, and, in fact, some patients find it impossible to change a habit at all. This common difficulty demonstrates the need for continuity in the moves employed.

Emphasise Ability. It is very necessary to develop positive attitudes in both patients and staff, and one important aspect in this is to see results from effort. By using the patient's existing abilities from the first the feeling of helplessness is minimised and hope is developed. The attitude to be encouraged is 'how can I do it?' and not 'I can't because ... '. The change from 'I can't' to 'I'll try' is one of the greatest steps forward that a disabled person can take, and the helper should be aware of its worth. It should be noted and built upon by the staff. Failure at this stage is crucial and so the staff should ensure that, whatever the results of his try, the patient should be left with a feeling of satisfaction for having made it. Small early gains play a large part in future motivation and the helper should be aware of their worth. The use of present skills ensures that they are not lost through neglect, and that time is not wasted waiting for movements which may not come, or which will be too weak or too poorly controlled to be of practical value.

The patient who demonstrates to himself that he can still do something to help himself is not likely to be the one who sits mournfully rubbing his hand while he waits for a miracle.

Use Simple and Direct Methods. Many dependent folk, and particularly those with overt brain damage, find difficulty in seeing the application of a skill learnt in one situation to its use in another. For instance, a patient who learns to roll and turn over in a mat class may still call a nurse to turn him during the night. This will remain his pattern of behaviour when he goes home unless he is reminded of the movement by the nurse, and encouraged to use it in the real situation. Similar difficulties apply to rising from a chair, using a bathboard, using the toilet and performing other daily moves. The task has more meaning than the exercise, although both involve the same movements. By using the task itself in retraining, the intermediate process of association of exercise with performance is avoided. The more direct the lesson, the more easily it is assimilated by people with learning difficulties.

Simplicity of subject matter and presentation is also required in teaching the elderly disabled. A complicated lesson is rarely learnt in a reasonable time, or retained once the learning period is completed. In the retraining drills the subject matter has been simplified by conscious elimination of inessentials and by emphasising factors concerned with safety and function. Adequate 'job breakdown', and the insistence upon 'one step at a time', are the main techniques used in the simplified teaching method.

Relate Activities to Future Needs. Positive motivation towards the effort involved in learning, and towards the sometimes frightening or painful moves which must be faced in the process, depends very much upon the patient's understanding of its relevance to his own needs. Few students are willing to give their best efforts to learning merely because someone else sees its value. The basic drills are usually accepted readily because of their obvious immediate value, but some of the less urgent retraining depends very much upon individual circumstances. The patient who lives alone will be easier to interest in dressing or cooking skills than the one who lives with protective relatives. It is important to know whether the statement, 'my daughter always does it' is factual or not, and whether the daughter is happy to do so. If in fact she prefers to do it, time can be wasted in teaching a reluctant patient. If she is unhappy about it, the lesson may make the difference between accepting responsibility for the patient and refusing to have him home. Helping the patient to see the relevance of what he is asked to do is part of the teaching process.

Involve the Patient. From his first day in retraining, the patient is involved both physically and mentally in the process. The drills themselves are based on the principle that the patient will be encouraged to do what he can, and be helped with what he cannot. The teaching method calls for explanations at whatever level the patient's mental status indicates. It also involves simple, step by step directions, and praise for effort as well as achievement. Even if a patient cannot be expected to understand an explanation, a simple one is given, as the tone of voice and the attitude displayed can give confidence even if the words are not understood. Involving the patient and working with him rather than on him, lets him see that something is still expected of him. It provides a goal, encourages positive attitudes, and helps him to maintain his self respect. A dramatic example of the value of involvement of the patient is the improved attitude of patients when toilet drill takes the place of the bed pan. Early involvement of the patient also helps to prevent unnecessary physical deterioration from inactivity, and so has both physical and psychological justification.

Be Consistent. The retraining programme covering many aspects of the patient's life, can seem arbitrary and disjointed if its various aspects are not linked by consistent aims and principles. Despite the variety of activities which may be used, the aims and principles are indeed constant. The principles outlined in this chapter apply to games, hobbies, crafts, social activities and the use of equipment, as much as they apply to the teaching of the drills. The activities may change, but the method of introducing them to the patient does not. In every case the teaching involves: (a) assessment of the patient's abilities and disabilities; (b) discussion; (c) simple explanations; (d) starting with something within the patient's powers.

With each activity he should receive help with what he cannot do, encouragement with what he can, and praise at suitable times along the way. From a simple beginning each patient is encouraged to progress at his own pace and to his own best level of performance. There is no absolute standard to be reached by all, but careful selection of tasks for the individual should mean that he can reach a high standard within his own limits. It is the responsibility of the staff to see that he does not fail at something he was not ready to tackle, and which was too difficult for him in the first place.

Acceptance and Management of Fear. A major obstacle to success in retraining is fear in one of its many forms. Fear of the unknown, fear of failure, and fear of the future can all make the patient hesitant to fight back against his disabilities. Such fears are just as potent inhibitors of action as the physical fears of pain, falling, or 'overdoing it'. The drills allow for these fears which are common and very natural. The teaching methods help to overcome them, by the emphasis on explanation and starting with the possible, by giving help where it is most needed, and by calm, step by step directions. The confidence of the helper and her understanding acceptance of the fears of the patient both play a large part in the successful management of this problem. They are discussed in more detail in Chapters 12 and 13.

Permanent Disability. The Newcastle Method is designed to help patients with many degrees of disability, and not only those who have good prospects for the recovery of full function. It accepts residual disability as inevitable in some cases, and helps those patients to adjust to it. The teaching methods for the drills depend upon accepting the patient as he is, demonstrating to him his present abilities, however small, and helping him to achieve satisfaction by small gains. Help which is given in areas where it is not reasonable to expect success is withdrawn progressively in those areas where improvement is shown. Psychological support and encouragement are complementary to the physical retraining and are focused upon possible goals and day to day achievements. Hope is not taken from the patient who is encouraged to keep trying and see how far he can get. On the other hand, he is not promised any specific result. In this way he learns to place value on small successes and to adjust to his disability.

In some cases modified equipment may be all he needs to make him independent. This will be provided as part of his retraining, so that he is familiar with it before discharge. If, after discharge, help from another person is needed, that person will be trained in the method and in attitudes suited to the patient concerned. Supportive services, if required, will be co-ordinated with his and his helper's known needs.

In these ways, success and failure are made relative to the patient's capacity, and not to an impossible absolute goal. The future mental well being of the patient who cannot make a full recovery depends in many cases upon his acceptance of his disability and his will to do his best in spite of it. The patient who has failed in a major goal finds acceptance difficult, but the one who has learnt to rejoice over small successes can usually continue to do so, and in so doing, will maintain his morale.

Continued Use After Discharge

The Newcastle Method is designed not only for application by skilled staff in the hospital or out-patient department, but for continuation in the home or community. The moves are such that they can be used effectively, however far the patient progresses towards full return of function. As he becomes able he may try short cuts for himself, but there is no need for him to do so. The drills as taught will give him a safe and simple method for independence in daily living, while the principles behind them will help him to find a way if he meets a situation not covered by the lessons.

Various Stages of Recovery. Psychological and physical factors are equally important in the decision concerning the patient's ability to manage at home. The grossly physically disabled patient who is well adjusted, cheerful, and responsive, is often less troublesome to his family than the depressed, agitated, or carping one with only minimal physical problems. Many formerly 'difficult' patients do respond to the psychological elements of retraining and the social content of the programme is included for this reason. Just as they need guidance in the physical sphere, the relatives often need help in understanding the 'bad' behaviour and in managing it. Psychological as well as physical gains may also need maintenance in the Day Centre, or by other supportive measures. Confidence is built in both the patient and the relative by the use of the same methods at home as those taught in the hospital. If help is still needed the relative will carry on where the nurse left off. Supervised practice with the patient helps in a smoother transfer of responsibilities to the relative. The provision of identical equipment to that which has been used also facilitates adjustment to the return home.

Because it is problem oriented, retraining has much to offer patients and relatives with many different problems in varying degrees of severity. The individual patient and his family must form a new team, and what is taught to them will depend upon their individual strengths and weaknesses within that team.

The Instruction of Relatives. It is not only the patient who has psychological problems in the face of illness and disability. Many kind and conscientious relatives are afraid of the responsibility of looking after someone who is ill or disabled. The fears take many shapes, and some are for the patient and some for themselves. Some of these are overcome by consultations with the doctor and medical social worker before and during the treatment period; some are minimised by the provision of supportive services in the maintenance phase; and some respond to instruction in managing the patient from the retraining staff. At these lessons the patient and the relative are taught to act as a team, and so to gain confidence in each other. Any difficulties experienced by the staff are openly discussed, and ways of dealing with them are demonstrated. Relatives are taught at the level they are able to accept, which for some means a thorough grounding in principles and theory, and for others simple repetition as is used for routine retraining. Some relatives will need only one explanation, while others may need to attend over a period of weeks before they are confident enough to manage at home. If after adequate training and practice the relative is still unable to do what is required for the patient's successful re-establishment at home, the possibility of nursing home care can be discussed realistically, because the relative, the patient, and the staff are all mutually aware of the real difficulties being faced.

Thus the teaching of relatives to use the drills can help them to overcome fear if they take the patient home, and can help them to feel less guilty if they are unable to do so. Similarly, it can build the patient's confidence in his relatives' ability to help if he goes home, and help him to understand and not feel rejected if he does not.

Use by Domiciliary Nurses. In the Newcastle Geriatrics Service, the visits of community nurses to the patient's home are an integral part of on-going care. These nurses continue to apply retraining methods in their work. As part of their orientation they learn the retraining techniques as used in the hospital, and use them when dealing with the patient and his relatives. This eases the visit, as everyone knows what to expect. It also means that the nurse reinforces the training and can observe and report deterioration and assess the need for a refresher course. Thus the stress to the patient of relearning is avoided, and confidence is bolstered in the maintenance phase.

Use in Nursing Homes. Because they are designed around daily routines, the retraining methods are eminently suitable for use in nursing homes. If they are so used the problem of maintaining patient morale is made easier, and more and more homes are realising that it is necessary to provide more than kindness and custodial care. There has been a tendency to believe that it is time consuming to help patients to maintain their independence and skills, but nurses who have learnt retraining methods do not find that this is so. The independence of some patients, and the more co-operative attitude of others, allow for extra time to be spent where it is really needed. Better staff/patient relationships, and greater job satisfaction for the nurses are side benefits which it is difficult to evaluate. The reduction in the volume of lifting is enough to recommend it to most staff members once they have mastered the Method, while the more sensitive and intelligent members will see the psychological advantages as well. Initial resistance, as in the introduction of any new method, can be expected, but this usually breaks down when the first results become apparent. The person introducing the Method needs to be secure in her own knowledge of and belief in the techniques, and to be patient with those who have yet to be convinced.

The patient who has received retraining in the hospital and goes to a nursing home where the Method is used, will make a much easier adjustment than the one who, having worked hard for a little independence, is returned to a completely dependent state because 'it is easier'. Fortunately more and more nursing homes are seeing the value of maintaining the independence of their clients, and where possible, helping them to build upon them still further.

Readmission. Readmission can be a depressing episode for the patient, who will see it as failure on his own part or that of his family. In the very nature of things it is to be expected that re-admission will be necessary for many patients, either for refresher courses, recurring illness, or a break for the relatives. Open discussion of its possibility during the original admission should not be avoided. Recognition and a welcome by someone can be very helpful, and the familiar routine of the drills can help in a positive way. If the patient has deteriorated the drills must obviously be applied at the present level, and not the one he had reached before. It is possible that some of his previous skills have been maintained and these should be encouraged. The continuity of the drills and their adaptability to many degrees of disability are invaluable in the early readjustment to hospital in the patient who must try again.

Job Satisfaction

The Newcastle Method of retraining has been discussed with reference to its psychological implications for the patient and his relatives, but when properly understood and administered by the staff it has value to them as well. There are many ways of viewing geriatrics, and some of them are completely negative in spirit. Those who work in the field are used to remarks and questions which demonstrate these ideas. 'Don't you find it depressing?', 'Of course you can't expect much at his age!', 'You must have a lot of patience to work with them all the time', 'I'd rather work with younger patients and see something for my work', 'Isn't it boring, just an endless round of washing, feeding and toilets?', and so on in a negative way or, equally falsely, the over-sentimental remarks such as 'making their last days happy', 'helping the poor old darlings', and many more.

There are a number of ways in which geriatric retraining helps the staff to avoid all these attitudes. Some of them are outlined below.

Integrated Aims

As those who play sport can attest, team-work is very satisfying to most human beings. Working together for a cause, and sharing successes and failures is satisfying in itself, leading as it does to the development of good inter-personal relationships, and elimination of loneliness and isolation. The mutual pleasure of two nurses who see a patient take a new step forward can be as rewarding to them as to the patient, if this is a mutual goal.

Unpleasant Tasks

Their training helps nurses to face unpleasant tasks without flinching, but an unpleasant task, or even a boring one, is never really undertaken from choice. Retraining techniques, while not necessarily making the task more pleasant, can make it more meaningful and acceptable. For instance, teaching a patient to be independent in using a commode is usually less distasteful than responding to constant requests for a bed pan. Most nurses, once they understand the reasons behind retraining methods, gain great satisfaction from seeing their patients' increased independence, knowing that the instruction they have given is largely responsible for it.

Achievable Goals

It is not only the patient who needs to see results from his work. The constantly recurring jobs of washing, toileting, feeding and moving passive patients can be demoralising to the intelligent nurse, to say nothing of her charge. Involvement of the patient, at whatever level he is able to achieve, guards against further deterioration, and in most cases leads to an actual improvement in physical and mental status. By aiming at small immediate goals the helper as well as the patient will gain interest and satisfaction. Even when a patient is not likely to improve enough to live at home, retraining methods can help to stop the onset of withdrawal and apathy, and give the staff the satisfaction of caring for alert and responsive people.

Staff/Patient Relationships

Fortunately the old rule that the staff should not talk to and get to know their patients as people has largely disappeared. In the retraining situation, explanations, discussions, and normal conversation are actively encouraged, and have therapeutic value. Being a good listener and encouraging patients to talk is one of the skills which is most useful in gaining co-operation from a reluctant patient, in discovering why attitudes have changed, or in stimulating a withdrawn patient to become aware of his surroundings. At the same time they can add new interest in her work for the helper, making her aware of the personalities of the people with whom she is dealing, and teaching her how to adjust her own approach to suit each individual. By involving her patients in routine retraining procedures she will herself become more involved and interested.

Useful Reporting

To the nurse who is involved in retraining as opposed to custodial care, the daily report takes on a new meaning. She will be looking for changes in her patients' abilities as well as their physical condition, and for difficulties which may need to be overcome before discharge can be considered. Such remarks as 'slept well', 'comfortable', and 'no change', are replaced by more specific information linked to his retraining programme. 'Up to commode once with light assistance', 'can now turn in bed unaided', and 'still cannot rise from chair', are examples of the more informative type of report which indicates further action or notes progress.

Reports of the latter kind are of interest to the team as a whole, while the former kind merely fulfil the letter of the law that a report must be written. Reports on long-term disabled patients who are not acutely ill can quickly deteriorate if retraining attitudes are not present in the situation.

The Patient's Response

Job satisfaction for the nurse or other helper of the patient will always depend to some extent upon the patient's response to her efforts. This may be an improvement in his condition, an improvement or development in his attitude and responses, or a combination of both. Retraining methods help in producing these changes, and also provide a frame of reference for assessing them. 'Last week he wouldn't try to do up his shoes, today he did it without being asked.' This kind of observation, demonstrating a positive response in the patient, is also very rewarding to the person who has been trying to achieve it.

In ways such as those outlined here, the nurse's interest in her work, and the satisfaction she gets from it can be enhanced if the attitudes and processes of retraining are added to the custodial role. In helping her patients to improve their skills, to preserve their intellects and maintain their interest, she will almost certainly be adding to her own satisfaction in her work.

Summary

The physical aspects of geriatric retraining are not complete in themselves, but are complemented by important psychological factors. These include the building of confidence and morale in the patient and his family, and involvement and enthusiasm in the staff. The method of presentation of the retraining procedures is as important as the content of the drills, and so teaching methods have been built into their design. Both the manner of presentation and the drills themselves should be taught to those who intend to practise retraining.

11 MOTIVATION

Good motivation is necessary for both staff members and patients. The mechanisms involved in motivation are discussed and related to the needs of the retraining process.

Introduction

Definitions

Strong motivation is one of the greatest assets of a person who faces a difficult goal; with it he will set out with enthusiasm, and go at least as far as he can, but without it he is likely to give up at the first difficulty he encounters. This applies just as much to the old person fighting a disability as it does to a climber facing a mountain.

A MOTIVE is defined as 'that which induces a person to act'. Thus to be MOTIVATED is to possess or to be given a motive, and MOTIVATION is the state of possessing a motive or motives. When we talk of 'good' or 'poor' motivation, however, the meaning is harder to define, because it includes an element of value judgement. It refers to internal motives which will keep a person moving in an acceptable direction, whether or not he is stimulated to do so by another person. Thus a patient who lives alone will need 'good motivation' if he is to maintain the standard of independence necessary for his safety and well-being. One who goes home to a relative may manage with 'poor motivation' if that relative understands how to motivate him, or is content to do things for him which, if better motivated, he could do for himself. It should be noted that in the second case the words good and poor refer to goals set by others rather than by the patient himself. He may be very well motivated towards actions which lead to his own goal of being waited upon hand and foot.

The Importance of 'Good' Motivation

The internal resource of 'good' motivation is one of the most vital factors in successful retraining. With it a patient will do everything he can to overcome his disability, involving himself in his treatment

134

and accepting the challenge it presents. Without it he will either accept treatment passively, because it is easier than refusing, or will reject it altogether. The motivated patient will probably maintain the gains he makes in hospital, and even improve upon them after discharge. The unmotivated will be very likely to regress into apathy and dependence as soon as he is away from the external support of the treatment team.

Staff Involvement

Because of the importance of good motivation to the patient, it is necessary for all those who treat him to understand its nature. It is part of their task to build up motivation in cases where it is in short supply so as to ensure that the patient will want to continue to function to the best of his ability when the time comes for him to go home. In more aggressive patients it will eliminate battles of will when the patient is required to act. Fortunately, poor motivation is not necessarily a permanent state, but is amenable to treatment. Discussion of the subject should be part of in-service training for all who are involved in the retraining programme as it is the basis of success or failure with the withdrawn elderly patient. In the critical early stages of treatment, a thoughtless discouraging remark, or an angry tone of voice from one person, may be enough to undo hours of careful building by the rest of the team. Each contact between a team member and the patient should have a constructive and not a destructive effect.

Staff Motivation

A staff which is not itself motivated towards retraining methods will have little chance of motivating the patients. The nurse who finds it quicker and easier to dress a patient than to see him battle to do it himself will need to be strongly motivated towards retraining goals if she is to resist the easier way. Successful motivation of patients depends largely upon staff encouragement and enthusiasm. Case conferences and staff meetings as described in Chapter 3 play a large part in staff motivation by ensuring that all team members understand the goals set for individual patients and their own responsibilities in achieving those goals.

The motivation of different team members will be as varied as that of the patients, as they too are individuals. Some relevant factors are as follows.

The Composite Nature of Motivation

The motive forces behind our work are not readily apparent, even to ourselves. In each of us a number of factors combine to make us act as we do, and each person will give them different priorities. Even in the same person the priorities will differ from time to time. Some of the factors may be antagonistic to each other so that we are pushed in two directions, and must decide between them. For instance, in mountain climbing the exhilaration of a challenge may be opposed to the fear of danger; in choosing a job a desire for more pay may be opposed by the lure of lighter or more interesting work, and as in a romantic novel, love may be opposed to ambition in the choice between an heiress and the girl next door. Conflicting motives cause uneasiness to the person who is experiencing them until the mind is made up one way or the other. The best way to make up one's mind is to understand the factors involved.

Thus the nurse who faces the choice between the quickest way and the retraining way needs to understand the pros and cons of both. The authority of the ward sister may be needed where there is wilful neglect of techniques which form part of treatment, but the nurse who understands the 'why' of retraining as well as the 'how' rarely needs compulsion to do what is best for her patient. Teaching her the philosophy behind its 'drills' is therefore as necessary in her training as teaching her the physical aspects of the 'drills' themselves.

Aims in Motivating Patients

As in other areas, staff motivation in encouraging the patient to act is probably mixed. It may be merely the wish to avoid discipline as mentioned above, but this is imposed motivation, and may well be abandoned as soon as the Sister is engaged elsewhere. More reliable and lasting motivation will be internal, such as:

(a) The will to help the patient, and fulfil a need to be useful and wanted.
(b) The desire to attract praise for a job well done, and to fulfil a need for the esteem of others.

(c) The satisfaction of seeing results from effort, fulfilling a need for self-esteem.

Internal and positive motivation of this kind should be aimed for by those in authority over the nurse, just as internal and positive motivation should be aimed for in the patient by those who treat him. Enthusiasm for the subject is necessary in the teacher before it can be elicited in the student in both situations.

Lack of Staff Motivation and its Results

If the staff is not motivated towards the programme, it is unlikely to be introduced with success, however well planned it may be in itself. Important details will be overlooked because their significance is not understood, enthusiasm will be lacking in its presentation so that the patients will not be stimulated, and camps may develop, for and against, leading to bad feeling and poor teamwork. Education of the staff is important, but good results with actual patients are even more so. In this respect, a demonstration with the staff's own patients by a competent person is invaluable. The staff themselves should be asked to bring forward those patients with whom they find difficulties. The person introducing retraining methods must be secure in her own knowledge and practical ability if she is to pass on her enthusiasm and convince other people that it works.

A practical demonstration followed by a good response from a 'difficult' patient is one of the most helpful tools for building staff motivation. Once the programme has been instituted and accepted such motivation should be reinforced by regular in-service lectures, demonstrations, and case discussions. New staff members need orientation, and basic talks on retraining so as to be able to take part with confidence and understanding of the regime.

Unsatisfactory Bases for Motivation

In working to help patients in their fight against disability, one should not expect gratitude as a right. Some patients will be grateful, some apathetic, and some antagonistic. None of these attitudes should be taken personally. They should be looked upon as assets to be used or difficulties to be overcome in the patient's retraining programme. The person who is motivated by sentimental reasons to 'do something for the poor old dears', and looks for gratitude for her efforts is likely to be disappointed. Many a start at introducing recreational activities into a nursing home has been abandoned because 'we tried it, but the patients weren't very keen'.

In almost any group of sick elderly people, poor motivation is the first difficulty to be faced. Until this is overcome response will be slow, and appreciation slight, but overcoming it is possible, and is in fact an integral part of the introductory period. For this reason the person introducing the scheme must have a much less personal and more practical motivation than her need for esteem to see her through the difficult early stages when no-one seems to want her. If she believes in what she is offering, understands how it can help those to whom it is offered, and is patient enough to make friends first, the response will come.

Mechanisms of Motivation

Motivation stems from the perception of a need, whether this be conscious or not. Thus the need for oxygen causes us to breathe, for the most part without conscious effort. If, however, a stuffy room makes us conscious of our need, we will act consciously to open a window. Some needs, such as the need for food and air, are instinctive and immediate, while others, such as the need for a certificate to practise in a chosen occupation, are distant and demand planning and well-directed effort. The simple and immediate needs of the rest of the animal kingdom are complicated in man by his ability to perceive needs which are likely to arise as well as those which have already done so, and to plan ahead for such contingencies. His motives are correspondingly complex as he tries to satisfy these needs. Although the basic human needs are the same for us all, the emphasis we place upon them can be very different, and so the motivation, produced will also vary from person to person, the poor motivations as well as the good. If we wish to help a person regain lost motivation it is necessary to get to know him as an individual, and to understand something of his view of the problem as well as our own. Although some of his needs may be very obvious to us they may not worry him at all, while others which are hidden may be his main motivating force.

Maslow's Theory of Basic Human Needs

The psychologist, Abraham H. Maslow has placed the basic

human needs in five groups, which he has then arranged in an order of urgency, postulating that those in the first group will always take precedence over those in the second and so on, when there is a conflict between them. Those who have worked at the treatment level with geriatric patients will be well aware of just how impossible it is for a patient who wants to go to the lavatory (group 1) to concentrate on a safe walking pattern (group 2), until the more primitive need has been met. Maslow's list, with some relevant examples is as follows:

(a) *Basic physiological needs.* Oxygen, food, and the elimination of waste products.
(b) *Safety.* Feelings of security and the ability to cope with physical and mental threat.
(c) *Affection.* The need for friends and a feeling of being accepted by one's peers.
(d) *Esteem.* The appreciation by others of ourselves, our merits, and our actions.
(e) *Self realisation.* Satisfaction with our life and a feeling that we have lived up to our own standards.

Application of Maslow's Theory in Retraining

As in all other aspects of retraining we must start at the patient's own level when we try to improve his motivation. From that point we build upon any gains we observe, however slight they may be. The patient who presents as being completely disinterested in his own future should not for that reason be denied retraining. It is part of retraining to help him regain that interest, and the first step is to make him comfortable by seeing to all physical needs. Maslow's 'Hierarchy of Needs' can be applied to retraining in the following ways.

Physical Comfort

The first step to be taken is to make the patient comfortable by seeing to his physical needs. This tends to build his confidence in the helper which will carry over into more advanced stages of treatment. Requests for a drink, toilet facilities, or a knee rug, should not be passed off as trivial or time wasting, for this valuable asset of trust can be quickly eroded.

Safety

Once the patient has passed this hurdle, more active measures may be introduced, but they should always be well within the patient's ability to achieve. Resistance, whatever the excuse given, is likely to stem from fear, whether physically or psychologically based. Fear of pain and fear of failure are two examples and such fears can make the patient decide that it is safer to do nothing. If, however, he has confidence that the person helping him will see him safely through his effort he will almost certainly 'give it a go'. This feeling of confidence in another person is not given automatically, but must be earned. It has many roots, but the main one is the helper's obvious interest in what she is doing and in the patient himself as a person. It is also essential that the helper should be well prepared for the job she is to do, and confident herself in her ability to do so.

Affection

Having been brought from a state of resistance to one of acting with help, the patient must be 'weaned' so that he is able to function independently. This must be done with kindness so that there is no likelihood of the patient feeling rejected. His need for affection will motivate him towards things which he knows will please his helpers and it is part of the mechanism that they should show appreciation of these efforts. His relationships with other patients will probably improve as he becomes less concerned with his own affairs, and he may form friendships among them. He may even be the one who tries to comfort a new and unhappy patient with reassurance such as 'I was just like you, and look at me now!' When this happens he will have graduated from needing affection to giving it.

Esteem

When this stage is reached the patient has moved into the phase where he needs less help, and where spontaneous and internally motivated action is possible for him. He should be encouraged in this as much as possible with generous praise and appreciation. This will aid his confidence, and reinforce his feeling that he is doing well. The expression of esteem is a strong force in the process of motivation.

Self Realisation

By encouragement and praise from others the patient is helped to feel pleased with himself as a person who may be battered, but is not bowed. The opportunity to prove to himself and others that he can still function as an adequate person is one of the values of retraining. To do one's best in the face of adversity demands character, and the patient who demonstrates this can achieve self realisation despite gross physical disability. Self realisation is reached if the patient can go home feeling that he has conducted a worthy fight against his problems, and intends to go on doing so. Whatever the disabilities he has learnt to accept he will be able to feel that life is still good, and that he himself still has a part to play.

No Watertight Compartments

Many patients, of course, do not begin at the bottom of this scale, and many others will not reach the top. At any stage, each will have needs which are similar to those outlined, and an awareness of these will be useful in encouraging the patient to progress. The needs will not necessarily present themselves in neat separate compartments. Praise, for instance, is possibly more necessary for the patient in the first stage who achieves a simple goal than for the one who has just produced a brilliant new idea. Many needs exist concurrently in us all. It is helpful to have some guide as to the order in which they should receive attention.

Causes of Poor Motivation

If the aim is to motivate people, we need to know the most common causes of difficulty, and to have guidelines for overcoming them. It is then possible to allow for them in planning our programmes, and so to leave only the more personal and unusual ones for individual attention. Good staff motivation is the first consideration and if this is achieved many problems will be avoided. Next it is necessary to produce a happy and enthusiastic group of patients who are willing to co-operate. Into this active group can be introduced a smaller number of initially reluctant patients, who will usually respond to the general atmosphere of optimism, and become part of the group. Occasionally there will be someone who does not so respond, and who remains resistant to retraining as a whole, or to some aspect of it which he feels unable to accept. The reluctant patient will be the subject of the rest of this chapter, but the strongly resistant patient will be discussed in Chapter 13 which deals with the 'difficult' patient. The more usual reasons for poor motivation, and some guidelines for overcoming them are as follows.

Medical Condition

Pain, dizziness, weakness, lethargy, incontinence, poor balance, defective sight or hearing, and loss of movement in a limb are all examples of factors arising from the patient's illness which may cause reluctance to act, to join a group, or to respond to friendly advances. If the complaint is new it should be reported to the appropriate team member for action. If it is already known and receiving treatment this fact should be explained to the patient (again and again if necessary). If no treatment is indicated, this too should be explained. The patient should be reassured that the matter has been discussed with the doctor, and that the activity offered is indeed part of his treatment.

Signs and symptoms may also be used as excuses when some other, less acceptable, reason is the real one. Whether or not such excuses are considered to be valid by the staff, the patient should not as a rule be made aware that he is disbelieved because this does not leave him a face-saving way out if he changes his mind and decides to co-operate after all. When it is quite plain that the problem presented is an excuse, the success of motivation will depend upon treating the underlying cause of the patient's reluctance to act. When this is done he will no longer need the excuse. Excuses and methods of dealing with them are discussed in more detail in Chapter 13.

Fear

A large proportion of reasons given by patients for not wanting to act can be traced back to fear, although this is rarely admitted to be the cause. To a generation which has been through one, and possibly two world wars, during which courage was seen as a prime virtue, it is extremely difficult to admit to being afraid. The face-saving physical excuse is a way out. The fears themselves are real, and reassurance is necessary before willing action can be expected. Fears can be divided into three main headings for the purpose of discussion, but combinations of these fears are likely to be present in many patients.

Physically Based Fears. These fears are natural, primitive, and common to most people. They include fear of pain, falling, damage to existing trauma, over-exertion of heart or lungs, going blind, and other such eventualities. To the person in hospital such possibilities can appear imminent. We are in fact asking him to act against his own judgement when we ask him to face them. Thus the trust he feels in us and our judgement is crucial to his willingness to do so.

DO

Listen to what the patient says about the symptom.

Ask relevant questions and show interest.

Give a simple explanation for anything in which an explanation may help.

Take the symptom into consideration in your activity.

Provide safety measures (such as an accessible chair or a second helper when starting a walk).

Let the patient say when he has had enough so that he feels that he is in control.

Begin slowly and quietly, with plenty of support and encouragement.

Ask the patient if all is well at frequent intervals.

Watch for signs of fatigue, and discontinue activity when they appear.

Give praise for a good try, whatever the outcome of the effort.

DO
NOT

Brush the patient's excuse away as irrelevant.

Let him think you do not believe him, or do not care.

Neglect to reassure him, even if you think he is unreasonable.

Force him to act before he agrees to try.

Ignore complaints of symptoms once he starts to cooperate.

Bully him into going further than he wants to.

Speak loudly, give peremptory orders, or seem to be putting on pressure.

Hurry the patient. Speed will come with confidence, but is dangerous without it.

Make early sessions too long.

Tell him he can do better and is not trying.

Leave him on a note of failure.

The fight or flight methods of dealing with fear are seen very clearly in patients who are facing activities and treatments of which they are afraid. Some will join the fight willingly and battle on, but others will choose flight by refusing to act. The helper's part is to be a trustworthy ally, giving physical and moral support as needed, thus helping the patient to find the courage to do his best.

Psychologically Based Fears. These fears affect most of us at some time. They have to do with the picture we have of ourselves and the ones we like other people to have of us. Because they are mental and not physical they are none the less real, and they can produce both conscious and unconscious results in our behaviour. Some of those which can cause difficulties in the motivation of the elderly sick are fear of failure, the unknown, disappointment, the future, or loss of dignity, self respect, or the respect of others. Because of such fears many patients will decide that it is safer not to risk any activity. No-one can say you failed if they have not seen you try!

Once again, trust in the helper is the key to overcoming these fears. This trust depends upon a good relationship, and all that has been written about the approach to the patient in Chapter 12 is relevant to this.

DO	Get to know the patient and give him a chance to know you.
	Let him tell you his problems as he sees them.
	Perform some small service for him if you can.
	Seat him near active and well-adjusted patients.
	Let him watch others to see that they are managing with problems very like his own.
	Give him plenty of time to observe, while giving praise and encouragement to others.
	If you feel he is ready, ask him to help another patient with a simple job at which he cannot fail.
	Watch for the slightest sign of interest and follow it up.
	Give appreciation for any activity undertaken.
DO NOT	Rush him into an activity without feeling your way.
	Make him feel under pressure to act.
	Seat him near patients with negative attitudes.
	Neglect to do anything you may have promised.
	Offer an activity which looks complicated.

DO   Offer an activity which looks childish or undignified.
NOT   Let him feel that you are too busy to listen to him.
       Tell him his problems are minor compared with someone
           else's.
       Show any signs of impatience or irritability, however you
           may feel.
       Threaten him with a report to someone of more author-
           ity.
       Leave him with a feeling of having failed you or himself.

If he makes a tentative beginning make sure you notice and give
him appropriate congratulations and encouragement to go further.
The way a small start is received can either confirm or allay his
fears, and future co-operation patterns may be set at this point.
Many patients need support of this kind at each new step in their
treatment. The key words are reassurance, support, and praise.

Socially Based Fears. Socially based fears are those which come
when a person perceives a threat to his established or chosen life
style. They vary greatly with the individual. A fear, such as that of
having to give up a home, may spur one person on to greater
effort, while causing another to give up the fight. The threat may
be real or imagined, but if it is real to the patient it is relevant to his
motivation. Social fears are often the basis of emotional and
unrealistic decisions by patients to go home too soon, to reject
help, or to refuse treatment. In these cases motivation is unwisely
directed rather than absent, and may in fact be very strong. Some
examples of social bases for fear are:

Danger, during the patient's absence, to a dependant, a pet, the
    garden, or to belongings by burglary or prying.
Loss of home, life style, independence, family support, respect or
    status in the community.
Being a burden to the family or neighbours, or receiving 'charity'.
Loneliness after enjoying the company in hospital, and feelings of
    insecurity in case of illness or emergencies.

Dealing with problems such as these is the task of the medical
social worker, but other members of the team must understand
them and make allowances for them in their treatment. If they do
not they may well find unexplained difficulty in motivating the

patient, or that they have been motivating him towards an unrealistic goal. When fears of this kind are known or suspected,

DO   Read the social worker's report if one is available.

Refer the problem to the social worker if it is not known.

Let the patient tell you his fears, and reassure him about minor ones.

Relate the treatment programme to known needs (toilet training, cooking drills, safety on steps, etc.).

Make the patient aware of the value of what you offer in relation to his problem.

Bring up the problem at the case conference, and suggest appropriate retraining action (home visit with the patient, training of relative, alteration to home, etc.).

Give positive support once a decision has been taken at team level.

DO   Act without the concurrence of the social worker.

NOT   Take sides against a relative, a friend, or any other team member.

Make promises beyond your usual duties.

Tell the patient what to do. It is not your decision.

Become emotionally involved.

Discuss the problem outside professional limits.

Argue with the patient. This usually strengthens his resolve.

Be negative about a team decision once it is made.

The goals of treatment for each patient are set by many factors. One of the most basic of these is his former way of life, and home conditions. Problems in this area can be potent causes of 'poor' motivation, sometimes because the patient wants to return so desperately that he sets unrealistic goals, and sometimes because he is afraid of returning to face his problems, and will set no goal at all. Such problems as these cannot be solved by individual team members, but by understanding them, and working together the team can build up the patient's motivation and help to channel it towards attainable goals.

Personality Problems

Poor motivation can be merely an extension of the patient's usual personality. He may be a person who has always expected others to wait upon him, make his decisions, and fight his battles, or he may be one who has spent more energy avoiding work than in doing it. He may be a 'loner' to whom placement in a group is foreign and frightening, or a 'drifter' who has chosen to let the world slip by. It cannot be expected that people with long-standing personality traits such as these will become strongly motivated fighters as a result of being ill. It is necessary to go gently with such patients, as they are usually very sensitive to any sign of disapproval, and react negatively to it. Positive reinforcement whenever they make an effort, and a friendly approach are usually our best tools, but even these can be turned against us if there is any hint of insincerity.

Ourselves

Although it is part of our job to motivate our patients, we ourselves can sometimes be the reason for their lack of motivation. We must always remember how easily our attitudes, moods, states of health, and careless remarks can influence our patients for good or ill. If we are tense and insecure in offering an activity, the patient is likely to feel the same way about it. If we are impatient, the patient is likely to become flustered, and if we seem bored the patient will feel that the activity is unimportant. Similarly positive attitudes such as enthusiasm, patience, confidence and belief in what we are doing will lead our patients in a more positive direction.

If we are not gaining the patient's co-operation, and are failing to motivate him satisfactorily, we should look at ourselves as well as the other factors which may be at work. Have we adjusted our approach to suit his needs? Have we chosen the right level of activity? Are we too business-like or too friendly? Have we let him down in any way? Have we given him full attention when he needed it? Have we brought our own problems to work? These and many questions like them should help us to see if we ourselves are the reason for lack of motivation in our patients.

Motivation in New Patients

Reluctance to make a start is more common among new patients than enthusiasm. This is natural, and usually lasts only so long as it takes the patient to get his bearings. It is for this reason that the initial interview (see Chapter 12) is so important. This initial reluctance is not 'poor' motivation, but merely a cautious approach to something new. Poor management at this stage, however, can cause poor motivation which may be difficult to overcome. If carried to extremes it becomes negative and resistant, and this aspect is discussed further under the 'difficult' patient (in Chapter 13).

Motivation of a Group

One of the greatest assets in motivating a new patient is to have a happy and well-motivated group in which to place him. When starting a new group it is wise to begin with a few enthusiasts, and not worry about numbers until a happy and positive atmosphere has been established. Whatever the activity, its success will depend more upon enthusiasm than upon any other single factor. Even after a good start the spirit of a group is easily deflated. One person who looks as if the current activity is beneath him can make the rest feel silly for enjoying it. If this one person happens to be a staff member who fails to join in, the result is particularly dampening, as other staff members are likely to be affected as well as the patients.

Further discussion of the management of groups will be found in Chapter 6.

Some Motivational 'Tricks of the Trade'

In motivating the elderly sick, some basic factors emerge. If these are carried out the majority of patients respond well, but if they are neglected trouble can ensue. They involve the following.

Giving the Patient Confidence

This involves the helper's belief in what she is doing and her ability to do it, a calm and confident manner, ability to adjust to the patient's disposition, and reliability in doing what she promises.

Managing Real Difficulties

Many of the reasons given by the patient for not acting can be treated directly or referred to someone else for action. If possible this should be done. Even if there is nothing to be done, the excuses should not be brushed aside. The patient should feel that we would help if we could.

Ensuring Success

Once a patient agrees to act it is essential to choose what we give him to do with great care. It must be well within his powers, and we should make sure it comes to a successful conclusion. If we misjudge his ability and he looks like failing we must take the blame and the responsibility upon ourselves. Praise for what he has tried to do is an essential part of motivation.

Positive Attitudes

Throughout the time when a patient needs motivation our own attitudes must be positive and appreciative. We must congratulate him upon what is good in his effort, and minimise his mistakes. We must point out the positive values in what he is doing and not its problems. We must expect success, as people usually try to live up to our expectations of them.

Conclusion

In geriatric retraining, motivation is an integral part of treatment, and not something which a patient just has or has not. If it is not present, it is the responsibility of the staff to do all they can to develop it, by the use of techniques which they themselves must learn. A patient must be motivated to do so if he is to achieve his best level of independence. Physical independence rarely lasts much longer than the patient's determination to use it.

It should be our aim to enthuse the patient so that he is strongly motivated towards his own goals. We are unlikely to succeed unless we ourselves are well motivated to do so.

12 PRESENTATION OF RETRAINING TO THE PATIENT

The relationship between the patient and the helper and the importance of this in the retraining process.

Introduction

The manner in which retraining is presented initially may make the difference between the patient's acceptance or rejection of the programme, while the attitude and teaching ability of the person presenting it will certainly influence the quality and speed of his learning. This takes courage, resolution, and an optimistic outlook at any age, and in any state of health. These qualities may be at a low ebb after the debilitating effects of illness, or the shock and distress of disablement. For this reason it should not be taken for granted that every patient will face the fight to regain his independence with enthusiasm. In many cases the first responsibility of the retraining team is to gain the patient's co-operation in the presence of apathy or even resistance. The team's ability to do so depends to a large extent upon the approach to the patient of every one of its members.

The New Patient

The Need to Make a Good Start

Early impressions tend to persist, and so every effort should be made to ensure that retraining is introduced in a manner which gives confidence and hope. A friendly welcome, concern for the patient's comfort, patient and honest answers to his questions, and clear explanations of what will be happening in the immediate future, are important details in helping him adjust to the new situation. Long, unexplained waits, staff members hurrying past as if he were not there, quick moves in a wheelchair to an unknown destination, and placement in the bustle of a ward, with no explanation of its routine can all leave him perplexed and frustrated. The new patient almost invariably feels apprehensive and alone,

150

and should never be left sitting in isolation, wondering whether he has been forgotten. If it is not possible to deal with him immediately, he should at least have this explained to him and be placed where he can see other people.

All patients adjust more quickly if their introduction is a friendly and helpful one, and this is particularly so for those who are confused, withdrawn, apprehensive, disgruntled or resentful. The impression the patient receives at the preliminary stage will determine what he will expect, and so what he will tend to perceive in the days that follow. An unhelpful attitude, by even one person, can cause distress out of all proportion to the incident. Therefore all staff members need to understand the emotional states of new patients, and the pressing need for simple human kindness.

Need for Adaptability in the Helper

The staff member is 'at home', but the new patient is in much the same position as a visitor. For this reason the staff member should cultivate a 'hostess approach', adjusting her manner and conversation to the needs of the 'guest'. Each patient must be seen as an individual with a different personality, different needs, different attitudes and different experience. A successful start to retraining depends very much upon the ability of staff members to adapt to these differences. However stereotyped may be the material which must be communicated, it should be presented to each patient in a manner suitable to himself.

Adequate presentation involves sensitivity on the part of the staff member, so that she can adjust her approach to suit the patient's response. Feeling one's way towards understanding the patient and learning how best to gain his co-operation is part of the preparation for treatment, and has nothing to do with the helper's own feelings as to whether or not she likes the patient. She is there to help him, and by making an effort to adapt her approach to suit him she will also make it easier for him to accept that help as it is offered.

Training and Experience Both Needed

Because of the nature of retraining, a special quality of trust is needed between the patient and the helper. At times the helper will have to ask the patient to do things which are frightening or painful, or which he does not see as being of use to him. Such things must be done with the patient's consent and co-operation, for compulsion has little place in the retraining situation. Even persuasion, if too forceful, may lead to increased resistance in many cases. This problem can only be overcome by patience and the re-establishment of trust.

Learning difficulties resulting from illness, lost confidence through past failures, or long-standing personality problems, are all likely to be encountered by the person who is engaged in retraining the elderly sick. Her own personality and experience may be either a help or a hindrance, but in either case she needs more specific skills than her own background is likely to supply.

The attitudes and skill needed for this specialised type of teaching can be acquired. They should be taught to the staff concurrently with their training in the physical aspects of managing the patient. The ability of many of the patients to learn will depend very much upon the staff's ability to teach.

The Initial Interview

The interviews discussed here are those of the team members who are actually involved in retraining procedures. It will be presupposed that administrative, medical and social worker's interviews have already taken place, and that relevant information from these is available in the patient's notes. Retraining cannot properly begin before the medical assessment and referral, nor can it proceed effectively without some knowledge of the patient's background. In situations where no medical social worker is available, it is still necessary for the team to know the retraining aims for the individual patient.

Most people entering a hospital face a number of interviews, and the same questions are often asked over and over again. Some of this is necessary, but team-work can minimise it to some extent if team members refer to the patient's notes before their first visit. In any case, the meeting is easier if backed by a little knowledge. Informed remarks give the patient confidence in the person approaching him.

A Two Way Process

The initial interview is a two way process in which the patient is assessing the staff member just as surely as she is assessing him. While one is looking for problems and assets, and beginning to plan suitable action, the other is assessing reliability, the value of what is being offered, and deciding whether to act at all.

The patient's introduction to retraining should be as relaxed and informal as possible, with the patient being encouraged to talk about himself, ask questions and express his fears and aspirations. It should not seem like one more interview with hard facts being entered on a form or into a note book, but rather like the initial meeting of people who are to work together in a team.

Apprehension in a New Situation

The new patient may feel lost or anxious, and much can be done in the initial interview to allay his fears. It is not always appreciated that the confused patient and the patient with communication problems are even more in need of a friendly word and reassurance than the aware patient who can ask his own questions. Even the patient who can understand may not have been properly prepared by those who sent him for retraining, may not have listened to what they told him, may have heard garbled accounts from other patients, or may have his own, strange, preconceived ideas. For these reasons the interviewer should:

(a) Greet him by name if possible, introduce herself, and explain her role.
(b) *Ensure physical comfort* — consider such things as a comfortable chair, whether he has had a meal, toilet needs, and other such comforts as may seem relevant.
(c) *Sit down beside him* — people tend to feel at a disadvantage in talking to someone who looms over them, and an easier relationship is produced by eye to eye contact. There is also a feeling of haste if the interviewer remains standing, and this can inhibit conversation.
(d) *Give him undivided attention* — however busy the interviewer, she must obviously spend some time on the interview, and if it is at all possible this should be given completely to the patient. The quality of the interview, at this stage, has more lasting consequence than its quantity. First impressions do count.

Management and Content of Interview

Encourage him to talk. Most patients respond best if allowed to say what they want to, rather than being plied with questions or fed a large number of facts. Some of the things he wants to say may not seem very relevant to the interviewer, but they are to the patient. If they are heard sympathetically at an early stage they are much less likely to be repeated over and over again later on, to the exasperation of the staff and the exclusion of more relevant material from the patient's mind. The first interview should be used to get to know the patient as a person. There will be time later to present the more practical aspects of retraining, and this will proceed much more smoothly if the two people involved understand each other. There is no better way to bring this about than to let him tell his own story.

Follow up his statements. A simple, direct question, which can be answered by one or two words is useful when facts are to be elicited quickly and efficiently, but it will do little towards producing an on-going conversation. If the aim is to get to know the patient, a more indirect method is helpful, and encourages him to expand his subject because it demonstrates interest in the listener. Invitations to proceed take such forms as, 'that's interesting, do tell me more about it', 'do you want to tell me about it?', 'how did you feel about that?', 'what was it like in those days?', 'you must have felt proud of that!', 'I've always wanted to know more about . . . I'm so glad to meet someone who knows'.

Implicit questions such as these help the patient to follow his own line of thought, and feel that he is really engaged in a conversation, and not another interview. For this reason they tend to bring out ideas, feelings and misconceptions which are difficult to elicit in a more formal situation. This method is useful in encouraging the hesitant patient. The over-talkative patient can also be a problem, but he too should be encouraged to have his say in the initial interview, so far as time permits. Having heard a patient once, makes it much easier to control the outpourings at a later date.

Listen to what he says. The person conducting the interview should be a good listener who does not press her own point of view. If she is in doubt about the patient's story (which is often the case), she should check it before acting upon it, but not let him see her doubt until she knows him better. If the contentious matter is a complaint, it should not be brushed aside. A non-committal response which leaves the door open for further discussion is usually helpful.

'That sounds unusual, I'll see if I can find out more about it for you.' There must of course be a follow-up to this, which satisfies the patient that you have, indeed, listened to him and taken action.

Take appropriate action. Small complaints, which could have been attended to quite easily, can become a focus of discontent if neglected. This applies to the group as a whole as well as to the individual patient. If this happens, it causes bad feeling quite out of proportion to the original complaint. A very small kindness can have the opposite effect. Many a noisy patient has quietened down when someone 'wasted time' listening to his needs and doing something about them. The new patient will not be spoilt by such small considerations, but will rather gain confidence in his un-familiar surroundings, and feel that he is in good hands.

More difficult problems may be outside the province of the interviewer, and should be passed on to a senior member of staff, or to the retraining team's case conference. The problem may already be known to the doctor, medical social worker, or other concerned person, and be receiving appropriate action. In such a case, interference could be intrusive and even dangerous.

Report back to the patient. If you have promised to do anything for the patient, it is vital that you should report back to him con-cerning your efforts. If you have been unable to carry out your promise it is even more important that you should make the effort to tell him so. This applies throughout his stay, but is specially significant after the first interview. The patient's confidence, not only in you, but in the programme as a whole, depends largely upon such courtesies. If you apologise, at least he knows you did not forget. If you do not, you are probably just one more proof to him that 'no-one cares, so what's the use of trying?'

Make no promise you cannot keep. If the new patient is distressed, there is a tendency to comfort him with vague promises. These 'comforting' statements may help to solve an immediate worry, but they are only deferring the problem, which may be even more devastating to the patient if events prove the comforter to be wrong.

Some familiar 'comforting words' are given here, with suggested alternatives. The latter, while making no definite promise, are designed to encourage hope at a practical level.

Unsuitable 'Comfort'	*Suggested Alternative*
1. You'll be home in a month.	The doctor will tell you when you are ready to go home. He does not keep people longer than they need to stay.
2. Of course you'll be able to go back to your own home.	It depends how well you can manage. We will let you try in our kitchen, to see how you go.
3. Don't worry! You'll be walking in a fortnight.	I don't know how long it will take, but you look like a good trier to me.
4. You do your exercises, and your hand will be as good as ever.	You can't be sure, but in the meantime we'll show you how to do things with one hand, to help you to become independent.
5. They make wonderful prostheses these days. When you get one you'll hardly know it isn't your own leg.	We'll start you in a walking frame, and see how you manage. Your arms are strong and should help you a lot.

Do not remove hope. In answering the patient's questions about his condition or prospects, honesty should be the first consideration, but the reply should be presented in a practical and optimistic way so as not to destroy hope. A direct lie, or even 'wishful thinking', can lead to much more difficult situations at a later date. At this stage it is wise to leave options open. The hopeful thing is to indicate a starting point. The patient will have more faith in someone who says 'I don't know, but I'll see what I can do', than in someone who gives him a false answer, even if it is the one he wants to hear.

Finish on a high note. Just as each patient is completely different, so is each initial interview. They should, however, have one feature in common: that is, that the patient should feel happier and more sure of himself as a result of being involved in it. If he has been distressed during the interview, there should be an attempt to lead him on to surer ground before terminating the interview. A short preliminary lesson, or a small physical service such as offering a drink of water, arranging cushions, or giving him a magazine is usually helpful at this point. A brief recapitulation of factual material, such as where he is, and what to expect next can also bring the interview back to a less emotional plane.

If he has performed any practical task during the interview, he should be told that he has made a good start. In any case, he should be told when to expect you again, and what you will be doing when the time comes. As has been stated elsewhere, explanations of this kind should be given, whether or not you think he will understand or remember what you are saying.

Foundation for retraining proper. By the end of the interview, the person conducting it should have some understanding of the patient, his view of himself, and his mental capacity. This, together with the physical assessment, forms the base from which retraining will begin. If the interview has really been a reciprocal viewing of each other, as the word implies, the next step in the patient's retraining programme should be faced by both participants with quiet confidence.

Subsequent Approaches

The principles and interviewing methods which have been outlined for the initial interview also apply to subsequent dealings with the patient. As in the formation of a friendship, the relationship should be a developing one built on trust and mutual respect. The patient's confidence must be earned. It will continue to grow as long as the helper proves reliable, but it can also be lost very quickly if she does not.

Later approaches to the patient are concerned with the practical aspects of retraining, and each step forward by the patient is likely to produce its own fears and hesitations. When these are severe, careful preparation is the main factor in helping the patient to face the thing he fears. This is discussed in detail in the section on motivation (Chapter 11).

Some points to be considered are as follows.

Be Confident and Well Prepared

Fear and confidence are both very easily transferred from one person to another, not so much by words, although these can help, but by the more primitive signals of 'body language'. Tension and insecurity are felt, even when the reason for them is not understood. For this reason, a confident and relaxed helper is most likely to be able to produce these useful qualities in her patients. In this context, confidence depends upon being well prepared. This means that she should have:

(a) Knowledge of the patient's physical status.

(b) Understanding of the psychological aspects of retraining.
(c) Knowledge of the subject she is presenting.
(d) Understanding of why she is presenting it and how it can help the patient.
(e) Sound preparation of all materials and equipment involved.
(f) Confidence in her own superiors and the rest of the team, so that she knows where to ask for advice if it is needed.

Gain the Patient's Confidence

A start in gaining the confidence of the patient should have been made in his initial interview, but the proof of this comes with the introduction of practical activities. In order to make a good start the activity should be presented simply, without pressure, and at a level at which success is assured. The course of events should make provision for the following stages.

Introduction. Greet him, and remind him of any previous contact, or tell him who you are.

Explanation. Tell him what is about to happen, explain your reasons, and answer his questions, and his doubts.

Reassurance. Assure him that you will be there to help, that you will start with something easy and see how he goes. Let him know that you do not expect him to be perfect at his first try.

Demonstration. Show him what is required of him, either by doing it yourself, or by asking a confident patient to help with a demonstration.

Presentation. Start where the patient is on something he can achieve. Let him know that you are there to help with any part of it which is beyond him. Do not give him too many choices until you are sure he is ready to make decisions, but have alternatives ready in case your own choice for him has not proved suitable. Start him on one simple process at which he is unlikely to fail, and see it to a successful conclusion.

Supervision. Supervision of what the patient has been asked to do should be given unobtrusively, but consistently. It should be at its maximum during the early stages of learning, and should be progressively withdrawn as learning takes place. Supervision should be given before mistakes are made, and at the end of each completed process before a new one is introduced. Good timing is the key to success.

Correction. Even with the closest supervision, difficulties and mistakes will occur. Nothing undermines a patient's confidence more surely than injudicious correction. If a patient makes a mistake, he may well be disheartened to the point of rejecting the task altogether unless it is well handled. Acceptance of some or all of the blame by his helper is often the best solution, although the individual patient's ability to accept blame must be considered.

Appreciation. Whenever a patient brings something to a successful conclusion, its value will be enhanced if it receives due recognition from those about him. If the conclusion is less than successful, the patient will be aware of the fact, and support is even more necessary. If praise cannot be given for the overall result, at least it can be given for a 'good try', or for some aspect which is satisfactory. Positive recognition of what is good will give the patient heart to try again at that part which he has not yet mastered.

Staff Attitudes and Manner

Probably the greatest factor in helping a patient to make the most of his treatment and his stay in hospital, is the attitude of the staff. If its members are friendly, positive, and enthusiastic, and can give the patient encouragement and a little fun, the treatment will be accepted, and even enjoyed. If the atmosphere is disinterested, negative, lethargic, and deadly serious, there will be great difficulty in gaining the patient's interest and involvement. Staff members should try to be, or at least should seem to the patient to be:

a. *Enthusiastic*   Believing in what they are doing and in what they are asking the patient to do.
b. *Positive*   Expecting success, and looking for ways to bring it about.
c. *Concerned*   Showing an interest in each patient, noticing progress, and doing something about problems.
d. *Involved*   Joining in whatever is going on with enthu-

siasm. This applies to group activities as well as exercises, etc.

e. *Interested* — Giving full attention to patients while working with them.

f. *Fair* — Not having favourites or black sheep. Personal likes and dislikes have no place in the treatment relationship.

g. *Appreciative* — Able to give sincere praise for a good job or a good try, and observant enough to notice them happening.

h. *Calm* — Ready to steady things if there is trouble, fear, or over-excitement. Self controlled in such situations.

i. *Reliable* — Being available when needed, never letting a patient down or making promises which cannot be kept.

j. *Confident* — Adequately prepared by study, thought, or preparation of necessary equipment for the job in hand.

k. *Unhurried* — Insulating patients from any feeling of haste experienced by the staff. Elderly patients rarely do well, and often go to pieces if asked to hurry.

l. *Sensitive* — Aware of changes in patients' moods, responses, interests, or health, and able to act accordingly.

m. *Trustworthy* — Being one to whom the patients talk without fear of having their confidences betrayed.

n. *Kind* — Laughing with patients, but never at them. Willing to do a small service 'beyond the call of duty'.

Empathy not Sympathy and Personal Involvement

Staff can help their patients best if they do not become emotionally involved in their problems. In 'sympathy' we tend to experience the feelings and emotions of those around us, and may even encourage them to exaggerate their woes. In 'empathy' we can let them know that we understand how they feel, and give them a steadier kind of support. In the first we cry with them; in the second we wipe their tears. The staff are employed to treat their patients, and it is not ethical to use this position to make personal friends of them. Even if it were acceptable to do so, it would not be possible to keep in touch with them all, and so selection and favouritism would result.

To try to keep in touch, except at the official follow-up level, would be both physically and emotionally exhausting, and would leave staff members less able to give their best to the new patients coming into their care. Thus rules against personal involvement of an on-going nature are in the interests of both patient and staff. On the other hand, it is doubtful if we could help our patients if we were completely detached. They need to feel that we really care about their progress and that we like them. We must be a friend to them while they need our help, but we must be able to give them up when they take up their own lives again. We have not succeeded if a patient remains dependent upon us, either physically or psychologically.

Conclusion

Those who deal directly with patients must recognise them as individual people with individual problems. Because the patients are there for treatment and help for these problems, many of which will be of a psychological nature, it is not the responsibility of the patient to make a good relationship and therapeutic atmosphere, but for the members of the retraining team to do so. The approach to the patient is part of his treatment, and should be designed to suit his particular needs. In this respect the therapist herself is the therapeutic tool.

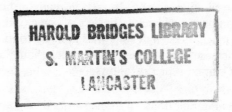

13 THE 'DIFFICULT' PATIENT

The patient who differs from the majority in attitudes and behaviour and some thoughts on his motivation and management.

Introduction

We all enjoy working with the pleasant, enthusiastic, well-adjusted patient who appreciates our efforts. He, on the other hand, probably does not need us as much as the bad-tempered, withdrawn, wandering old 'nuisance' who resists us at every turn. We prove our real concern for people, and our professionalism, when we accept the latter as well as the former, and give to both our best attention. 'Difficult' behaviour has many different causes and attention to these is part of the treatment programme. Certain attitudes and skills are necessary in helping these patients, and the most important is to accept that we have no right to return anger for anger, or to become personally upset by the patient's behaviour. Our reason for working with the patient at all is to help him to adjust to his problems, of which 'difficult behaviour' is merely one.

Attitudes

Staff attitudes are even more important to the 'difficult' patient than to the well-adjusted one. In fact, in many instances, difficult behaviour can be traced back to neglect of some of these principles by someone who has been dealing with him. To continue to neglect them will increase the problem still further. Some aspects which need special emphasis are as follows.

Acceptance

We must accept the patient as he is, and never let him feel that we are judging him. It is not for the helper either to condone or condemn his behaviour, but to help him towards a frame of mind in

162

which he can make the most of his retraining, and enjoy the process. If his behaviour is not generally acceptable, there will already have been many people who will have told him so, obviously without effect. One more will not help. A rational attempt to discover the cause of the behaviour, as the patient sees it, is usually the best way to begin. If something can be done about the cause, so much the better, but even to discuss it calmly can help the sufferer. The sure way to aggravate the problem, and to reinforce the patient's feeling that no-one understands, is to join the chorus of disapproval which usually meets 'difficult' behaviour. 'A friend is one who knows our faults, and loves us just the same.'

Concern

We should always remember that the 'difficult' patient is an unhappy person with a problem. It is hard to visualise a happy and secure 'difficult' patient, so it seems logical to deal with the causes of unhappiness if we want to moderate the behaviour pattern. Concern for how the patient feels rather than how he acts should be encouraged in all who are dealing with these patients. It is not enough to be concerned for him if the patient is not aware that we want to help. Small services, and the ability to listen are both useful in helping him to understand that this is so.

Concern for the individual should not exclude concern for the group as a whole. If one patient's behaviour is upsetting others every attempt should be made to protect them from excessive exposure to his problems. For instance, the patient whose noisy behaviour has disturbed other patients at night, should not sit with those same patients by day, but should be introduced into a different group. Such simple expedients show concern for both the individual and the group. Seating patients with regard to their problems also shows practical concern. It is usually a simple matter to sit the patient who worries about his bowels close to the toilet exit, the one who complains of glare with his back to the window, and the one who is afraid of draughts away from the passage way. Such small privileges bring large dividends in contentment, even if the original complaints are known to have little basis in the patient's medical condition. They can eliminate unnecessary grumbling and fussing, which can destroy a pleasant atmosphere and consume much valuable time. The fact that staff are seen to 'care' is one of the strongest factors in preventing 'difficult' behaviour, as well as in treating it once it is present.

Patience

It is not easy to be patient with 'difficult' behaviour, and yet patience is essential in helping someone through his problem. Firm handling of a difficult patient may be necessary, but this should always be the result of assessment of the need, and not of exasperation on the part of the helper. Most difficult behaviour only becomes worse in the face of impatience, and so we must have enough self discipline to appear outwardly calm when a patient is disturbed. This applies to such problems as aggressiveness, weeping, wandering, and demanding behaviour as well as to less dramatic ones like slowness, lethargy, poor concentration and verbosity. Impatient treatment of a minor irritation can easily precipitate the insecure patient into really 'difficult' behaviour.

Restraint

This form of patience demands restraint in the expression of the helper's own feelings, and so it is essential that it be seen as part of the technique of handling the difficult patient. It should be accepted as an attitude which must be adopted consciously in difficult situations, and not as a personal trait which some possess and others do not.

Honesty

Lack of faith in his family, his treatment, or those who are trying to help him, can produce difficult behaviour. Where this is so, the building of trust is a major factor in controlling it. An untrue statement or an unkept promise will undermine the confidence of anyone, but it can be particularly damaging to the unhappy person who has come to expect to be let down. To solve an immediate problem by even a 'white' lie is only to defer it and give it time to grow. To say 'I'll be back soon', unless we intend to do so, may help us to get away from a demanding patient. It will also make him try harder than ever to hold onto the next person who deals with him. Trust is the surest foundation for continuing co-operation.

Understanding

'To understand all is to forgive all', is a proverb which comes close to the truth when we are dealing with difficult behaviour. It is enlightening to see the change in staff attitudes towards a 'difficult' patient once the background to his problems has been explained at a case conference. Basic personality, rejection by others, poor handling in the immediate past, fear of failure, frustration, attention seeking, insecurity, self pity and many more such factors can be involved. These produce complicated patterns of cause and effect which may never be completely unravelled. They should, none the less, be allowed for in our dealings with the patient. If we make an effort to understand why a patient behaves as he does, it is easier both to accept him as he is and to help him to overcome his problems for the future.

Fairness

The 'difficult' patient can be very time consuming if his helpers do not take a realistic view of the situation. We have all seen the whole staff gathered round an already disturbed patient, trying to help by words or actions. The situation is much better managed by one person who can remain calm unless dangerous aggressive behaviour is involved. This leaves the other staff members to go about their job as normally as possible, and to attend to the needs of the rest of the patients. One person should remain within call to help if needed, but the fewer people actually involved with the patient, the more likely he is to settle down, and the less likely other patients are to become disturbed.

The disturbed patient may need a great deal of attention during an acute outburst, but he should not be led to expect this as a right when the need has passed. He should receive as much, but not more attention than his neighbours except during times of real distress. In geriatric retraining there is no place for black sheep or favourites. Attention should be in accordance with need, and not personal feelings and interests. Needs will vary between patients, and in the same patient from time to time. The patients themselves need to understand this, as any hint of favouritism can create its own problem behaviour.

Humility

Few 'difficult' patients respond favourably to the authoritarian 'I know what's good for you' approach. It is not usually the Sister's greater authority, but her greater experience which helps her to handle a difficult situation more expertly than the junior nurse. Some patients, indeed, are only further incensed by any show of authority of this nature. Whatever our position, we need to be able to meet the patient at his own level, so that he feels he can talk to us. If we are asked a difficult question, it is better to say 'I don't know, but I'll try to find out', than to give an evasive or incorrect answer. If the patient fails at a task and is upset about it, we can help by taking the blame. If a junior member of staff is getting through to the patient she should be encouraged to continue to do so. She may have some quality to which the patient can respond and which we lack. The patient's need should always take precedence over our own pride.

Never 'Give a Dog a Bad Name'

Many patients come to the hospital or retraining unit with a report of difficult behaviour in another place. Such reports may be by word of mouth, or written in a case chart, but in either case they should be noted, but not acted upon uncritically. A move to a new situation, with new helpers and new companions, is often just what the patient needed to make a new start. This opportunity should never be lost because of a 'bad' report. Much will depend upon his management in the first few days of his stay, and immediate friendly acceptance is essential. It is common human practice to live up to what is expected of us, and so it is common sense to expect the best of every new patient. The adverse report should alert us to the need for special care. It should not influence us towards prejudging the patient's potential.

Common Reasons for 'Difficult' Behaviour

Reasons for difficult behaviour are almost without limit, but they do tend to fall into categories for the purpose of discussion. Some of these groupings are as follows.

The Illness and its Symptoms

'Difficult' behaviour is not usual in people who are happy, and are receiving kindness and attention, but sickness itself can make people irritable, frightened, lonely, and uncomfortable. Difficult behaviour can be the result. Such behaviour may be a response to the illness, but it may also be a recognised symptom of the illness itself. In either case it should be seen as a matter for treatment and not anger. Some symptoms, by their very nature, can lead to 'difficult' behaviour, so the patient needs help to put up with them, and not criticism for failing to do so. Skin irritations, bad nights, general weakness, continuous nagging pain, and unaccustomed dependency are examples of such symptoms. Not all patients will respond to the discomforts and frustrations inherent in their illness with difficult behaviour, but some will, and these should not be penalised so that their morale is lowered still further.

Social Problems

Social problems are often behind difficult behaviour, and if not already known to her, should be referred to the medical social worker when this becomes evident. Some typical examples of such problems are:

Resentment against those who arranged admission to hospital.
Worry about the welfare of a spouse, pets, or the garden.
Worry about valuables left in an empty house.
Financial worries — the rent, the gas, or electricity, the tradesmen.
Worry about a disabled, retarded or alcoholic relative who has relied upon their care.
Fear of returning to live alone and being unable to manage.
Fear that this admission is preliminary to placement in an institution.

There are endless variations of these problems, and many patients will be able to express them, organise measures to deal with them, or rely upon their families to see that all is well. Some patients, however, will not have the necessary resources to solve their problems, and will become unhappy, and sometimes distraught as a result. The problems resulting from their worries may include poor concentration, restlessness, wandering, demands for premature discharge, refusal to become involved in treatment and aggressive behaviour against those whom the patient sees as opposed to his interests. It is common in these situations for the patient to be unable to think clearly about treatment, or to be realistic about his disability until the social problem to which he has given priority is overcome.

Misunderstanding

Misunderstanding can lead to difficult behaviour if communication with the patient is poor in the early stages of treatment. This may be due to his illness and its effect on his mental ability, or to insufficient attention to the subject by his helpers. Half heard conversations, misinterpreted explanations, unrealistic expectations can all cause trouble. For instance, preconceived ideas about going to hospital 'for a rest', may lead a patient to expect a nurse to dress him, when in fact, part of his treatment is to learn to do it for himself. Such misunderstandings can lead to anger, resistance, reports of staff neglect, trouble stirring, and general dissatisfaction. In most cases they are unnecessary, but they are never unimportant. Similar reactions may occur if the patient has been encouraged unwisely and has been led to entertain false expectations of cure.

Anxiety

Anxiety is an element in most 'difficult' behaviour. It will vary from mild unease to a severe state in which the patient can think of nothing else. Most of the causes of bad behaviour outlined in this chapter lead to anxiety which in its turn produces the problem reactions. The anxious patient may be restless, demanding, noisy, inclined to wander, unreasonable, unable to concentrate, and either tearful or aggressive. While the cause of his anxiety may be real and deep seated, or imagined and superficial, it should be remembered that it is real to the patient and is causing him distress. His anxious response is likely to continue as long as this is so.

Frustration

Frustration is an almost inevitable companion to disability. The ability of the patient to adjust to it will play a large part in forming his attitudes and patterns of behaviour during treatment and later if there is any residual disability to be faced. Frustration may come from his own inability to act, or from other people's failure to do as he wants them to. Communication problems are often involved as well as physical difficulties. Impatience, anger, aggression, and rejection of difficult aspects of retraining are some of the problems which can result. The temptation to 'give up' is very real, and so continued frustration can go beyond anger to resignation and withdrawal.

Confusion

There are various reasons for confusion in the elderly sick, and many of them respond to treatment. Whatever its cause, confusion can lead to 'difficult' behaviour, and good management is essential while that cause is being investigated and treated. Restlessness, wandering, forgetfulness, resistance, strange toilet and personal habits, disturbed sleep patterns, loss of belongings, looking in other people's lockers, unprovoked aggression and many such unpredictable actions can result.

Depression

Whether depression is a response to real external difficulties, or a feeling of hopelessness generated from within, it can still cause problems of management. Withdrawal from activities and social contacts, disturbance of sleep pattern, negative attitudes, weeping, refusal of food, and general unresponsive behaviour are common. Such patients may also have a dampening effect on the morale of others in the group, depressing some and irritating others.

Fear

Fear is a major cause of resistant behaviour. It can be physical (pain, falling, over-doing things), psychological (failure, looking silly, the unknown), or social (going home alone, rejection by family, loss of belongings). Fear can result in refusal of treatment, noisy behaviour, panic situations, and dangerous unexpected movements. One problem is that it is so easily communicated and may affect other patients who are not usually fearful people.

Psychological Needs

All the basic human needs if left unfulfilled can lead to 'difficult' behaviour (see Chapter 11). Feelings of discomfort, feelings of insecurity, feelings of rejection, loss of face, and loss of pride can all cause trouble. Two common causes of 'difficult' behaviour which are based on such needs are outlined below.

The Need for Attention. Just as some children would rather be spanked than ignored, so some patients would rather be known as a nuisance than not be known at all. There is usually a feeling of insecurity behind this kind of behaviour, which is usually modified once the patient learns to trust his helpers. Some difficulties it produces are excessive requests for toilet facilities, noisy behaviour, refusal to co-operate without a fuss, demands for special privileges, and attempts to engage every nurse who passes in lengthy conversation.

The Need for Self Assertion. The self assertive patient can cause problems if he feels a lack of opportunity to express himself. He will usually resist any sign of coercion, and probably lead other patients into following his example. He will be the self-appointed expert on everyone's treatment including his own, and his opinions will not necessarily coincide with those of the staff. If his energies can be turned into acceptable channels they can be an asset. If not, they can lead to disgruntlement and spreading resistance to the established programme. The patient's need for esteem is involved, and his behaviour is often over-compensation for the loss he feels as a result of his disability. He needs to prove to himself and others that he is still a force to be reckoned with.

Personality Clashes

Differences between people seem to be inevitable in the human condition, and they usually bring difficult behaviour in their wake. Fights between patients are not unknown, and if not well handled these can cause continuing problems in either or both of the rivals. Bad feeling between a patient and relative, patient and patient or patient and staff member can lead to deterioration in the patient's attitudes and behaviour. These are difficult to eliminate unless the personality problem is known to the team. 'Difficult' behaviour which these patients may exhibit includes anger, crying, rejection of activity, demands for discharge, stirring of resentment in other patients, playing off staff against staff, reports (factual or embellished) to relatives, and other reactions depending upon the personality and ability of the patient.

Medication

In many cases, 'difficult' behaviour is precipitated by the patient's medication. This may be an unavoidable side effect of a necessary drug, or the result of unsuitable medication, prescribed or otherwise. Any idea that medication may be involved should be discussed with the doctor in charge of the case by a responsible team member, or reported at the case conference. Some of the problems encountered are lethargy, giddiness, confusion, irritation, aggression and complaints of other unpleasant symptoms. These may be severe enough to stop the patient co-operating, or they may be used by an already uncooperative patient as an excuse for putting off his treatment. In either case, discussion with his doctor is the first step to be taken.

The Management of 'Difficult' Behaviour

Some people have a natural sensitivity to the feelings of others, and the ability to respond to them in an appropriate manner, but good management of the patient should not be left to the fortuitous presence of such rare skills. These skills should be explained to all who are engaged in geriatric retraining, learnt by them, and practised consciously as part of the treatment of difficult behaviour. It should be understood that 'difficult' behaviour is often only the exaggeration of a natural response, and that a sensible approach to the patient brings a more moderate attitude (see Chapter 12).

Generally speaking, the patient should be approached calmly and non-judgementally. He should be encouraged to tell his story as he sees it, and attended to with patience and courtesy. Argument should be avoided and any necessary explanations should be given quietly and factually. Any helpful action which can be taken should be done as soon as possible, and the patient should be made aware that it has been accomplished.

In more specific situations additional techniques may be necessary. Some examples of difficult behaviour and some techniques which have been found helpful in overcoming them are as follows.

Refusal to Join In

This is only 'difficult' behaviour if carried to excess. It does not usually persist if the precepts outlined in Chapters 11 and 12 are observed. The patient is presumably in the group because his doctor or someone who knows his problems has decided it can help him. To gain this benefit he himself must believe that this is so. Strong resistance usually comes when he is unwilling or unable to see the relevance of the programme to his needs, or sees some other course of action as of more importance. To exert pressure without convincing him that the activity is in his interests will only lead to further resistance, and even aggressive actions.

DO   Encourage him to explain his point of view.

Follow up legitimate complaints.

Incorporate as many of his own ideas as possible in the original plan.

Make sure he knows why you want him to act.

Remain calm, reasonable, and non-judgemental.

DO   Give direct orders which will lead to a confrontation.
NOT   Appear to know best what is good for him.
          Become emotional over the issue.
          Raise your voice, argue strongly or threaten dire results.
          Neglect to leave him a face-saving way of complying.
          Treat him like a naughty child.

If he remains determined, make sure the activity is really necessary, by discussion with whoever referred him, or with the rest of the team.

Withdrawal

Many patients who come for retraining are withdrawn and unresponsive. This may be the result of illness, medication, problems of communication, depression, fear of facing their problems, attempts to manipulate others or 'social neglect'. If something becomes too difficult for us it is very tempting to 'opt out', and usually the withdrawn patient is responding in this way. These patients are not a 'nuisance', as they tend to sit quietly, seeing little and demanding less. As a result they tend to be forgotten, and left to dream away their time unless the staff is aware of withdrawal as a problem demanding their attention. Retraining is an active process involving the patient, and withdrawal is the very opposite of involvement.

DO   Discover why the patient is withdrawing, and deal with any matters which can be helped.

          Make sure the patient is stimulated as frequently as possible, by a friendly word, attention to comfort, recognition that he is there.

          Touch him to gain attention when talking to him.

          Come to his level literally when talking to him. Sit or kneel and look directly at him to hold his attention.

          Be aware of even slight responses, and follow them up.

          Remember that personal contacts are needed to stimulate him, and too large a group or a noisy background will only give him an easier place to hide.

          Sit him near 'motherly' patients or those he can respond to as helpers.

          Put something simple but interesting in front of him, and use it as a basis for conversation (e.g. book, flowers, simple job picture, etc.).

Make sure he is not left out of what is happening around him.

Give explanations of activities whether he seems to be listening or not.

DO
NOT
    Put him in a corner and wrap a rug around his knees, letting him doze while you deal with more alert people.

Turn up the television and hope it will get through to him instead of making the effort yourself.

Overpower him with too large a group, too difficult a task, too much background noise, or too much pressure.

Forget that he may not notice meals, danger (radiators etc.), toilet calls, his own clothing (fastenings). You should talk to him about all such things and use them to stimulate interest.

Neglect to show appreciation of every small effort he may make.

Underestimate his intelligence and treat him as childish or beyond hope of reactivation.

The withdrawn patient is usually in need of human contacts, and a feeling of being wanted and respected. There are no mechanical means for giving him these. If left to himself he will be more than ever convinced that he is unwanted and 'finished'. 'Fussing' over him should be avoided, but regular, reliable, friendly exchanges should be encouraged.

Excuses

Patients produce many excuses for not co-operating in their retraining programme. Behind the excuses will be their reasons, and these may or may not coincide with each other. The excuses should be heard so as not to antagonise the patient, but the reasons should be sought out and acted upon. If an excuse is valid, action should be taken to solve the problem or to reassure the patient that allowances will be made appropriately.

Some common excuses are heard repeatedly from new patients. No-one who has worked at geriatric retraining will be unfamiliar with such statements as 'It's my eyes', 'I only have one hand', 'I'm waiting for my bath', 'I won't be here long enough', 'My daughter does all the housework for me', 'I've worked all my life, and deserve a rest', 'I pay to be here and have things done for me', and many more. If managed in accordance with the precepts in Chapters 11 and 12 the excuses will fade as the patient gains confidence. When they are too vociferous, or continue too long, they can be seen as 'difficult' behaviour.

DO   Use all the mechanisms of motivation as outlined in Chapter 12.

Remember that the patient is trying to say no without giving offence, or admitting he feels inadequate.

Treat him and his excuse with respect so as not to lose his good will, which is your best tool in gaining his co-operation.

Present something well within his powers, which makes little use of the asset he claims to have lost.

Remember to check his progress and ask if he has struck any difficulties at fairly frequent intervals until you are sure he feels secure.

DO   Let him feel you do not believe him.
NOT   Make his excuse sound silly to himself or others.

Offer any task which may lead to failure, particularly if it involves the weakness he has claimed in his excuse.

Be authoritarian in your approach. The most common reply to 'you must' is 'I won't' and once this point has been reached one or the other must give in.

The patient who gives excuses to the point of being 'difficult' is usually either afraid of the new situation he must face, or a person to whom effort is distasteful. The former needs support and confidence in the person helping him, while the latter may respond to 'jollying along', or even firm handling. We must discriminate, and deal with each case according to its needs.

The Demanding Patient

While some patients need encouragement to accept their retraining, others expect constant attention, even at the expense of other patients. In managing this type of behaviour it is necessary to be firm, but fair. The reasons behind the behaviour range from having been spoilt at home, and so expecting too much service, to having been neglected and feeling the need to demand it, expecting none. Some of these patients are merely enthusiasts who want to get on quickly, and others like the feeling of importance when they are having notice taken of their needs. Some have regressed so that they do not exercise control over natural impatience, but others are just selfish and unaware of the needs of others. It is impossible to manage these patients well unless the motivation behind their demanding behaviour is taken into account.

DO   See to immediate needs, and be sure that all legitimate calls for attention are promptly met.

Be fair in allocation of time, and deal with each patient in accordance with need and not nuisance value.

Explain that others need help too, but be factual and not impatient in your explanation.

Make sure that he does get his share of attention to build up a feeling of trust.

Have a private talk to him about the problem, and ask for his patience and co-operation. If he is quieter, show appreciation.

DO   Tell him to be quiet, or let others do so.

NOT   Give him extra time just for the sake of peace.

Give him less time because you are irritated.

Make a promise you do not intend to keep just to get away.

Sit him near other patients if they are getting irritable and telling him to wait his turn.

Patients who have needed a good deal of persuasion to begin work often seem to become those who demand too much attention once they start. It is necessary for them to know that you are not giving them less because you have lost interest, but because they have improved, and other new patients now need the care you gave them. They need to develop pride in their independence, not a feeling of rejection if their improvement is to continue.

Aggression

Aggression is usually seen in patients who are confused, frustrated, frightened, or feeling under pressure. It may take verbal form, or extend to actual hitting out at somebody. That somebody may be the one who has upset the patient, but usually it is just the one who is nearest when the patient finally loses control of his emotions. That person may have been unskilled in her management of the situation, but this is more likely to have been a last straw than the true cause of the aggression. The best management of aggression is preventive, and when the risk is recognised the patient should not be pushed beyond his capacity. Arguments, loud voices, too many people taking a hand, and physical restraint all tend to increase the patient's determination to fight for freedom. He needs peaceful surroundings in order to find a little peace within himself.

DO   Leave the situation to one person who can remain calm.

Have someone quietly nearby if there is danger of an actual attack, but let them be as unobtrusive as possible.

Let him let off steam, and say anything he likes about the situation, however much it might normally be offensive.

Speak quietly and sensibly. A loud voice encourages a loud response, just as a whisper is usually answered with a whisper.

Give him as much freedom of movement as possible. As long as he is not endangering himself or others, physical activity will help.

Make sure other patients are not at risk.

Remember that aggressive behaviour is part of the patient's problem, and needs as much help and understanding as his other symptoms.

Ask for help if you feel you have lost control of the situation. It won't help anyone if you are knocked out.

Report serious degrees of aggression to the doctor, or at the case conference. They are relevant to treatment.

DO   Take anything the patient does personally.

NOT   Appear to be afraid, angry or upset.

Join a group of people all talking to the patient at once.

Argue with the patient, however wrong you think him to be.

Continue with any pressure upon him to conform, unless it is absolutely essential.

Try to make him 'sit down and be quiet'. A little 'pacing' will probably help him.

Stop him stating his case, however unreasonable it may seem.

Use any physical restraint, except as a last resort.

Try to move him somewhere else before he calms down.

Attempt to hold him, or pull and push him against

his will unless his safety is involved.

Show any signs of resentment the next time you meet him. If he remembers the episode he will probably be ashamed. If he does not he will wonder why you seem cold towards him. Be the friend who 'knows our faults and loves us just the same'.

Aggressive behaviour can be distressing to all concerned, and not least to the patient. It is never improved by over-reaction from the staff. Even if physical restraint is necessary this should be applied as efficiently and quietly as circumstances allow, without raised voices and a panicky atmosphere. Safety for the patient and those around him must be considered, but the more freedom the patient is given the sooner he is likely to settle down. To fight back at one's tormentors or captors is a very primitive response, and to the distressed patient that is what those around him usually appear to be. For this reason, physical restraint is often the factor which changes aggressive attitudes to aggressive action.

Forgetfulness

The forgetfulness of many of the elderly sick can cause difficulties in their management, and so be seen as 'difficult' behaviour. It may vary in intensity from occasional lapses to almost complete loss of the skill. For each person there is a point at which the degree of loss becomes significant, depending upon his responsibilities, his way of life, and his family support. In some cases the loss is reversible, improving with the patient's condition and state of awareness, while in others it is permanent, and must be accepted and allowed for.

Memory defects are inconvenient and a source of worry to those patients who have insight. They can be a real source of danger to those who live alone and must manage their own medication, heating appliances, shopping, cooking, keys, and business affairs. They may, in fact, determine patients' ability to continue in their homes. Where there are lesser degrees of loss, the domiciliary services may provide the necessary support.

DO   Make sure that all that can be done has been done for problems of communication (spectacles, hearing aids, etc.). We cannot remember a message we have not received.

Speak simply and clearly and ask the patient to repeat what he needs to remember.

Work with routines which are repeated at regular intervals.

Provide aids to memory if the patient is able to understand them. (A clockwork alarm for regular toilet visits, tablets placed where the patient has his meals, etc.)

Use repetition rather than explanation in the teaching method.

Give the patient a simple daily responsibility in the group (changing a wall calendar, saying when it is time to clear up for lunch, watering pot plants, etc.).

Reassure the patient if his forgetfulness is causing him concern. Tension only makes it more difficult to remember.

Concentrate any memory practice you give on recent events.

Include simple memory practice in the games programme.

DO
NOT
Make too much of a lapse of memory, particularly in front of other people.

Brush it aside if the patient himself wants to discuss it.

Do things automatically for the patient. He should have the opportunity to think for himself.

Leave the patient too much in the past. You should try to encourage him to relate his past to his present. (Ask if he still enjoys some related activity, whether his grandchildren take after him, if the old place is still there, etc.)

Send him home with a gross memory defect without making some supportive arrangements.

Neglect to mention these problems in any activity assessment or report to case conference.

Give the patient too many different instructions at once.

Give too many different reasons or explanations. One good one repeated as often as necessary is better.

Become impatient if you are asked the same question or told the same story many times. You should answer the questions with patience and sidestep the story with tact.

As with most problems in geriatric retraining, we must treat the treatable causes of memory defect, and accept the untreatable, helping the patient to manage the problem with the provision of equipment or services.

Disorientation

Disorientation in the physically active patient is one of the causes of difficult behaviour, as it can lead to the patient wandering away, becoming lost, going to the wrong bed, or locker, or becoming agitated. It may affect his understanding of time or space, or both.

DO	Tell him where he is at regular intervals, and whenever he shows that he does not know.
	Point out simple, reliable landmarks to him.
	Make sure the necessary daily moves are kept to a minimum.
	Use distinguishing marks on his equipment (e.g. a special coloured label or bow).
	Give him as much freedom as is safe. In some cases an alert patient can act as guardian to the benefit of both.
	Let him lead you when moving from one place to another, so that he must think, giving hints as necessary, of course.
DO NOT	Agree with him and so reinforce his misapprehensions.
	Let him feel you think he is stupid. You should accept his mistakes as natural, but correct them gently.
	Argue with him to the point where either of you feels upset.
	Leave him unattended, or near open doors.
	Treat him like a baby, so that he gets no chance to improve.

Disorientation is an important factor in whether or not a patient can live alone. It can also create great problems of management for relatives, as the disorientated patient usually needs constant supervision. The blind and the confused patients are particularly likely to need special orientation programmes.

Wandering

Wandering is seen as 'difficult' behaviour, because it is both time consuming and worrying to the staff. It may be a vague and unintentional, or purposeful and aggressive thing. In the former case it is usually the result of disorientation and confusion, and in the latter a response to frustration, fear, or misunderstandings.

DO Allow the patient to wander unhindered so long as he is within sight, and not in danger.

Be a friend, not a gaoler. Meet him and offer your arm instead of following him and taking his.

Lead him on and around rather than trying to make him turn back.

Be concerned for his comfort. Offer a chair, cup of tea, 'nice warm heater' in the place you want him to go, and see he gets it when you get there.

Remain calm and do not seem over-anxious that he should comply.

Give comfort and support if he is lost and frightened. Scolding will not help.

DO
NOT
Insist upon him sitting down every time he gets up unless there is a medical or safety reason for doing so.

Make any more restrictions than are absolutely necessary.

Use physical restraint, or force except in extreme cases.

Allow a crowd to gather, or noisy argument to develop.

Give direct orders which may sound like a school teacher or policeman.

Tell lies to gain his co-operation. It may work once, but will only create problems for the future.

Forget that wandering is a symptom of disease or distress, and in either case needs understanding care.

Wandering is often closely associated with dementia and confusion and becomes less troublesome as the patient adjusts to his environment. The main problems which are attributable to it are those of safety, and home management.

Bowel and Bladder Problems

Incontinence is one of the most distressing of the problems faced by many of the elderly sick. It is a major cause of withdrawal from the social scene, is embarrassing to the patient and abhorrent to many relatives. It is often the factor which determines the need for nursing home care, particularly when the patient is no longer able to manage the washing and cleaning it necessitates. Its causes are medical, physical, psychological and social, and all these aspects need investigation and remedial action before it is accepted as inevitable.

(a) Medical investigations should not be neglected because of age or reduced mental capacity. The retraining team needs to know why the patient is incontinent, what type of incontinence is present, and something of the prognosis if they are to treat the reversible elements and plan management of the irreversible ones. Diuretic and aperient usage should be checked.

(b) Physical disability may make the patient slow in getting to the toilet, or it may prevent him from doing so without the help of another person. He may be unable to rise or sit on the toilet pedestal, manage his own clothes, or reach the toilet roll. Patients with problems such as these may be reported as incontinent when this is not strictly true. Retraining and suitable equipment are needed to relieve the difficulty. For instance, extra practice in chair drill may teach the patient to rise and sit more easily, or a built up toilet seat may achieve the same end.

(c) Incontinence based upon psychological causes tends to improve as the patient is integrated into the group, and made aware of his surroundings. Attention seeking, withdrawal, poor motivation, reduced awareness, loss of hope, and even the wish to punish or manipulate a relative can all lead to incontinence, and treatment must be aimed at the cause rather than the symptom.

(d) The social causes of incontinence include the factor of 'social neglect', where the patient is not stimulated by human contacts, feels rejected, and asks himself 'why bother?' Architectural barriers may make it difficult for him to reach the toilet in time, or he may be unable, through his disability, to manage his clothes appropriately. Emotional factors involving his social situation may also be important.

DO   Report incontinence to the doctor as soon as it is seen to be a problem (unless it is already being treated).

             Be open and natural in dealing with the patient. Any embarrassment you show will increase his distress.

             Discuss the problem with him and work out a plan to suit

his particular case (seating near the toilet facility, a chair on wheels if he suffers from stress incontinence, a clockwork timer, a bedside commode, adapted trouser fasteners, routine toileting procedures, the linen service, etc.).

Respond to toilet requests at once, and without a show of reluctance.

Use groups where the sexes are mixed for patients who are withdrawn, or whose attention is defective.

Think of the patient's feelings rather than your own if you have to clean him up.

Remember that it is mentally and physically cruel to deny toilet facilities when they are needed.

Be reliable in adhering to toileting programmes. This is habit building, and part of treatment. It is not merely a convenient way to keep the patient dry.

Remember the importance of control in this area to the patient's whole life style.

Consider the patient's dignity as a human being in all your dealings with him and his problem.

DO
NOT
Be judgemental. Discipline, anger and expression of disgust only add to tension, and make things worse.

Neglect any common-sense measures which can be taken.

Use appliances thoughtlessly and undermine the patient's dignity. (Catheters, receptacles, bags, etc. should be covered by clothing or under a rug.)

Make a fuss about incontinence in front of other patients.

Refuse to take a patient to the toilet because 'he has just come back'. The best way to stop incessant demands is to make the patient confident that he will not be kept waiting when really in need.

Forget regular visits for patients receiving habit training.

Promise to come back 'in a minute', and neglect to do so.

Leave a puddle any longer than you must. It is an embarrassment to one patient and a walking hazard to many.

Fail to report incontinence, particularly if it is new, increasing, or offensive.

Some of our earliest training, with punishments and rewards, was in control of bladder and bowels. It is no wonder that loss of ability in this area in our later years is so involved with feelings of shame and embarrassment. Medical diagnosis and treatment will proceed appropriately in most cases, but over and above this the patient needs understanding and support from all who are in contact with him and are aware of his problem.

Obsession with Bodily Functions

Some patients, who are not necessarily incontinent, become obsessed with their bodily functions, and particularly with the process of excretion. Conversation will revolve around whether their bowels have or have not worked, excessive medication will be demanded, requests to go to the toilet will be numerous, and usually unproductive, and excuses for not joining in routine activities will abound. Diagnosis and treatment are the responsibility of the doctor, but, as with incontinence, the management of the patient is in the hands of the retraining team as a whole.

DO   Make sure the problem is known to the doctor and the
                ward sister.

          Give quick access to the toilet when asked.

          Listen the first time, and then remind the patient tactfully
                that he has already told you if he brings it up too
                often.

          Make him mentally comfortable, by seating him near the
                toilet exit, telling him to call when he is ready, and
                reassuring him that the ward sister is aware of his
                problem.

          Find him a simple but interesting job to occupy his
                thoughts.

          Be aware that this obsession is annoying to many other
                patients, and try to seat him near those who will not
                be upset by it.

DO   Show impatience or annoyance yourself.

NOT   Leave the patient out of the group to sit and concentrate
                still harder on his obsession.

          Allow him to 'entertain' the group with vivid details of
                his problem. Lead the conversation into more general
                subjects.

> Ignore his request to go. It may be really necessary this time.
>
> Promise to come back and fail to do so. Building his confidence is essential to overcoming his anxiety.

This is one of the least endearing forms of 'difficult' behaviour, and is irritating to staff members and other patients alike. The patient's acceptance by his fellows, and his enjoyment of their company is at risk. We can help him best by encouraging other interests, and minimising the outward signs of his preoccupation. The obsession itself is unlikely to be overcome until its deeper causes are eliminated.

Attention Seeking

Attention seeking has many causes, most of which can be related to feelings of insecurity. These feelings may spring from deprivation in any of the common human needs. The patient himself is usually quite unaware of the reason for his behaviour, and sees his attention seeking as justified in its own right. It becomes 'difficult' when it disrupts the programme, or interferes with the equal rights of other patients to a share of the attention.

DO   Listen the first time, and deal with any real physical need you can find. Get to know him and his background.

Be sure the patient feels secure in your promises, fairness, acceptance of him as a person, and appreciation of his achievements.

Give him an outlet for his talents (inventiveness, ability to sing or play an instrument, skill at a trade or hobby, knowledge of a sport, and so on).

Emphasise his abilities and not his disabilities.

Be friendly, even if exasperated.

Give the real reason if you cannot give him as much time as he demands.

Appeal to his sense of fair play.

Explain his problem to others who find him 'difficult' if you understand why he is behaving in this way.

DO
NOT   Ignore his requests and hope he'll give up. He will probably only 'call out the more'.

Give him more or less of your attention than other patients receive.

Neglect the attention he really needs (toilet calls, positioning in his chair, tea to his liking, reassurance as needed, and a friendly response from you).

Join the chorus of those who call him selfish, a nuisance, demanding, and other derogatory things.

Let him think that attention seeking is either annoying you or gaining his ends.

Attention seeking takes many forms, from incessant calls for the nurse, to bad language, trouble stirring, noisy rejection of treatment, dramatic 'turns', and noisy weeping. It usually becomes manageable if the patient becomes confident that he will receive attention when he really needs it, and is offered a job which is 'specially chosen', and can be seen to have some real value and importance.

Inter-patient Animosity

A group of patients is made up of people whose only certain common ground is that they are ill. They represent every social, intellectual, political, religious and occupational background, and bring with them all their prejudices, taboos, customs, and preconceived ideas. It is surprising how well most of them adjust to each other, and make friends across established lines. Occasionally this does not happen, and old battles or personal dislikes produce behaviour which can disrupt the activities and equanimity of the group. In such situations the staff should not act as judges, but as peacemakers.

DO   Talk to both patients quietly and separately and hear both sides of the question.

Iron out any unnecessary misunderstandings.

Give factual and unemotional explanations if they apply.

Let both patients 'get it off their chests' to you, without taking sides.

Arrange a reconciliation meeting if differences can be ironed out.

See that the antagonists are not placed too close to each other in the group, at the dinner table, or in the allocation of beds if cross purposes persist.

DO   Take sides, or show any favouritism.

NOT   Allow factions to develop if you can avoid it.

Place the patients together so as to annoy each other still
further.

Shout at either of them. There is enough anger already.

Condone disruptive behaviour. You should point out
how it is upsetting other people, disrupting treatments, etc.

Ignore early signs of discord. Prompt action may prevent
the trouble developing at all.

Disagreements between reasonably rational patients usually
settle down fairly quickly. Unfortunately, other patients, and even
some members of the staff, tend to take sides, and the less popular
patient tends to be isolated unless conscious efforts are made to
bring him back to the fold. 'Ganging up' can quickly lead to feelings of rejection, unhappiness, and consequently to further 'difficult' behaviour.

Confusional States

The many different problems which are loosely covered by the
term 'confusion' can and do cause behaviour which is seen by
many as difficult. Many see treatment of these patients as a waste
of time, 'don't bother too much with him, he's confused!' but much
can be done to help both the patient and his relatives if the task is
tackled with adequate medical treatment, good management,
optimism and common sense. Some basic precepts for managing
these patients are:

DO   Address the patient with title and name. Christian names
        should only be used at the patient's request.

        Give the patient the same respect as you give to non-
        confused patients.

        Explain all moves and actions simply and clearly,
        whether you think the patient understands or not.

        Be patient and calm, however unreasonable the patient's
        actions may seem.

        Keep the environment as simple as possible. Eliminate
        background noise, bustle, cluttered furniture, too
        many different people dealing with the patient, too
        many choices of activity, complicated activities,
        too many instructions, etc.

        Answer questions clearly, simply, and honestly.

Keep to reality, and do not reinforce the patient's fantasies.

Look for rational content in an irrational speech, and build upon that.

Show concern for physical comfort and well-being.

Remember that it is not the confusion, but superimposed agitation which produces 'difficult' behaviour, and try to eliminate frustration, irritations and fear.

DO NOT   Treat a confused patient as a child. Whatever his response, you should talk to him as you would to any adult in the same situation.

Neglect to talk to him at all. 'Social neglect' is the cause of much confused behaviour, and will certainly not help to cure it.

Lower standards of cleanliness, tidiness, grooming, etc. in care of the patient. Spilt food should be wiped from his clothes, fastenings done up, and hair attended to if the patient is unable to manage such things for himself.

Say derogatory things about the patient in his hearing. Your words may mean little, but your attitude and tone of voice will be registered.

Scold the patient like a child for lapses of memory, touching other people's belongings, incontinence, etc. Give a calm factual explanation if necessary. Keep it simple.

Neglect praise for anything the patient does well.

Take it for granted that everything the patient says is confused. There is usually a basis of truth which has been misunderstood. Confusion, like memory, can be selective and patchy.

Much so-called 'confusion' is the result of toxicity related to disease or its treatment or to misunderstandings concerning drugs. Much is due to environmental factors of mishandling by other people. All these factors need attention before a patient is labelled as 'confused'. If they are treated, the residual 'confusion' is likely to be mild enough to be readily managed at home. If the patient cannot be cured, it is still very likely that his condition can be improved.

Playing Off

This form of behaviour is usually produced by the patient's personality and not his disease. It is mentioned here because it can be disruptive unless the staff are aware of what is going on. The patient tries to gain advantage for himself by exploiting jealousies and differences between staff members. 'Miss X doesn't do it nearly as well as you do', is a danger signal as well as a compliment. It may be innocent, and it may be manipulative.

DO   Make sure differences of opinion over treatment are worked out at case conferences.

Discuss the problem with the other member of staff if you suspect trouble making.

Resist the temptation to feel pleased and never encourage the patient to make comparisons in your favour.

Remember that what you say will be repeated, even if it is only tacit agreement with what the patient has said.

Try to be a good team member, even if you really agree with the patient's remarks. Disagreements should be resolved within the team.

DO   Listen to gossip about another member of staff, what-
NOT   ever you may think of her yourself.

Favour a patient because he flatters you, particularly if it is at someone else's expense.

Be disloyal to a team member or team decision in discussion with the patient.

Forget that the manipulator probably says the same about you to the other person.

The manipulative patient is only a danger where staff communication is poor, or when treatment aims are not clearly understood. 'Playing off' will only continue so long as the manipulative patient sees some advantage to himself in using it.

Bad Language

Patients who use bad language may do so for many reasons ranging from habitual use as part of normal conversation to really aggressive use in anger. The precept 'don't condone and don't condemn' is usually of help in this situation. If taken aside and reminded that there are ladies in the room who could be offended, most of the first group will apologise and try to remember to leave out the offending words. When a patient is swearing in anger the suggestions for restoring calm listed under 'Aggression' should be carried out. If anything can be done to remove the cause of the anger it should be undertaken. The patient should not be made to feel that he has lost respect as a result of the incident, but the rest of the group must be protected from an unpleasant situation.

To ask the patient to sit down and tell you his troubles quietly may have the desired effect, but telling him to be quiet or raising one's own voice will not. Patients who have lost control of their emotions and are beyond reasoning should if possible be taken to a quiet place, and given the opportunity to say whatever they please without upsetting other patients. Outbursts of this kind should be seen as demonstrating the need for help, not punishment.

One type of swearing is quite beyond the patient's control. Certain aphasic patients lose their speech with the exception of one or two words which come out spontaneously whatever the patient intends to say. Occasionally these words are expletives which can cause misunderstanding with other patients and uninformed persons. Relatives are often surprised or embarrassed by this and say 'father was never a swearing man'.

Anyone in contact with the patient who is likely to be offended or upset by the oft repeated word should have the situation explained to them as being the patient's misfortune and not his fault.

No staff member should ever take a patient's swearing personally. It may be that she has angered him, and it may be that everything has just become too much for him. In either case there is need for understanding and calmness in her attitude. It is very true in most cases that 'a quiet answer turneth away wrath'. When things quieten down it is important that the patient should not feel that he has put himself in anyone's bad books.

Combinations and Variations of Many Problems

In this chapter specific aspects of 'difficult behaviour' have been discussed separately, and some means of managing them have been suggested. Unfortunately, difficult behaviour rarely comes separately in the individual. Various degrees of severity, and various combinations of difficulties will be presented, and each case must be treated on its merits. Experience is the best teacher in dealing with these problems, but it is hoped that the guidelines offered here may help while experience is being gained.

Conclusion

In dealing with difficult patients we must remember that we are employed to help them, and that their 'difficult' behaviour is as much part of their problem as their physical disabilities. By patience and understanding we can usually reach them, and become allies instead of enemies. In doing this we ourselves often find greater satisfaction than in helping the patient whom everyone loves from the beginning. The retraining staff should be well equipped to deal with these patients and to help in their readjustment. They should remember that the patients' problems can best be overcome by treating them as symptoms instead of faults. We must help these patients, not add to their difficulties.

PART FOUR
The Physical Aspects

Part Four describes the movements
used in the Retraining Drills. Detailed
step by step directions are given for
the basic drills and for the variations
needed for some common specific
disabilities.

14 ROUTINE RETRAINING METHODS

The use of daily routines as treatment media, relating needs for independence to treatment and resettlement programmes. The design of appropriate 'drills' is discussed.

Routine retraining is the original concept of Dr R.M. Gibson and his team, who planned and instituted the Royal Newcastle Hospital's Geriatrics Service in 1955–8. It is the basis of the Newcastle Method of Geriatric Retraining, and although there have been additions to some of the original techniques and modifications of others, the original concept has stood the test of time. It is based on recognition of the fact that daily activities, which must be performed at regular intervals, are an ideal medium for training the disabled in personal mobility and independence, and that the nursing staff, who traditionally play a helping role, can encourage independence by assuming a teaching role as well. Dr Gibson has written,

It was appreciated from the beginning that the student nurse must learn the techniques used by the ancillary specialist and bring these new methods and attitudes into her patient care, adding them to the disciplines of her nursing training. It is emphasised that in the end it is the patient who must learn and the staff who must teach. This fact must be constantly kept in mind through the procedures of dressing, bathing, shaving, etc. If these activities are not brought within the scope of nursing care they stop when the ancillary specialist is not present, and the nurse has left only custodial care which is dull, non-rewarding and depressing. It has been traditional for nurses to nurse sick people and in some situations this means doing things for them. Activity nursing emphasises the role of the nurse as a teacher who shows — helps — encourages her patients to learn to do things for themselves.

Routine retraining, using carefully selected and codified techniques, is designed to develop confidence and independence with

193

safety in the geriatric patient, and can be justified in physical, psychological and social terms. It allows for great variation in the learning ability of patients, and when necessary, for compensation for residual disability.

Integration of Retraining and Ward Routine

The daily activities which we learn to do for ourselves as children, and perform throughout life almost automatically, are the very activities which create most difficulty for relatives if an adult becomes unable to do them for himself. They include such basic things as feeding, toileting, bathing, grooming, dressing, transfers and ambulation, and in cases where people live alone, household tasks, shopping and cooking. Both physical and psychological illnesses can deprive us of these skills, and it is not surprising that they play a large part in the management problems of the elderly disabled. They may be lost progressively over a long period as in rheumatoid arthritis, Parkinson's Disease, or dementia of gradual onset, or suddenly as the result of a stroke, a fracture, or an acute psychiatric episode. Whatever the cause, it is often the loss of these skills rather than the illness or accident which brought about their loss which creates the patient's problem in returning to his home. It seems logical therefore, to help him to regain them, or to become competent enough to manage with whatever help is available to him.

Problems Faced by Relatives

If a patient becomes dependent upon others for his daily needs, the stress upon those others can become unbearable. Relatives, who may themselves be neither young nor strong, can become exhausted by the constant demands for help as well as the physical effort of lifting, often without any knowledge of safe methods of doing so. The nurse who must lift a heavy patient is usually able to obtain help from another nurse or a wardsman if the task is beyond her, but the relative is often quite alone with the problem. Some of the main problems which may be faced by relatives in this situation are:

a. Being 'on duty' 24 hours per day.
b. Heavy lifting without skill in the subject.
c. Lack of confidence by patient or helper, or both.
d. Lack of readily available help.
e. Pre-existing frailty in the helper.
f. Badly designed or badly placed equipment through lack of knowledge.
g. The physical strains of lifting, fetching and carrying, and disturbed rest.
h. Conflicting advice from well-meaning but uninformed friends.
i. Emotional ties with the patient who may be more difficult with family than with strangers.
j. Loss of outside interests as a result of being tied to the house.
k. Feelings of isolation and rejection by those who no longer keep in touch.
l. Family stress as to which member is helping and which is not.
m. Stresses between the patient and the helper which are inherent in the whole situation.

Routine retraining of the patient and training of the relative in using the same methods as the hospital staff can ease many of the problems outlined above, lightening the load at both the physical and psychological levels.

The Patient's Point of View

Although there are some people with dependent personalities, most people are proud of their independence and ability to cope for themselves. It is very difficult for these to accept a dependent state, and anyone who has worked among disabled people will know of countless instances where tremendous odds have been overcome by determination 'not to be a burden'. Encouraging and helping people to use this drive to its full advantage can bring only beneficial results, while neglect to do so may well mean the difference between a return home and a future spent in a nursing home. Some of the problems faced by the patient who has become dependent upon others are:

a. The physical discomfort of being 'lugged about'.
b. Fear of being dropped or hurt during lifting.

c. Fear of being too heavy and hurting the helper.
d. Fear of the future, of being alone and helpless, of being a burden, of going into a nursing home, of financial stringency, and more.
e. Feelings of inadequacy and loss (loss of dignity, independent action, life style, authority, respect, and control of his own affairs).
f. Disinclination to ask for help. 'Putting up with things'.
g. Boredom.
h. Resentment of the whole situation.
i. Frustration, with difficult behaviour arising out of the above, possibly hurting his helpers against his will.

Routine retraining can help the patient both physically and psychologically in many of these problems, because it uses the abilities he still has, involving him actively in his own care. It encourages him to be proud of what he can do instead of being depressed over what he can not, and it sets goals which are possible, and so worth striving for.

Involvement of the Nurse

Because of the learning difficulties of many elderly people and the teaching methods necessary to combat them, it is essential that any scheme designed to improve independence in these patients should provide ample opportunity for repetition at short intervals. As the transfers and movements under discussion are regularly helped or supervised by nurses in the normal course of their duties it is logical that they should be asked to use the appropriate method every time they attend to a patient.

In their training nurses are taught safe and scientific methods of lifting, but they are not generally taught how to encourage a patient to help in the movement himself in such a way that he will eventually be able to carry it out unaided. This demands movements which are specially designed for the purpose, and training of nurses in the use of these movements. It also requires that nurses understand the importance to the patient of involvement in his own care so that they learn new attitudes to his management and carry out the moves accurately and conscientiously as part of his treatment programme.

A demonstration project carried out at St Joseph's Hospital, Yonkers, NY, USA, established the value of training the nurses in the skills necessary to teach their patients to be independent. A class of 36 freshman nursing students were given such training, and their performance was recorded against that of a group of 38 senior nursing students who had not received it. Some significant findings from the nursing point of view were:

a.   The experimental group used correct body mechanics 66 per cent of the time, while the control group used them only 27 per cent of the time.
b.   Back strain and injuries were reported by the control group (numbers are not stated), but none were reported by the experimental group.
c.   The experimental group was concerned for safety factors and took effective action 81 per cent of the time and the control group 37 per cent of the time.
d.   In 40 out of the 50 daily activities observed the experimental group gave patients more opportunity for self help than the control group.
e.   Supervisors estimated that the experimental group students saved one hour each per day's assignment.
f.   Where four students were assigned, one assignment could be distributed to the other three, thus releasing one from a self care oriented area to a situation involving intensive care.

That the staff is too busy is often given as an excuse for not encouraging self care by the patients. This may apply when retraining is first introduced, because all patients will need help and careful instruction from the nurses. It must be remembered that as the original patients gain in independence the help can be withdrawn from them, leaving the staff more time for new patients, those who are sick, or the slow learners of the group. Once momentum is established, the more hopeful feeling in the ward, and the stimulus of seeing the patients progress, will mean that the work becomes not only physically lighter, but also more interesting and rewarding to the nurses themselves.

Training in the Techniques

Not only the nurse, but everyone who moves the patients should be trained in using the same method for doing so. In this way the patient receives his repeated lessons, and is not confused by varied and conflicting instructions. The Newcastle Method has evolved with this as an important consideration. The chosen method must be simple enough to be used by lay people such as relatives and voluntary helpers as well as by all grades of staff. This factor is a help rather than a hindrance, as simple methods are also better understood by the patients themselves.

Ideally, there should be one person responsible for teaching the chosen techniques to the staff, and to the patients' relatives, so that variations are kept to a minimum, but all senior personnel should be responsible for seeing that they are carried out in their own areas. It could well be more important for the night sister to insist that her nurses encourage independent use of a commode than that the day sister should do the same for the toilet. Lectures on self help will not produce results unless they are backed by insistence upon their practice in the wards.

Retraining Priorities

There is no hard and fast rule as to which activities should be introduced first, either to the programme or to the individual patient, but if the aims are well considered, the most important activities will tend to choose themselves. Fortunately, the most valuable group of activities, the 'drills', are also the least demanding of extra space, equipment, and staff, and so can be introduced as soon as there is one person who understands them and has the ability to pass on her knowledge to others. The drills, which are described in detail in Chapter 15, are designed for use with normal household furniture and a few simple aids (see Chapter 18). The most usual problem in hospital or nursing home is not too little equipment, but too much of unsuitable design. Examples of this are high beds, low chairs, and elaborate walking aids which are unsuitable for use at home.

Even if no other activities are possible, the drills can be started in the ward, and they are probably the best introductory activities in most situations.

Assessment of Independence in Activities of Daily Living

An assessment form which lists the activities which are needed for independent living is helpful as a guide to programme content as well as being essential for assessment of a patient's need for services before he goes home. It can be used to indicate weaknesses in a patient's performance at the start of treatment and to demonstrate progress when repeated at a later date. The form needs to be simple and practical, and to make it easy to see problems at a glance. Many such forms have been designed, varying from one to twenty pages in length. The one which is used in conjunction with the Newcastle Method of Geriatric Retraining was originally simplified and adapted for local conditions from that of Dr Howard Rusk of New York, and it has been further modified at intervals in response to changing conditions and team discussion. A copy of the present form is included in Appendix B. It has been kept to two quarto pages in size, in keeping with other records on the patient's charts. The ratings have been made as objective as possible, indicating the amount of help required. It eliminates verbal reporting except where the scale does not give adequate information, as in the description of walking ability. Page 1 deals mainly with the patient's performance in the ward, and page 2 with his daily activities in the retraining area, and his interactions with other people. The first is usually completed by the retraining sister, and the second by the occupational therapist, both conferring with other members of the team and with each other as necessary.

While delineating the areas in which independence is necessary, and so setting goals, the main use of the form is as a guide to the patient's status before discharge. The final test is used by the doctor and medical social worker in planning discharge and determining what equipment and services will be required for resettlement at home. For this reason marking is hard, and when doubt exists the lower grade is recorded. It will be noted that both physical and psychological areas are covered. The purely physical questions may well show a patient to be capable of doing everything for himself, when in fact his motivation, his ability to organise himself, or his personality may indicate that he is most unlikely to achieve his physical potential. Such a patient would be quite unsuitable for unsupervised living, although well able to manage in a family setting. Problems of motivation, a tendency to withdraw if not stimulated, and similar difficulties are among the reasons for asking relatives to attend for instruction in retraining. Personality difficulties are just as important in the patient's management as the residual physical problems. Possible difficulties in both areas are clearly demonstrated by an accurate completion of the Activities of Daily Living Assessment form (ADL).

Design of the Drills

The 'drills' of the Newcastle Method have been designed, simplified and codified specifically for use with elderly patients. Certain principles were laid down, which took into consideration the needs of the patients and their relatives as outlined earlier in this chapter, and the teaching methods best suited to their learning capacities. Some of the principles are controversial, chiefly because the method aims for general competence in the patient's own situation rather than specific recovery of function in individual limbs. The drills teach independence in necessary daily activities, and in performing them the patient gets exercise and so gains in strength, balance, co-ordination and so on. This is the chief difference in emphasis from more traditional methods where specific exercises are given to produce strength, balance, co-ordination, etc., so that he can perform necessary daily activities. The two methods are not mutually exclusive, and exercises are prescribed for specific problems when suitably qualified personnel are available to give them. The drills, on the other hand, are simply redesigned methods for performing routine tasks, and so can be used to improve the patient's performance by any staff member who is called upon to help him.

The drills themselves are described in detail in Chapter 15 together with a job breakdown so that they may be followed step by step. The main principles behind their design are as follows:

a. Retraining should come through performing a task, such as rising from a chair, rather than through formal exercise.
b. Retraining should begin without waiting for specific muscle re-education or the problematical return of function in damaged limbs.
c. Emphasis should be on ability and not disability.
d. Safety and good balance should take precedence over the traditional emphasis on good posture.

e. Methods should be simple enough to be learnt and applied by first year nurses.
f. Methods should be suitable for teaching the patient's relatives so that they can continue to use them when the patient goes home.
g. Trick movements are acceptable if they make a task easier for the patient.
h. Each activity should lead on to the next so that there is no need for relearning.
i. Lifting should be eliminated or kept to a minimum, the helper's job being to direct and guide.
j. The patient's weight should be taken as far as possible through his own body or limbs.
k. In each movement the patient's weight should be distributed as evenly as possible over his strong limbs.
l. Pushing up and leaning should be used rather than pulling up and holding on.
m. The patient should be helped with what he cannot do, but not with what he can.
n. Help should be progressively withdrawn as the patient improves, in such a way that he eventually performs the original move unaided.
o. Each move should be suitable for a step by step breakdown, so as to be presented to the patient 'one step at a time'.

The Chosen Movements

By careful analysis it has been found that a person can achieve all the moves needed to transfer the body in ordinary activities if he can make the following basic movements:

a. Sit up from a lying position.
b. Move along a flat surface.
c. Stand up.
d. Balance.
e. Turn around.
f. Sit down.

If these moves are allied to walking or the competent use of a wheelchair, a person can be independent in his mobility. All these movements are incorporated in bed and chair drills (Chapter 15), and a simple, direct method for retraining in walking is given in Chapter 16.

The drills other than bed and chair drills are made up of the same movements arranged in a different order. These are usually achieved quite readily once the two basic drills have been chosen in preference to other well-known methods because they contain all those necessary moves.

Areas Other than Mobility

Retraining is necessary for the elderly disabled in areas other than mobility. The nurse's role as teacher is just as important when the patient is dressing, bathing, or eating, as it is when he is transferring from his bed to a wheelchair. The amount of skill he needs to get home will depend to some extent upon how much help is available to him, but the more he can do for himself the better, even if he has a loving family ready to wait on him hand and foot. In fact, such a patient may have more need, psychologically, than the one who will be left to struggle for himself.

As in the mobility drills there are basic ways of teaching these tasks so as to minimise the effects of disability. Variations may be needed for individual patients, or their problems may best be solved by the provision of aids and equipment (see Chapter 18).

There are many books on this subject if the reader wishes to go into it in more detail, and for this reason only equipment which has been found generally useful in routine retraining, or which has been developed in the Newcastle programme is described in this book.

The more qualified and experienced staff members there are available, the more sophisticated the training in activities can become. Even so there is a limit to the acceptance of complicated gadgets by the elderly, and to the time it is reasonable to ask them to spend learning difficult skills. In the Newcastle Method the basic needs are seen to first, and then those patients who have the will and the ability to progress further are referred to continuing treatment as out-patients after their return home.

Individual Patients' Problems

Because people differ so markedly in their responses to any situation, and because of the prevalence of multiple disabilities in the geriatric patient, routine retraining as described must make provision for the patients whose problems are not covered by the usual methods. These must receive individual attention from qualified members of the team until their special problems are solved. When a suitable plan of treatment has been worked out, it is passed on to the rest of the staff, and adopted by all. Patients who fall into this category most often are those with gross deformity from long-standing rheumatoid arthritis, lower limb amputations combined with hemiplegia, and contractures with various degrees of fixed deformity as a result of periods of immobility before referral for retraining. The principles of retraining usually still apply, but help from specially designed equipment (see Chapter 19) and some variations to the drills may be necessary.

The Training of Relatives

Unless the patient's relatives understand what the patient is able to do for himself, and what help he really needs, there can be dangers of either over- or under-protection. The accurate ADL Assessment can be used in the final discussion before discharge to make them aware of minor needs. If the problems are seen to be too complicated for this, or if the relatives themselves lack confidence, the relatives are asked to attend the hospital to work with the patient. A selected member of the staff teaches, observes and encourages them until the problem is solved, or a decision is made that placement in a nursing home is necessary.

Some of the situations in which the training of a relative is indicated are as follows.

a. When the patient has been unable to remember the details of the drills, but is able to manage them if reminded of the details.
b. When the patient is able to manage the drills, but is unsafe because of sensory disturbance, blindness, or poor concentration.
c. When the patient is poorly motivated and tends to ask for help unnecessarily.

d.   When the patient performs well when stimulated by company, but withdraws if left to himself.
e.   When the patient has some residual disability which makes some special technique necessary to his easy handling.
f.   When a patient has some specially adjusted piece of equipment which needs to be understood by the relative.
g.   When the patient or the relative is nervous about their joint ability to manage.
h.   When it is thought that the patient will slip back unless he is given continued encouragement or firm handling.
i.   When it is expected that the patient will slip back, and the relative is required to ask for help when a refresher course seems necessary.
j.   When there is doubt whether the relative will be able to manage the physical strain, and needs to prove it to herself one way or the other.

In cases such as these, the person teaching the relative should obviously be one who has worked closely with the patient, and can manage him well herself. The aim is to help the patient and the relative to become a team of two, and to be able to work smoothly and calmly together at whatever drills will be needed in their own situation. In most cases it is wise to include a safe method for getting a patient up from the floor after a fall in which there has been no damage. This is a fear which neither the patient nor the relative likes to express, and there is usually great relief when it is brought up in a matter of fact way in the course of the lesson. If the relative is obviously too frail or too frightened to be able to cope, the usual advice is to provide blankets and pillows, and to call a strong neighbour or the local ambulance.

Going Home

Routine retraining has been given to the patient so that he will be able to manage at home, and has been modified to suit known variations in his own environment. There may also need to be changes in that environment to compensate for skills he has not been able to achieve. It is essential that such skills as he has should not be wasted because a bed is too high, a chair too low, or a passage too congested. It is also necessary that the patient should translate what he has learnt in one place to his way of living in another. Patients who are likely to find this difficult, and those who show apprehension as the date of discharge approaches, can sometimes be helped by a preliminary visit with a confident member of the retraining team to prove themselves on their home ground. This applies particularly to those who live alone or who will be alone for part of the day. If unforeseen problems do present themselves at this stage they can be dealt with before the actual discharge takes place.

The standard equipment which the patient has used in hospital, and any special aids which have been made for him, should be delivered before he returns home, so that he will be able to function properly from the beginning. Referral back to his family doctor and the organisation of domiciliary care services are also completed at this time to make the home-coming as smooth and safe as possible.

The routine retraining will then go forward under the supervision of relatives and the maintenance team until further help is needed from the other phases of the geriatrics service.

15 ROUTINE RETRAINING 'DRILLS'

Directions are given for the basic movements required in independent mobility by people with some use in all four limbs.

Introduction

The Newcastle retraining drills are given in this chapter in the form of a step by step job breakdown. It is in this form that they should be presented to the patient. The actual physical movements cannot give their best results unless those who teach them understand their purpose and principles as well as their mechanics. It is recommended that before presenting the drills to patients the staff should read and discuss the principles. They should then follow the movements step by step themselves, simulating the appropriate disability. This is probably best done by working in pairs but it can be done alone. The aims, principles, and recommended teaching methods are explained in Chapter 14.

Summary of Principles for Revision

In the Design of the Drills

(a) Repetition and habit forming.
(b) Maximum use of strong limbs.
(c) Distribution of body weight over strong limbs.
(d) Involvement of the patient in all movements.
(e) Gradual progression towards independent use of the movement.
(f) Emphasis on safety factors.
(g) Balance before beauty.
(h) Elimination of heavy lifting.
(i) Use of ordinary home furniture.
(j) Use of simple equipment which can be used at home.

In Teaching the Drills

(a) Know as much as you can about the patient before starting.

(b) Have all necessary equipment at hand.

(c) Give a simple explanation to the patient of what you intend to do.

(d) Give directions slowly and clearly, one at a time.

(e) Give the patient time to think and act before giving the next direction.

(f) Avoid hurrying the patient. Work at his speed.

(g) Encourage the patient to use what strength he has, giving help only when needed.

(h) Withdraw help progressively as the patient improves.

(i) Encourage nervous patients by being calm, starting with an easy task and giving praise.

(j) Hold lightly and let the patient feel what happens as he moves.

(k) Talk and explain as you work, even if the patient does not seem to understand.

(l) Use mimicry and hand gestures as well as speech for patients with learning problems, receptive loss, etc.

(m) Remember you are teaching by repetition. Do not expect the patient to learn at the first try.

(n) Give plenty of praise for a good try, a step forward, or achievement. If sincere, it will encourage the patient to further effort.

(o) Leave the patient on a note of success. Finish with something you know he can do, and praise him for doing it.

Although the drills themselves are formalised and carried out in a routine way, remember that each patient is an individual and will have individual reactions to his illness, his retraining, and his helpers. The ability to understand what is being done, and the speed and ability with which he can do it will set the learning speed of each patient. We must adjust our lessons to suit these individual needs.

Content of the Drills

The basic drills of chair and bed provide all the movements necessary to the patient for transfers from one seated position to another, and for standing and sitting safely. When allied to safe walking the same moves make him independent in his mobility, whatever the degree of recovery in his damaged limbs. It is possible to begin these moves as soon as the patient is considered medically fit to do something for himself. The first time he sits by the bed an attempt should be made to involve him, however slightly, in the move. Thus the psychological content of the drills will come into play. If the recovery can only be partial, the gains the patient makes will still be valuable in lightening the load for whoever will eventually help him. The practical, home-oriented nature of the drills should be remembered when working with the patient.

The Basic Drills for Patients Using all Four Limbs

The basic drills, using four limbs, are suitable for frail patients with weakness rather than specific disability in individual limbs, or with evenly distributed bilateral problems. If any limb is markedly weaker than the rest, the patient should be taught the drill as modified for that condition (see Chapter 17). In all the movements the helper should remember the distant aim of independence as well as the more immediate one of moving the patient. This will lead naturally to giving physical help only when it is needed. As much of the patient's weight as possible should be transmitted to the ground through his own body or limbs. In the early stages the nurse may have to take most of it, but she should still put the patient through the prescribed movements. As his strength and understanding improve, her help should be progressively withdrawn. In the case of these basic drills, all four limbs should take their share of the weight.

Indications for Use of Drills Using all Four Limbs

(a) Weakness in limbs from long periods of immobility, however caused.
(b) Weakness due to specific diseases, e.g. Parkinson's Disease, rheumatoid arthritis, malnutrition, Paget's Disease, multiple sclerosis, etc.
(c) Stiffness or pain, e.g. rheumatoid arthritis, osteoarthritis, senile osteoporosis, early weight bearing after fracture, etc.
(d) Problems of balance, or history of falls.

(e) Impaired vision and other sensory loss if not associated with hemiplegia.

Preparation for Introducing the Drills to the Patient

Equipment. Check that all necessary equipment is at hand. Ensure that it is the correct height for the patient. Check safety features such as brakes, rubbers, and stability before use.

The Helper. Make sure you know the patient's medical status from his chart or a senior member of staff. Assess which drills are needed, and make sure you know them yourself. Be ready to adapt the drills to the patient's needs and ability to co-operate (see Chapter 17).

The Patient. Tell him what is going to happen, show him any equipment which will be used, demonstrate the moves, and re-assure him that he will not be asked to do the impossible. Once he knows what to expect it is still necessary to talk to him about what is about to happen. He must be involved in every move.

Introduction to Chair Drill

Its Importance

Great stress is placed on this drill, not only for the useful movements it incorporates, but also for its safety value. Careless moves in and out of chairs are a major cause of falls among the frail elderly who have not been well trained in this area. This drill should be started, with such help as is needed, the first time the patient gets out of bed, and continued throughout his retraining. It should be used every time he stands up or sits down. At best it will lead to full independence in mobility, and at worst it will minimise lifting problems in his care. The chair drill teaches the patient to:

(a) Rise from a seated position.
(b) Balance, leaning on the hands.
(c) Turn on the spot.
(d) Sit down safely, without a 'flop'.

These moves form the basis of the other drills. They are used in various combinations in the drills for bath, shower, bed, toilet, and car. These other drills come easily once chair drill has been mastered.

The Equipment

For successful chair drill the patient needs a seat of suitable height, whether it be a bed, a chair, a wheelchair, a commode, or a toilet seat. Suitable footwear should be insisted upon from the start. Leather soles are important, as rubbers tend to stick, and plastics to slip. Sloppy slippers, including the 'cosy' lambswool type, and stockinged feet (including bed socks), are particularly to be avoided. If the patient is to walk, his walking aid should be at hand. Most patients who use the basic chair drill will start their walking retraining using a walking frame. For more details about equipment see Chapter 18.

Basic Chair Drill — Job Breakdown

(a) Seat the patient comfortably in a suitable chair.
(b) Place a similar chair opposite, approximately 12 cm (5 inches) from his knees.
(c) Tell the patient he is going to stand up, turn right around, and sit down slowly in the other chair. Explain that you will give him the necessary directions one at a time, and ask him not to move until you ask him to.
(d) Giving help and support as needed, and time for each move to be completed safely, ask the patient to proceed as follows:
  1. Wriggle forward so that both feet are firmly on the ground.
  2. Place feet so that they are about 11 cm (4-5 inches) apart, with the heels in line with the front legs of the chair on which he is sitting.
  3. Place his hands forward in a comfortable position on the arms of his chair, keeping his elbows in to his sides.
  4. Lean forward, and look over his knees to see his toes.
  5. Still looking down, push forward with his hands and straighten his knees, so that his body weight is brought directly over his lower limbs as he rises. (The arms should not push him straight up, leaving the weight behind the lower limbs as this results in poor balance, and a fall back into the chair.)

6. Stand, feeling as tall as possible, and balance.
7. Place hands on the arms of the second chair, and lean on them. The palm of the hand should take the weight, and there should be no need to grip tightly.
8. Turn round whichever way feels most natural, letting go with the leading hand, and placing the other one in its place.
9. If necessary, use the arms of the original chair to support the leading hand during the turn, but keep the other hand on the chair in which the patient will sit.
10. Keep turning until facing squarely the original chair.
11. Reach back so that both hands are on the arm of the new chair.
12. Lean on the hands, with the head forward, and hips and knees slightly bent.
13. Lower down gently into the chair, bending hips and knees and watching the toes as in rising.
14. Move back in the chair if necessary, and relax.

Note 1. This movement should be done in the early stages as an exercise with patients who are not yet adept at it. Two or three good efforts have more value than a number of ones in which too much support is given. It should also be done routinely whenever the patient is moved.

Note 2. If the patient needs help he should be supported through the arc described in movement 5 above. He should not be lifted straight up from the seat and then put on his feet. Habit forming begins at this stage, and correct patterns should be applied, so that relearning will not be needed.

Note 3. If the patient is very heavy, very weak, or unpredictable, two people should help until he becomes more proficient, as would be necessary in lifting. It should be remembered that when the staff cannot manage, it will also be too much for the relatives and a hoist may be the best solution. This should not be decided before the patient has been given ample opportunity to learn the drill.

Introduction to Bed Drill

Its Importance

Bed drill teaches the patient not only to get in and out of bed safely, but also to move along a flat surface, as on a bathboard, a sofa, or a car seat, and to sit up from a lying position, as may be necessary after a fall. It is particularly useful for the patient who is to return home, either to live alone, or to be cared for by his family, as it obviates the need for lifting by an attendant or relative. Bed drill has three main divisions. These are:

(a) Moving in bed, including sitting up from a lying position.
(b) Moving along the side of the bed.
(c) Getting in and out of bed, including swinging up the legs.

All these moves have value as exercise as well as in actual bed-time use. As in chair drill, the principles involved are those of keeping the weight over the patient's own limbs, and pushing up rather than pulling up. The first principle eliminates heavy lifting, and the second leads to safety and greater freedom. The latter comes about because the patient is not restricted to places where rails, overhead rings, and other aids are provided.

Not the least important aspect of bed drill is that when combined with chair drill it makes it possible for patients to use a bedside commode independently. Night care is often a decisive factor in assessing whether a patient will be able to manage at home, and his ability to stay once he has gone there.

The Equipment

Geriatric patients, except when acutely ill, should sleep in a bed of ordinary domestic height. This bed drill has been designed for such beds. The height of the bed on which the patient is retrained should be the same as the one he will use at home, and both should be adjusted to a height he can use with safety. If for some reason a high bed must be used, a walking frame may help the patient get in and out, and a chair on which he can place his feet may help him to move up and down the side of the bed. These should only be a temporary measure until a suitable bed can be arranged. It cannot be stressed too strongly that high beds are both inefficient and dangerous for geriatric patients and for those who nurse them.

The patient should have his own walking aid available by his bed, and should wear suitable footwear. It is safer to have bare feet than bed socks, stockings or sloppy slippers. If the patient is not yet walking, the bed drill should be combined with chair drill using a wheelchair, a commode, or a bedside chair with arms. For details about equipment see Chapter 18.

Basic Bed Drill — Job Breakdown

(a) Sitting up in Bed from a Lying Position

This drill is indicated for patients who are unable to sit straight up from their pillows in bed because of weak muscles or obesity. It should not be used if the patient complains of pain in his back. In such cases, a pull up rope, tied to the end of the bed should be used.

1. While lying on the back, bend both knees, placing the feet flat on the bed.
2. Roll over to the side on which the patient usually gets out of bed, bringing the opposite arm forward across the body, as the bent knees come down onto the side of the bed. Shoulders and hips should turn together, so there is no twisting at the waist.
3. Place the hand which has come across the body on the side of the bed.
4. Place the arm which is under the body so that the elbow is as close to the body as possible, and the forearm runs away from it at a right angle over the edge of the bed.
5. Bring the shoulders forward over this elbow, and push up on it.
6. Using the top hand for support, push up off the elbow until the underneath hand can be placed flat on the bed and the elbow straightened.
7. Move back to a sitting position, with both hands behind the body for support.
8. Straighten the legs.

(b) Moving Back to the Pillows Method I (Figure 15.1)

The patient should sit up as described above. Both hands should be placed flat on the bed, about 10 cm (4 inches) behind the hips, and slightly wide of them.

1. Bend the knees, and place the feet flat on the bed.
2. Push up on the hands to lift the buttocks slightly clear of the bed.
3. At the same time, straighten the knees to push the body back so that it is seated between the hands.
4. Replace the hands 10 cm behind the hips as before, and lean on them.

5. Repeat the manoeuvre as often as necessary to achieve the required distance.

Note 1. The top of the body and the neck should be bent forward during this drill. If the patient sits upright or leans his head backwards, his whole body will tip back instead of his buttocks moving back between his hands. No ground will be gained this way.

Note 2. In the early stages it is easier for the patient to get well up on the pillows if they are removed, and put back in position after he has moved back.

(c) Moving Back to the Pillows Method II

Some patients find it easier to put their feet out of bed, and move along the side of the bed. If this is the chosen method, the bed clothes should not be tightly tucked in on the operative side. For this method the patient sits up as described above, up to, and including move 4, then proceeds as follows:

1. Put both feet over the side of the bed.
2. Lean forward to bring the shoulders over the supporting arm.

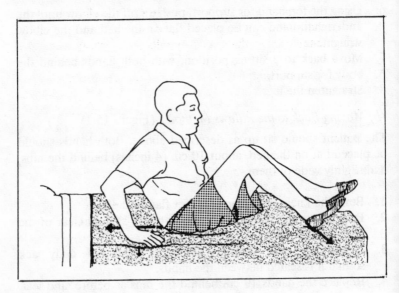

Figure 15.1: Moving Back in Bed: Method I

3. Push up on the supporting elbow, and then the wrist to sit squarely on the side of the bed.
4. Move along the bed in the required direction, using all four limbs.
5. Swing the feet back onto the bed.

This method is the method of choice if a patient is likely to need help from another person, as it eliminates the need to drag the patient across the bed, and depends upon positioning rather than lifting. If the bed is too high for his feet to touch the ground, a chair or a stool may be used and moved along beside the bed as he progresses.

(d) Turning Over in Bed

The patient who has difficulty in turning over in bed finds the nights long or uncomfortable. He is also gravely at risk, through the danger of pressure sores. Turning is very like the beginning of sitting up. The patient should proceed as follows:

1. Straighten himself as well as he can.
2. Bend both his knees to use as a weight to help him roll.
3. Reach forward with the arm which will be on top, bringing the shoulder over towards the direction in which he wants to roll.
4. Bring the knees down onto the bed, while reaching forward with the top arm, so that the body rolls over without twisting at the waist.
5. Place the top hand flat on the bed close to the underneath shoulder.
6. Push up with this hand, to take the weight off the shoulder.
7. Draw the underneath elbow back under the body.
8. Relax.

To turn back, the patient should:

1. Straighten the top leg, but leave the lower one bent.
2. Reach back with the top arm in the required direction.
3. Push simultaneously with the underneath limbs to roll his body onto its back.

Note 1. This movement can be practised best by the patient lying on his back with his knees bent, and rolling from side to side alternately. It is incorporated this way in the mat class drills.

Note 2. To give the patient confidence, and also to help if necessary, the person teaching this drill should stand on the side towards which the patient is turning. There is often fear of rolling right out, and occasionally the danger of it.

(e) Getting out of Bed

This movement is a combination of the other aspects of bed drill with the beginning of chair drill. The patient should be helped out of bed by this method from the beginning, instead of being lifted bodily. It is less frightening for the patient and less dangerous to the backs of those who lift. The patient should:

1. Roll towards the side from which he wishes to get out. (See paragraph (a) moves 1-4 inclusive.)
2. Put his feet over the edge of the bed.
3. Lean forward to bring the shoulders over the supporting arm.
4. Push up on the supporting elbow, and then the wrist, to sit squarely on the side of the bed.

Note 1. If the bed is the right height his feet should be placed firmly on the floor at this stage, making him confident and safe. If it is too high he will not be adequately supported, and may slip. If it is too low the next stage will present the same problems as rising from a low chair.

5. Place both hands on the edge of the bed with the palms flat on the bed, and slightly away from the body.
6. Place both feet back so that the heels are in line with the edge of the bed, and about 11 cm (4–5 inches) apart.
7. Lean forward and push up as in basic chair drill.

Note 2. If the patient is to get into a chair or wheelchair or use a commode, he completes the second half of chair drill. If he is going to walk, his walking aid should be appropriately placed before he rises.

(f) Getting into Bed

This is a modified form of chair drill. The patient who uses a pylon stick or walking cane should walk up facing the bed at the level at which he wants to sit. He should 'park' his stick safely, and transferring his hands to the bed, should do a complete turn and sit down as in the second half of chair drill. If he uses a walking frame, he should back up to the bed until he can feel it with the back of his legs, and then placing his hands back on the bed, let himself down slowly to a sitting position. Finally, if he is returning from a chair, wheelchair, or commode, he should be seated facing the bed, and proceed as with basic chair drill. The basic difference is that, the bed having no arms, he must lean directly on the bed. If a patient is having trouble in holding too tightly to the arm of a chair, it is helpful to practise bed drill first to encourage leaning instead of gripping.

When the patient has completed the 'chair drill' part of the movement, he should check to see that he is seated as far back as possible, and at a place where his head will come down onto the pillows when he lies down. The place varies with the height of the patient and the number of pillows he uses, and so must be decided individually for each patient. If the patient still needs practice in moving along the side of the bed, it is helpful to ask him to sit too close to the foot of the bed deliberately, and to move up before swinging in his legs. When he is seated well back, and in the right position, the patient should:

1. Rock himself over sideways, taking his head down onto the pillows, and raising his feet to the level of the bed with the same movement.
2. Bend his knees to bring his feet onto the bed. Some patients find it easier to bring up one leg at a time, and some prefer to cross the feet and bring up both together. The best way is the one which proves easier to each individual.
3. Roll over onto his back, or take up whatever position is needed.

Note 1. All that has been said about low beds applies here too. If it is too high the patient will not be able to sit back far enough, and will finish the movement too close to the edge. He will also be in danger of slipping as he tries to swing up his legs. In some cases he will be unable to manage at all, and will have to be lifted, thus endangering the backs of his helpers.

Note 2. It is essential to the principles and practice of the Newcastle Method that bed drill be understood and used by the night staff. If the patient is trained during the day only, he will not as a rule associate that training with the real situation in the ward. Just as he receives help from the night staff, so he will expect and need it from his family. Night calls and heavy lifting are two of the common causes of a breakdown in family care.

Introduction to Commode Drill

Its Importance

Commode drill is an aid in managing nocturnal toilet problems which are distressing to the patient and to his relatives. If the patient is not independent in this area the relative must cope with either a wet bed or a disturbed night. Both can lead to friction and distress. In the Newcastle Method all female patients are taught to use bedside commodes at night, and male patients are taught to use a urinal and empty it into a bucket. If it is still needed, the domiciliary care service will provide similar equipment when the patient goes home.

It is necessary for commode drill to be taught by the night staff, and reported by them on the final assessment form, because many a patient who is quite capable of performing the moves in daylight and when fully awake, is quite unsafe in the different conditions which occur at night.

The Equipment

The equipment is a commode with arms for the women, and a urinal and plastic bucket for the men. The commode must sometimes be built up, as the commercial products are lower than an ordinary chair, and many elderly people find it difficult to rise from them. The commode should be placed opposite the bed, not beside it, on the side the patient uses for getting in and out. The patient should be taught not to get out on to a slippery floor in bed socks. Bare feet or leather soled slippers are both safer.

Commode Drill — Job Breakdown

(a) Sit on the side of the bed, using the method described above under 'Getting out of Bed' (e), moves 1–4.
(b) Stand up as described in paragraph (e), moves 5–7.
(c) Place the hands on the arms of the commode and lean on them for balance.

(d) Complete the second part of chair drill to sit down (paragraph (d), moves 7–14)

Note 1. The return to bed is a basic chair drill, except that his opened hand should be placed flat on the bed instead of on the arms of the chair.

(e) Complete beginning of chair drill (paragraph (d), moves 1–6).
(f) Place palm of hand furthest from the pillows on the bed, and lean on it for balance.
(g) Turn towards the pillows, moving the supporting hand to a position 30 cm (1 foot) closer to the pillows.
(h) Complete the turn and put the second hand back on the bed.
(i) Lower the body, resisting gravity so as not to 'flop', and sit on the side of the bed.
(j) Complete bed drill (*Getting into Bed*, paragraph (f)).

Note 2. Commode drill needs to be well practised, and to become automatic, because people in a hurry tend to forget safety precautions. The urgency to which elderly people are prone tends to have this effect when the commode is needed.

Note 3. When the chair drill itself is established, practice should be given in managing the clothes.

Introduction to Bath Drill

Importance of Bath Drill

There is often a certain amount of fear of falling in the bathroom among the frail elderly. There is also nervousness about managing this area on the part of their relatives. Many have already had frightening experiences with difficulties in getting out of the bath, and have already decided that it is safer to wash at the basin. Those who have no such problems can certainly continue to use their own method, but for the majority of patients who present for retraining a safer method is needed. The simple bathboard has proved its worth in the Newcastle Method for the following reasons:

1. The patient completes the drill on one plane, avoiding the need to raise or lower his body.
2. The basic moves of the other drills are all that is needed to

complete bath drill. This means less extra learning time.

3. The standard bathboard can be adjusted for most traditional baths. Unfortunately some 'modern' designs are creating problems, but other equipment has been developed to solve these (see Chapter 19).
4. The lifting of the patient is eliminated to the advantage of patient, nurse and relative.
5. Tension is reduced, and bathing is no longer seen as a hazard. This helps to solve the problem of reluctance to bathe which can be the result of fear.
6. As with all the Newcastle equipment, the bathboard is simple and standardised, so that it is possible for it to be used in the domiciliary care service.

The social worker's report is important, as it is a waste of time to train a patient for a situation which does not exist. If the home has a shower recess only, or a bathroom which is inaccessible to the patient, that patient should be taught a method suited to his own needs. 'Shower Drill' is described here, but the problem of the inaccessible bathroom must be worked out on an individual basis (see Chapter 19).

The Equipment

In considering the equipment necessary, the existing equipment in the home is the basis from which we must work. The traditional bath, mounted so that its rim is approximately 48 cm (19 inches) from the ground is ideal. Baths which differ markedly from these will probably need adjusted boards. Other equipment besides the bath itself may include:

1. The bathboard, adjusted to fit the individual bath. A firm fit is essential for safety and confidence.
2. A chair beside the bath, equal to the height of the top of the bathboard when in position.
3. A hand shower attached to the taps, if not already installed as a shower.
4. If a hand shower is not available, a dipper or two-pint jug.
5. If water is not laid on, a second board in front of where the patient sits, to hold a wash basin.
6. A towel over the seat and back of the chair.
7. A suction cup rubber mat in the bottom of the bath, or on the

floor in front of the chair if the patient is inclined to slip.

8. All the patient's usual toilet needs.

9. In the Newcastle Method, rails are not generally needed, and should only be provided in exceptional cases. They tend to encourage patients to revert to dangerous methods relying on the grip of a soapy hand.

10. A hand grip on the wall near the bath may be useful for a frail patient with poor balance to stand safely for the washing and drying of the sacral area.

Bath Drill — Job Breakdown

Preparation

1. Assemble equipment as needed.

2. Place the chair beside the bath so that the patient's stronger limbs are nearest the bath. It should be well back so that there is plenty of room to put his legs in without bending his knees.

3. Place the bathboard in the bath so that the front is about 7 cm (3 inches) ahead of the front of the chair.

4. Run water into the bath and test the temperature before helping the patient onto the board. If a hand shower is to be used, remember to test the temperature away from the patient before applying it. Bring these precautions to the patient's notice, and let him test it himself as soon as he is able, to build a habit for when he goes home.

Job Breakdown

1. Seat the patient on the chair to undress, using the appropriate chair drill.

2. When undressed ask the patient to place one hand on the bathboard, and one on the chair, lean forward, and stand as in chair drill.

3. Ask him to turn away from the bath so that his back is towards the angle made by the bath and the chair.

4. Ask him to sit down well back on the bathboard.

5. The foot nearer the bath is raised and placed in the bath.

6. The outside foot is raised and put in the bath. It may be necessary for the patient to move along the bathboard a few inches (using the bedside movement, page 214) before putting the second leg into the bath.

7. Using the same movement the patient should move into the middle of the board.
8. Make sure that the patient's feet are firmly placed to give him balance. They should be slightly forward, and about 15 cm (6 inches) apart.
9. The patient should be washed by whatever method has been decided upon, and given time to do as much of the washing as he can for himself.
10. Patients should wriggle forward in order to wash the genital region. In some cases it is better for the patient to stand in a walking frame or holding a hand grip for this procedure. The use of a bathboard can sometimes lead to carelessness in this matter, and the problem should not be ignored.
11. When washing is complete the patient should move back to the outer end of the board.
12. Ask him to place one foot out of the bath.
13. Ask him to move a little further towards the chair.
14. Ask him to place the second foot outside the bath, and wriggle forward until both feet are on the ground.
15. Ask him to move over until he is sitting safely on the chair.
16. Dry the patient, or let him dry himself, while seated, and help him to dress as needed.
17. Ask him to rise from his chair and return to his walking aid or wheelchair, using the routine chair drill.

Note 1. Precautions — because of the real and imagined dangers of the bathroom it is necessary that the helper should be very aware of the need for sensible precautions, and should let the patient know that she is so. Soapy water on the floor, the patient's own balance, the heat of the water, should all be matters of concern. Until a patient is well and independent he should not be left alone in the bathroom.

Note 2. Stiff and painful hips — many patients with stiff and painful hips need the drills outlined in this section, but find putting their legs up and over the rim of the bath to be a difficult move. (See Bath Drill in Chapter 17 for help in this situation.)

Introduction to Shower Drill

Its Importance

Shower drill is necessary for those patients, who through preference, or the facilities provided at home, are unable to use a bath. The older fixed showers can cause problems if the angle is unsuitable, but with the modern hose type showers there is little to choose between the bath and the shower for retraining purposes. The one which suits the individual patient should be chosen. The main advantage of the shower is that it is very direct, and easy to understand. It is merely a routine chair drill combined with a wash. Its disadvantages are that the helper often gets very wet if the taps are badly placed, and that other architectural features can cause trouble. Amongst these are hobs placed in front of the recess to stop the water from flowing out. They also can stop a disabled person from walking in. The danger of slipping on a wet soapy floor is increased, and so patients with poor balance are usually safer with bath drill.

The Equipment

The equipment for shower drill is simple, but its arrangement is important. It includes:

1. The shower itself. If possible a hose type shower should be placed so that it can be reached by the patient from a seated position. When used from a fixed position, the water should come down just in front of the patient's head when he is seated in the shower chair.

2. The taps. These should be where the patient can reach them from his chair, and the helper can turn them on and off from outside the recess without having to stand under the flow of water.

3. A hand grip should be placed so that the patient can stand safely and support himself for washing and drying of the sacral region.

4. A shower chair. This should be a sturdy chair which will not be affected by constant wetting. Glued wooden chairs and metal chairs likely to rust are not suitable. Plastic has been found satisfactory. The chair should be placed facing the entrance, and close enough for the patient to reach the taps. He should also be well positioned for the spray if the shower is of a fixed variety.

5. The usual toilet requirements of the individual patient.

Shower Drill — Job Breakdown

Preparation

Collect and place all equipment as above. Bring the patient to the recess, and, using routine chair drill, sit him on a chair just outside it to undress. If he is in a wheelchair he may undress whilst seated in this.

Job Breakdown

1. Whether walking or in a wheelchair, approach the shower chair as for routine chair drill.
2. Transfer to the shower chair, using routine chair drill.
3. Wash the patient, letting him do as much for himself as possible.
4. Using chair drill, ask the patient to stand and hold the hand grip for washing and drying of sacral area.
5. If no hand grip is provided, the patient's walking aid, or the arms of the well-braked wheelchair may be used for support in this process.
6. Place the dry chair, or the wheelchair so that the patient can sit down to complete drying and dressing procedures.

Note 1. Dangers and difficulties — the shower is not only a place where falls are likely to happen, but because of the confined space the patient is more likely to hit his head, or fall in an awkward way. For these reasons it is essential that the helper should be alert and ready to help while the patient is at risk. The other dangers and difficulties, outlined above, should receive attention if there is any possibility of making them safer and easier to use.

Note 2. Method must be appropriate at home. However much the helper feels that it would be easier to use one method than another in the hospital, it must be remembered that the shower is part of retraining, and not merely a way of keeping clean. If the method used is unsuitable for the patient's home, it is a waste of time.

Introduction to Car Drill

One of the main pleasures enjoyed by many otherwise house-bound people is a drive with relatives. Others can go shopping, so long as someone will pick them up and bring them home. Getting the patient in and out of the car, however, is often a problem if the would-be driver does not know the easy way to manage it. Many have hurt their own backs by opening the driver's door, and attempting to pull the patient into the car from there. If the correct combination of routine drill movements is used, this is quite unnecessary.

Car Drill — Job Breakdown

Preparation

1. Decide which door the patient is to use. Unless there is a good reason against it, the front seat is usually the easiest and best.
2. Open the door as widely as possible.
3. Let the patient come as close to the car seat as he can using his walking aid or wheelchair if necessary.
4. Ask him to complete his usual chair drill to sit sideways on the car seat.
5. Ask him to move as far back as he can as in bed drill.
6. If he finds this difficult, ask him to place his hands behind him on the seat to keep himself sitting upright.
7. Someone in the back of the car can help by placing a hand behind the shoulders to keep them forward if this is a problem.
8. Ask the patient to bend his legs and place his feet against your legs just above the knee.
9. Working together, with a sentence such as 'Ready, set, push!' ask the patient to push against your legs as you push forward against his feet. This should move his seat backwards towards the driver's seat, with very little effort, and no risk.
10. Ask the patient to swing his feet down to the floor, and straighten himself on the seat.
11. Adjust seat belt.

Job Breakdown to Get Out

1. Ask the patient to move as close to the door as he can, using bed drill method.
2. Open the door and remove seat belt.
3. Ask the patient to swing his legs out the door, turning so that he faces outwards.
4. Stand using routine chair drill, and return to his wheelchair or walking aid.

Getting Down to the Floor and Up Again

Because falls are a relatively common problem in the elderly, it is desirable that all patients should be taught a suitable method of rising from the floor with as much independence as possible. If some help is needed, the patient's relative should be instructed before the patient goes home.

The training begins with a method for descending to the floor. The greater the part the patient plays in this movement, the greater will be his confidence. The patient should learn to relax on the floor and to check to see whether he has been hurt before trying to rise from a fall.

To Go Down to the Floor

1. Face a chair or other item of similar height (bed, sofa).
2. Bend the knees until kneeling on the floor in a 'praying' position against the chair.
3. Put one hand on the floor.
4. Come slowly to a sitting position on the floor.
5. Lie on the floor and relax.

To Rise Again

1. Sit up using the method employed to sit up in bed.
2. Move to a chair by the patient's method for moving back in bed.
3. Place hands on the seat of the chair and come to a kneeling position.
4. Bend the hip and knee of the stronger leg, placing the foot firmly on the ground.
5. Stand, pushing up firmly with the arms as well as the lower limbs.
6. Straighten up, turn and sit in the chair.

Summary

In this chapter the basic retraining drills for patients who can use all four limbs, albeit weakly, have been described in detail. The basic movements which must be learnt first by the helper are as follows.

Chair Drill (page 209)

1. Stand up.
2. Turn.
3. Sit down.

Bed Drill (page 211)

1. Move along the side of the bed.
2. Put feet in and out of bed.
3. Roll over.
4. Sit up supported on own limbs.

Once these moves have been mastered, all the other drills are simplified, as they are merely made up of these moves in different combinations.

16 ROUTINE WALKING PRACTICE

Retraining in walking, with discussion of the techniques, teaching methods and equipment involved and some methods for negotiating steps.

Introduction

Walking problems are common in the elderly, with causes ranging from a neglected corn to the gross deformities of long-standing destructive disease. The more dramatic walking problems produced by a fracture, an amputation or a stroke, will probably receive attention at an early stage. The more insidious problems related to arthritis, Parkinson's Disease, vertigo or the aforementioned corn may not. Awareness of each patient's walking ability is a necessary part of retraining, whatever the degree of disability or the pathology involved. The use of routine retraining methods applies to walking as much as it does to the drills already described. As with those other retraining movements, elderly folk learn by repetition and by linking their lessons with everyday needs.

The Developmental Sequence

Without labouring the point too much, routine retraining in walking resembles the way we all learnt to walk in infancy. This involves progress from movement in bed as in bed drill, through standing with support at the wall bar, practice in weight bearing and balancing at the bar, and walking with a helper and a walking aid, to going unaided if and when this can be accomplished with safety.

Strengthening

This is the equivalent of the baby's kicking and moving in his cot. It is provided through bed drill which is introduced from the beginning of retraining, and prepares the patient for weight bearing in his chair drill and at the wall bar. More specific exercises of this kind may be provided in a 'Mat Class' under the direction of the physiotherapist. Patients with Parkinson's Disease and some stroke patients find this particularly helpful.

An exercise which is not recommended, and which can lead to difficulties in rising from a chair, is quadriceps training while the patient remains seated. This includes the use of springs and pulleys, and at a more general level, the kicking of balls and the playing of floor games with the feet. These activities may strengthen the quadriceps, but they also teach the patient to anchor his body and kick his leg forward when his need is to anchor his foot and raise his body. Those patients whose feet slide forward when they go to rise, and who complain that the floor is slippery, have usually developed this habit as a result of seated exercises for the quadriceps.

Note The quadriceps receive strengthening in standing at the wall bar and in the movements involved in chair drill. These movements link in a practical way with those needed in real situations.

Weight Bearing

This is the retraining equivalent of the baby pulling up on the side of his cot or a piece of furniture and trying out his legs. Safe and confident weight bearing is an essential preliminary to walking. It is encouraged in chair drill when the patient pushes up on his chair to stand, and more specifically when he rises and sits at the wall bar. Standing exercises at the wall bar have been adapted from Dr Marjorie Warren's *Bed End Exercises*. They have been varied by placing the hand bar near a window so that the patient can look out at something interesting when he stands, and by pushing up with the legs rather than pulling up with his hands.

The patient's capacity for weight bearing will dictate the type of walking aid he will need. As a general rule it is necessary to have some such capacity in both lower limbs in order to use a pylon or walking cane. A walking frame can be used with only one leg able to bear weight. The walking frame demands two weight bearing upper limbs, but the pylon and cane need only one. A flaccid limb such as is common in early hemiplegia, may need to be supported by a back slab or caliper until some tone returns, or until it is decided that a permanent caliper will be required. The back slab should be applied only when the patient is to walk, and should be removed while he is sitting down.

Pain on weight bearing should never be taken lightly. If the cause has not been investigated, this should be done before further attempts at weight bearing are made. If the cause is known and weight bearing must proceed despite discomfort, understanding and encouragement are essential. If after appropriate investigations it appears that the patient is exaggerating his pain, this should still be seen as a psychological need, and not as 'difficult' behaviour (see Chapter 13).

Balancing

Learning to balance follows the baby's attempts to stand without support. Retraining has its equivalent but not to the point of sitting down suddenly as the baby does. Balancing is a component of routine chair drill. It is practised every time the patient transfers his hand from the original chair to another chair or to his walking aid. In some cases this routine practice in balancing needs to be reinforced by more deliberate efforts. These include:

1. Practice at the wall bar. The patient stands in the approved way, and is encouraged to remove his hands from the bar and to stand unsupported, bearing weight through both limbs if possible.
2. Practice with his walking aid. The patient stands up, leaning on his walking aid with such support from his helper as is necessary. His limbs are positioned to give him balance, and the support is slowly withdrawn.

Note 1. In these balancing sessions the patient should be allowed to feel the results of standing incorrectly. He will not learn if the helper takes his weight the moment he goes 'off centre'. She should explain to him that she will let him go down as far as can be done with safety, but that she will help before he reaches the point of no return. Reassurance that you are still there is necessary, but given this, few patients find this procedure particularly threatening. A second helper should be asked to help if the patient is too heavy for one, or if it is not possible to predict the side to which he will fall.

Note 2. The patient who needs the support of a helper should always be walked in such a way that his posture is suitable for walking alone. Habit forming is basic to learning a walking pattern, and once learnt, any habit is difficult to eradicate. For instance, a patient who has been supported in the early stages by a helper placing a hand on his back will learn to trust that hand and lean against it. When the time comes to walk alone he will still tend to lean backwards, even to the point of falling. Learning to balance using his walking aid for support should begin the very first time he tries to walk, and he should be reminded to do so whenever he starts to lean on his helper instead. Safe independent walking at a later stage depends upon achieving balance in the early stages.

Walking with Support

This is the equivalent of walking around the cot holding the rail, or walking by holding mother's hand. The walking aid represents the cot rail, while the helper takes the place of 'mum'. The patient must learn to rely on his own strength, and until he can do so the walking aid should be his primary support. The helper should be there to encourage, to instruct, and to protect him from danger. She should not be there as his major support or a leaning post.

Important skills are involved in assessing the amount of help actually needed, and in withdrawing that help progressively as the patient improves. The over-protective 'mum' can lead the learner to dependence rather than independence, however kindly she gives her help.

Going Alone

This means independent mobility for both the baby and the patient. In the patient's case the continued use of an aid such as a walking frame, a pylon or a cane may be needed, but the patient will not need the presence of another person. The helper who has withdrawn support progressively as described in the previous paragraph will, in most cases, bring the patient to a point where physical help is no longer needed. The patient who reaches this point should still receive supervision until his safety is beyond doubt. The helper should no longer touch the patient, but should walk beside him or behind him in such a position that help is possible if it is needed. She should watch the patient's feet as he progresses, so that the signs of a fall can be recognised. In this way she can be aware of trouble and give help in time to prevent the fall.

During this stage of supervision the patient's path should not be cleared of hazards, but he should be encouraged to note them and take appropriate action. There will be many hazards in the outside world, and the patient should be prepared to meet them.

Routine Method for Using a Walking Frame (Figures 16.1A and 16.2)

The walking frame is used in the early stages of ambulation to give the patient confidence and to prepare him for progression to a pylon or walking cane. If the patient needs more support than is given by these one-handed aids he will probably continue to use a walking frame after discharge. The patient who uses a walking frame must be able to bear weight through both arms. For this reason it is unsuitable for most hemiplegic patients. Its value is mainly in helping those with problems of weight bearing or poor balance. For elderly patients a walking frame is preferred to crutches because it has been found to be safer, and to give more confidence. It does not slip on wet floors, nor does it fall to the floor when not in use, and it will not put the patient at risk of nerve damage through pressure in the axilla. It is also more practical in the home, as a tray can be fitted to allow articles to be carried while the hands are in use.

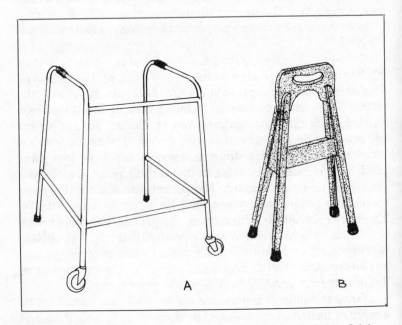

A   B

Figure 16.1: A. Walking Frame (standard pattern); B. Pylon Stick (standard pattern)

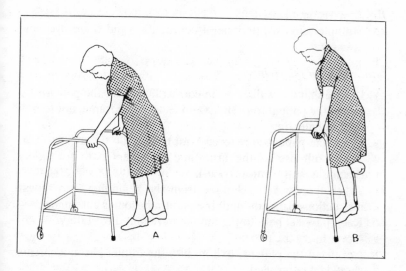

Figure 16.2: A. Patient with Balance Problem Leans down on Walking Frame; B. Patient with Weight-bearing Problem Pushes up on Walking Frame

Indications for Use — Weight-bearing Problems

1. Non-weight-bearing fractures.
2. Partially weight-bearing fractures, and those who are afraid of falling again with a pylon or cane.
3. Pain in either or both lower limbs.
4. Osteoarthritis of hips or knees.
5. Rheumatoid arthritis.
6. Poor circulation in the lower limbs.
7. Ulcers and vascular disease of the lower limbs.
8. Single amputation, with or without a prosthesis.
9. Double amputation with a prosthesis.
10. Paraplegia (usually with calipers).

Indications for Use — Balance Problems

1. Impaired balance mechanism.
2. Ataxic gait.
3. General frailty.
4. Dizzy spells.
5. Parkinson's Disease (selected cases).
6. Bilateral hemiparesis.

7. Poor vision.
8. Multiple sclerosis, peripheral neuropathy, and other disabling diseases.

Guidelines for the Helper

1. Ensure that the walker is the correct height for the patient.
2. Teach the patient to push up and lean on the frame, not to pull up and hang on.
3. Teach the patient to relax and not to grip too tightly.
4. Teach full use of the arms and shoulders both for safety (balance), and comfort (pain).
5. Teach the correct technique from the beginning, and repeat instructions patiently until the pattern becomes automatic.
6. Keep physical help to the minimum required for safety.
7. Never hurry the patient.
8. Never tell the patient to 'hop' into the frame. His movements should be controlled.
9. Help the patient to accept and be pleased with the walker, and do not encourage him to look forward to a more advanced aid until it is certain that he has the capacity to use one.
10. Be sure that the pattern will not involve relearning if the patient graduates to a pylon or crutches.

Uses for Walking Frames Besides Ambulation

1. To help the patient stand and balance for toilet attention, washing and drying, pulling up pants, etc.
2. To help a chair-bound patient stand and take his weight off his buttocks with minimal lifting.
3. To help patients get in and out of high beds.
4. To help bed to chair transfers with minimal lifting.
5. To help a patient balance while adjusting a prosthesis.
6. To act as a trolley in the kitchen and to help with housework (a tray is attached for this purpose).
7. To dry clothes by the fire in winter (there is no need to teach this).

Some Adaptations and Attachments to Basic Frames

Many adaptations and attachments have been designed for the standard walking frame, and others will no doubt be developed in response to individual needs. Some that have already been used are:

1. A tray for domestic use.
2. Various bags and panniers to carry personal belongings.
3. Single or double elbow rests for use when one arm or both arms are unable to take enough weight.
4. Glides instead of rubbers on the back legs when the back cannot be lifted.
5. A 'pistol grip' for use with weak wrists. (Partial return of function in a hemiplegic arm.)
6. Built up sides for specially tall patients.
7. A single side built up for hemiplegic patients to maintain the lean they will need to use a pylon.
8. A knee restrainer for patients who tend to fall backwards. (Some patients with Parkinson's Disease.)
9. A foot plate for paraplegics to help them lock the knees of their calipers.
10. 'Skis' for use on sand drifts and the beach.

Some of the more commonly used adaptations are illustrated in Chapter 19.

Choice of the Correct Size

It is very important that the size of the walker should suit the patient. When he is standing as straight as he can, his hands should rest on the arms of the walker while his elbows are slightly bent. Generally speaking, those with balance problems should lean down slightly, and those with weight-bearing problems should push up. If there is only a choice between too high and too low, choose the low one for balance and the high one for weight bearing. If the discrepancy is too great, an adaptation may be necessary. The width (27 inches or 69 cm) fits through standard domestic doors, but occasionally a particularly narrow door is found. In this case the walker may be altered. In small homes problems may be encountered with cluttered furniture or difficulty of access to certain rooms. If possible, any necessary adjustments should be made in the home before the patient's return. Strategic hand grips may be required in narrow places, and sometimes two walkers may solve the problem — one can be used each side of the bottleneck.

Method of Use for Non-weight Bearing

The following directions should be given to the patient, who completes each stage before proceeding to the next.

1. Stand on your strong leg with your foot just behind the back legs of the walker.
2. Lean on your hands.
3. Push up from the shoulders to lift your whole body, swinging your strong leg forward.
4. Let your body down gently onto your strong leg.
5. Bring your body over the strong leg and make sure you are safely balanced.
6. Lift the back of the walker and wheel it forward rather like a wheelbarrow.
7. Put it down and lean on your hands.
8. Continue repeating steps 3 to 7 as often as necessary.

Note 1. It sometimes helps to repeat the following words as the patient moves:—   Pick it up, put it forward.

                            Lean on it, up and over.

                            Land gently, balance.

Note 2. Many elderly patients find it hard to understand how to take their weight on their hands. Sometimes they will see what is required if told to 'swing through like Tarzan'. In other cases a preliminary drill is helpful. This is described below.

Method of Use for Control of Pain in Weight Bearing

By using this method the patient can take as much or as little weight on the painful limb as he can tolerate. The painful limb is moved first and placed in line with the hands so that it can be supported by them to a greater or lesser degree as the condition demands. The patient should be instructed as follows:

1. Stand with your feet just behind the back legs of the walker.
2. Place your hands on the walker just in front of its back legs.
3. Lean on your hands.
4. Place your weak foot forward and ground it under the line between your hands.
5. Push up on your hands, taking as much weight as necessary while you lift your strong foot forward.
6. Ground your strong foot just ahead of the toes in your weak foot.
7. Bring your weight forward until you are standing firmly on your strong foot.

8. Lift the back of the walker and wheel it forward rather like a wheelbarrow.
9. Put it down and lean on your hands.
10. Repeat steps 4 to 9 as often as necessary.

Note 1. It sometimes helps to repeat the following words as the patient moves: Pick it up, push it forward.

                                   Put it down and lean on it.

                                   Weak leg between your hands.

                                   Up and over with strong leg.

Note 2. Small steps are usually less painful than large ones. They should be permitted, but care should be taken that both steps are of the same size and equally spaced. In this way a limping habit is not developed, and larger steps can be taken as pain is resolved and confidence returns.

Method of Use for a Balance Problem

Because he walks on two feet man has greater problems of balance than the four-footed creatures when afflicted by injury or disease. He can, however, compensate by the use of sticks or other walking aids which bring his 'forefeet' into play. The walking frame is such an aid. The patient balances himself by using the back legs of the walker as extensions of his arms.

The back legs have rubbers attached to them to act as stoppers or brakes while the patient moves himself, but they are raised so the walker can be moved forward on its front wheels while the patient stands steady. This easy flowing movement is not possible if the patient stands too far forward with his hands in the centre or at the front of the frame. For this reason the patient should start by standing just behind an imaginary line between the two rubbers on the feet of the frame, and should place his hands on the padded grips towards the back of the frame.

He should be instructed as follows:

1. Hold the walker lightly without gripping too hard.
2. Raise the back about $\frac{3}{4}$ to $\frac{1}{2}$ an inch (2 cm) from the ground.
3. Push it forward on its wheels, like a wheelbarrow. Approximately 9 inches (23 cm) is enough.
4. Ground the feet of the walker, and lean on the frame.
5. Take two steps into the frame, still balancing yourself with your hands. The second foot should be placed just ahead of

the first one but about 6 inches (15 cm) wide of it.
6. Transfer your weight to your front foot, and stand steadily.
7. Repeat steps 1 to 6 as often as necessary.

Note 1. This process should be repeated until a rhythmical movement is developed. It sometimes helps to repeat the following words as the patient moves: Pick it up, push it forward.
                                                                                          Put it down and lean on it.
                                                                                          Left foot.
                                                                                          Right foot.

Note 2. The steps taken by the patient should not be too large. The first should ground the foot in line with the hands, and the next should bring the heel of the second foot very slightly ahead of the toe of the first foot. If both lower limbs are of equal strength it is best to teach the patient to move off with the left foot every time so that all staff members will give the same directions. If one lower limb is painful or weaker than the other the weak or painful limb should move first so as to gain support from the hands.

Preliminary Drill for One-legged Use of the Walking Frame

Paraplegic patients or amputees, or those who are non-weight bearing in one lower limb, must learn to take all their weight on their hands. Many old people find it hard to understand this, or are too weak in their upper limbs to achieve it. Obesity can also make it difficult. The following drill has proved helpful. The lesson should proceed as follows:

1. The patient stands in the walker with his hands on the hand grips and one helper on either side. The helpers' arms are placed between the patient's arm and his body.
2. The patient is asked to push up with his hands, and at the same time the helpers lift gently, so that the three are working together as a team.
3. When the patient has pushed up as high as he can he is asked to try and stay there as the helpers slowly withdraw their support.
4. After this has been done two or three times the patient usually begins to understand how to support his own weight. He learns more easily by resisting gravity in coming down than by trying, without success, to lift himself up. As his arms strengthen with

practice and his confidence improves, the upward movement will usually be mastered.

Some Unhelpful Patterns

It is better to give adequate training in the early stages and to encourage a correct movement than to let the patient progress any way he can at the expense of learning bad walking habits. 'Hopping' should be firmly discouraged because it is strenuous, dangerous, and a poor preparation for good walking patterns when the patient's strength returns.

At this stage if it is necessary to move in a hurry it is better to use a wheelchair than to build up a bad walking pattern which must later be overcome. The most common of these unhelpful patterns is to push the frame forward with its back legs grounded and to ignore the purpose of the rubbers and the wheels. The patient can progress quite easily in this fashion on smooth hospital floors, but it is quite unsuitable for his home where there are likely to be carpets, mats, small steps, and garden paths of varied texture. If a patient cannot understand the importance of lifting the back of the walker he should be taken for a walk on a lawn or other rough surface. A small mat kept in the retraining area and placed in front of the walker may also provide a good object lesson.

Routine Method for Using a Pylon Stick (Figure 16.1B)

The pylon stick is the wooden version of the quadripod, and is preferred to it for elderly patients because of its greater stability. It gives more support than a simple cane but is less cumbersome than the walking frame. The minimal physical requirement for its use is one reasonably strong hand and full weight bearing in the lower limbs, with or without a caliper.

Indications for Use as Retraining Equipment

1. Hemiplegia.
2. General frailty with a mild balance problem.
3. Elderly patients with a single lower limb amputation and a prosthesis.
4. Elderly patients with full weight bearing after a lower limb fracture.

Indications for Use as a Permanent Walking Aid

1. Hemiplegia.
2. Elderly or infirm patients who need more support than is provided by a walking cane.

Guidelines for the Helper (see Figure 16.3)

1. Ensure that the pylon is the correct height.
2. Stand on the patient's weak side.
3. Teach the patient to bend slightly to the strong side and lean on his pylon. He should not push up and away from it.
4. Encourage him to relax and not to grip the pylon too tightly.
5. Teach him to see that all four legs of the pylon are on the ground before he takes a step himself.
6. Teach the correct movements from the beginning, repeating instructions patiently until the pattern becomes automatic.
7. Hold the patient as lightly as possible consistent with safety.
8. Never hurry the patient.
9. Help the patient to be pleased with the pylon and do not encourage thoughts of a cane until sure that he has the capacity to use one.

Adaptations and Attachments to Pylons

1. A tray for carrying belongings.
2. A handbag or 'panniers' for personal belongings.
3. Padding on the handle if the patient complains of discomfort.
4. A specially designed handle if the patient cannot learn not to turn the front of the pylon inwards in front of his foot.
5. A wooden platform under the feet of the pylon for use on sand.

Choice of the Correct Size

For safety and ease of learning, the size of the pylon must suit the individual patient. When he stands on his stronger leg with his other limb relaxed he should be able to lean comfortably on the pylon in a relaxed attitude. If choice is limited it is better to use a pylon which is slightly too low rather than one that is slightly too high. The shorter pylon can be exchanged for a slightly taller one once the patient has achieved good balance.

The Basic Method for Using a Pylon (Figure 16.4)

1. Start with the patient seated in his chair. Place the pylon ahead

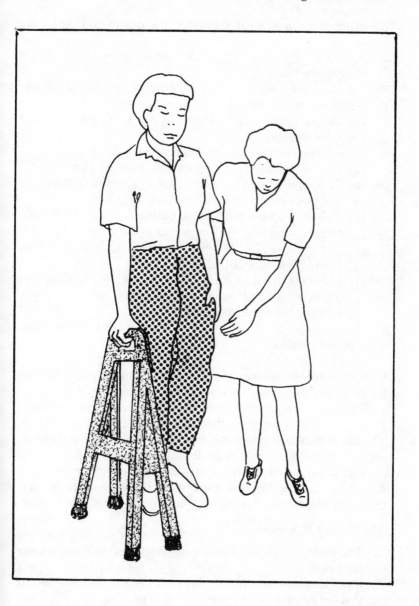

Figure 16.3: Use of Pylon Stick. Encouragement of the patient to move his weak lower limb

of the chair and to the side on which it is to be held by the patient.

2. Stand on the patient's other side, usually the weak one, ready to help as needed.

3. Ask the patient to move forward on his chair so that his feet are firmly on the ground.

4. Ask the patient to perform the rising part of his chair drill and check his balance.

5. Give the patient step by step directions as follows:
    (a) Place your hand lightly on the pylon and lean on it.
    (b) Step forward with the foot which is further from the pylon and place it opposite the handle of the pylon.
    (c) Balance yourself between the outside foot and the pylon.
    (d) Step forward with the foot nearer to the pylon and place it so that the heel is just ahead of the toe of the outside foot.
    (e) Check your balance and stand steadily.
    (f) Move the pylon forward so that the back feet of the pylon are in line with the toe of the inside foot.
    (g) Lean on the pylon to ensure balance.

6. Repeat steps (b) to (g) as often as necessary to achieve the required distance.

Note 1. Many patients find it helpful to repeat the following words as they progress: Pylon, lean on it, left, right

or

Pylon, lean on it, right left.

The first pattern being correct if the pylon is held in the right hand, and the second if it is held in the left.

Note 2. If one side is stronger than the other the pylon should be held in the hand on the strong side. If there is little difference it is usually more practical to hold it in the hand on the dominant side.

The Method of Support Until Confidence is Gained

1. The helper stands sideways to the patient on the side opposite the pylon.

2. She places her arm loosely between his arm and his side so that her forearm rests against his rib cage.

3. Her arm is used to give confidence, and to position the patient gently so that he leans towards the pylon, and not away from it.

4. The patient should not be permitted to lean on her arm and so

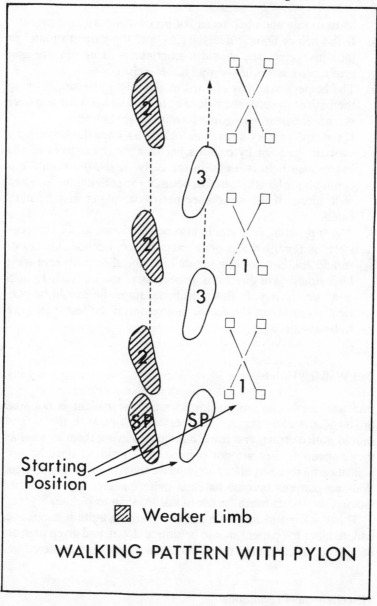

Figure 16.4: Walking Pattern — left sided weakness. SP, Starting position 1. Place pylon ahead of feet. 2. Place weak foot opposite pylon. 3. Place strong foot slightly ahead of pylon. Repeat steps 1, 2 and 3, as often as necessary

learn to rely upon her instead of his own arm and the pylon.

5. If the helper finds it necessary to hold the patient up and to take his weight she should discontinue walking practice and give more chair drill and wall bar exercises.

6. The helper's arm may be used to give slight pressure, pushing the patient towards the pylon, or to help to keep the shoulder on the side near her slightly forward to aid balance.

7. If the patient has difficulty in locking his knee the helper may support the joint by cupping her hand over the front of the knee. Such help is useful in the early stages, but should not continue for lengthy periods, because the patient must learn to walk alone. If the weak knee persists a caliper may be indicated.

8. The supporting arm should also be withdrawn as soon as possible, but until the patient gains his confidence the helper should continue to walk beside him. She should observe what he is doing, give directions as necessary, and be ready to help in an emergency. In this transitional stage she should be particularly aware of the correct placement of the feet if falls are to be avoided.

Bad Walking Habits

Bad walking habits are quickly learnt if the patient is not well drilled in the early stages. Any person walking with the patient should notice errors, and teach him how to avoid them as soon as they appear. If they are not pointed out to him at once he will almost certainly resist efforts to improve the pattern at a later time. Walking patterns become habitual quite quickly, and if unsatisfactory, they seem much harder to discard than to pick up.

This does not mean that a harsh or carping attitude should be adopted, but the patient should be slowed down, and given patient, detailed instruction until the correct pattern has been mastered.

Miscellaneous Precautions

(a) Make the patient conscious of the need to be properly balanced before moving his stick or taking each step.

(b) Make sure he is conscious of the placement of his feet. Do not add to his difficulties in this by insisting that he should look up. In the elderly, safety and confidence are more important than elegant posture.

(c) Watch for fatigue and do not push a patient beyond his limits.

(d) Notice if a patient loses concentration, forgets his walking pattern, staggers, shakes, becomes breathless or says he is tired. A rest is indicated. It is advisable to have chairs placed conveniently in the walking area so that they can be reached quickly if necessary.

(e) Be conscious of the patient's problems as a whole, and make allowances for them. Watch for fear, changes of mood, distractability, embarrassment, problems of understanding, sensory impairment, poor vision, deafness, loss of body image, and giddiness. Remember that the presenting problem such as a fractured femur, a stroke, or an amputation may only be part of the picture.

(f) Never hurry a patient. Let him take as long over a movement as he needs to do it accurately. A few moves done well are more valuable than many done incorrectly. Speed will come with learning and confidence but not with pressure. If haste is necessary before the patient is ready for it he should be taken in a wheelchair.

(g) Make any help you give as light as it can be with safety. Too much help encourages dependence.

(h) If the patient is too heavy for you do not be too proud to ask for help from another person. There is no value in an accident to the patient or damage to your own back.

(i) Give plenty of praise and encouragement. Make sure the patient sits down after his walk with a feeling of accomplishment.

(j) Report any difficulty you encounter to a senior member of staff.

STEPS AND STAIRS

Introduction

Basic methods for teaching a patient to negotiate steps will be discussed here, but more specific methods for patients with different diseases or injuries will be described more fully in the chapter dealing with the disease in question.

Patients are usually afraid of their first attempt at negotiating steps. In order to give confidence the helper herself should feel and appear confident. Understanding of what is to be done and why, is necessary for this, and preparation is necessary for the helper as well as the patient. If in doubt she should try out the movements herself, acting out the patient's problem before taking the patient near the steps. Another helper should always be at hand until the patient's abilities have been demonstrated.

No attempt should be made until the patient is competent at walking on flat ground. The drill should be attempted early in the day when the patient is fresh. The helper's directions should be given in simple terms and in a calm manner one at a time. 'One step at a time' is the watchword.

Method of Holding the Patient

The helper stands sideways to the patient, placing her forearm between his arm and his rib cage. The patient should feel it as a strong and steady bar which he can use for support if necessary. He should not feel it as a restraint, transferring her tension to him. The helper's hand should be relaxed, but ready to move in response to the patient's need should he lose his balance. She should not grip his arm with her hand as this will be of no help to him if he should overbalance, and will probably result in bruising.

When the top step is reached the helper stands sideways with her leading foot on the lower step, and the other on the step on which the patient is standing. The patient should be told that he will only be asked to do one small thing at a time and that he may go as slowly as he pleases. If a second helper is present she should not give added instructions as this divides the patient's attention and makes understanding more difficult.

The Basic Method for Negotiating Steps

The general rule for a disabled person negotiating steps is that the weaker limb takes the lead on each step going down, but the stronger limb takes the lead going up. This is because the weight is supported by the back leg in descending, and the stronger limb is better able to control the movement. In going up the leading limb must lift the body to the step above, and so the stronger limb is placed first to perform this task. The helper should be on the weaker side.

Many people, including the relatives, find it easy to remember this order if reminded that the good go up to heaven, but that the bad go down below.

The patient is given the following instructions:

Going Down

1. Walk up to the top step. Stand with the toes of both feet just over the edge.
2. Stand on the stronger leg, or the one on the side away from the helper if both are of equal strength. Put the other foot forward over the edge of the step so that the heel clears the edge.
3. Bend the knee of the stronger leg, and lower the foot of the weaker one to the step below. This should be a steady movement controlled all the way down.
4. Make sure you are balanced, and take the weight on the lower foot as you bring the back foot down to stand level with the first one.
5. See that both feet are placed with the toes over the edge as in step 1.
6. Repeat steps 2 to 5 on each step until the bottom is reached.

Going Up

1. Walk as close as possible to the bottom step.
2. Stand on the weaker leg, and place the strong foot (or the one on the side away from the helper if both are equal) onto the step above.
3. Lean forward and raise the body by pushing up with the leading lower limb.
4. Place the second foot beside the first on the higher step.
5. Repeat steps 2 to 4 as often as necessary to reach the top step.

The Use of a Hand Rail

Most patients find it too dangerous to manage more than one or two steps without a companion or a rail to steady them. The rail should be on the side which allows the patient to stand sideways to it with his weak foot towards the lower side. The patient should be given the following instructions:

Going Down

1. Stand sideways to the rail and hold it with both hands.
2. Move your feet as close to the edge of the step as you can.
3. Put your weaker foot over the edge and place it on the lower step by bending your stronger knee.
4. If necessary move it out to make sure there is enough room for your strong foot between your weak foot and the step.
5. Bring your strong foot down beside your weak one.
6. Move your hands down on the hand rail.
7. Repeat steps 2 to 6 as often as necessary.

Going Up

1. Walk as close as possible to the bottom step.
2. Stand sideways to the rail so that your strong leg is near the high side.
3. Hold the rail with both hands.
4. Place your strong foot on the first step. Make sure it is far enough on to leave room for the weak foot.
5. Straighten your strong knee and help with your hands to raise your body and bring the weak foot up beside the strong one.
6. Move your hands further up the rail.
7. Repeat steps 4 to 6 as often as necessary.

Variations when Using a Walking Frame

Most patients can manage one or two steps with a walking frame without a helper, but more than two steps usually demands help from another person. If a helper is not available, some can overcome the problem with a hand rail and two walkers. The indoor walker is brought to the top of the steps and left there. The outside walker is parked ready at the bottom of the steps. The patient descends using the method described above, and takes up the outside walker on reaching the bottom. The process is reversed on returning to the house.

If a helper is available the following procedures are used.

Going Down

1. The helper stands on the third step down, facing the patient, and places one foot on the step above it.

2. She encourages the patient to walk up to the edge of the top step, and to place the toes of each foot just over the edge. The helper supports the front of the walker while this is being done.

3. The patient and the helper move together in lowering the walker so that its rubbers are safely on the first step down and its front supported by the helper.

4. The helper steadies the walker as it moves forward and places its front bar on her bent knee.

5. The patient takes his weight on his hands at the back of the walker and steps down with his weaker foot.

6. He brings his strong leg down besides his weak foot and sees that the toes of both feet are just over the edge.

7. The helper moves down one step and takes up the original position with one foot on the step above and the walker supported on her knee and steadied by her hands.

8. Repeat steps 5 to 7 as often as necessary.

Going Up

1. The patient approaches the bottom step by turning round in the walker, so that its wheels are behind him.

2. He walks as close as he can to the bottom step.

3. He raises the rubbers and places them as far back as possible on the first step.

4. The helper steadies the walker as the patient rises. The patient puts his stronger leg up on the step above, and pushes up with his strong leg and his hands.

5. The patient places the weaker foot beside the stronger one, stands steadily, and lifts the walker until he can put its rubbers up onto the next step.

6. The helper places the front of the walker on her knees as in 'Going Down', and steadies the frame as the patient moves up to the next step.

7. The moves are repeated steps 4 to 6 as often as necessary.

Note 1. Unless the patient has previously proved himself able to carry out this procedure it is essential to have two helpers. The one who supports the frame cannot help the patient if he loses his balance or his nerve. The second helper should stand sideways beside him as in the basic method until his competence is proved.

Note 2. A patient with only one weight-bearing lower limb can master steps provided that he has learnt to push up on his hands on the walker. (See page 238 'Preliminary Drill for One-legged Use of the Walking Frame'.)

Variations for Using a Pylon or Walking Cane

The patient should have gained reasonable competence with the pylon or cane walking on flat ground before attempting the steps. It is advisable to have two helpers present at the first try, even if he seems safe, in case he loses his nerve. Details of managing more specific problems are discussed in Chapter 17. The patient is instructed as follows.

Going Down

1. Walk up to the front of the top step.
2. Stand with the toes of both feet just over the edge.
3. Place the pylon sideways on the step below.
4. Lean on the pylon, and feel your weight through your hand.
5. Put your weak foot forward over the edge of the step.
6. Bend your strong knee and lower yourself gently onto the weak foot.
7. Make sure your weak foot is placed wide enough to leave room for the strong one between itself and the pylon.
8. Make sure of your balance and lower your strong foot to the second step.
9. Make sure that the toes of both feet are just over the edge of the step.
10. Repeat steps 3 to 9 as often as necessary.

Going Up

It is useful to have a chair at the bottom of the steps to allow the patient to take a short rest before starting to ascend again. When ready the patient is directed as follows.

1. Walk as close as possible to the bottom step.
2. Place the pylon sideways on the first step. It should be well to the side to allow room for the feet to be placed beside it.
3. Place the strong foot up on the step beside the pylon.
4. Make sure the whole foot is well on the step.
5. Lean towards the pylon, and raise yourself by pushing up with

the strong knee and strong hand.
6. Make sure the weak foot clears the top of the step as you bring it up beside the strong one. (The helper may need to assist in this in early attempts. If the patient is unable to clear the step by bending his knee he may be able to manage by raising the shoulder and hip on the weak side to lift the foot clear.)
7. Make sure you are properly balanced.
8. Repeat steps 2 to 7 as often as necessary.

Rewards for Effort

Negotiating steps for the first time after illness or accident demands courage from the newly disabled person. The helper should be calm and confident to help them tackle the task, and appreciative of their effort when they have done so. In the Newcastle Retraining Unit a flower is placed on those who achieve this as a badge of honour. This is worn with pride by the recipient, and brings congratulations from others. It is well worth supplying some other simple award if flowers are not available so that the day he first managed the steps is to the patient an important milestone.

17 SOME SPECIFIC DISABILITIES

A description of the methods used to vary the basic retraining programme to suit the needs of patients with some common disabilities.

A. GENERAL CONSIDERATIONS

Introduction

While routine retraining is designed to solve the transfer and mobility problems of the majority of patients, it is obviously necessary to adapt it to the actual needs of those with special problems. Some of these needs are quite individual, as for example in the presence of multiple pathology, where the particular combination of problems is unique to one patient. Others are problems which recur through a group with similar disabilities, such as those with Parkinsonism, arthritic disorders, amputations and painful weight bearing. These are the problems which are the subject of this chapter.

Aims of Retraining

The primary aim of retraining is to fit the patient for a return home, with as much independence as he can achieve, and if necessary, help with those things he cannot do. Residual disability is accepted realistically, and retraining looks for ways to help the patient deal with it if a cure will take a long time, or cannot be expected at all. Because 'home' is the final goal it follows that retraining must be fitted to the patient's own home, and to the needs of his family as well as his medical status.

Principles of Management

The principles behind the methods used for these patients are the same as those behind routine retraining (see Chapter 15). In the

252

context of this chapter the most important of these are:-

(a) Procedures should follow medical investigations, and fit in with any treatment prescribed.
(b) A positive attitude should lead to the question 'how?'
(c) The patient's strengths and assets should be used to advantage.
(d) The patient's weaknesses should be minimised.
(e) Equipment should be custom built or adapted for the individual if basic equipment does not suit his need.
(f) The patient's co-operation should be sought at each step because little can be achieved without his co-operation.
(g) The whole team should be made aware of the details of new or altered treatment.
(h) It should always be remembered that the family is part of the team.
(i) The patient should be helped to adjust to his own actual home conditions rather than an imaginary ideal.

The Immediate Needs of the Patient

With the advances in medicine and allied treatments many long-term disabling diseases are not so devastating in their effects as they once were. Nevertheless, we still see in the geriatrics unit the sufferers from former days who are already permanently disabled, patients who for some reason have not responded to treatment, patients with the complicated problems of multiple pathology, and those who must wait long periods for their treatment to take effect. All these patients have problems of mobility in the present. They must use the lavatory and go to bed this very night. Retraining methods can help such patients immediately and will be no load to carry if and when special methods are no longer needed. This practical approach is very helpful in maintaining morale and preventing the patient from accepting a passive role in his treatment, whatever the end result may be.

Some General Concepts

Trick Movements

A trick movement in this context is one which may be used by a patient to perform an action in a manner he would not usually employ. This is generally discouraged when the aim of the treatment is complete recovery of function. It is welcomed and encouraged when the aim is independence despite residual disability. These two opposing concepts can lead to conflict within the team if there are divergent aims for the patient concerned. In geriatrics the trick movement is much more readily accepted than in younger age groups, because of differing life styles which lead to different emphases on the needs of the patients. In the older age group residual disability is more prevalent and must often be accepted. In most cases independence at home is preferred to lengthy in-patient treatment which may or may not bring practical results. Trick movements can make an early return home possible in many cases and are acceptable to the patient, though not necessarily to the purists.

Alternative Methods

Patients who cannot manage the routine drills still need to perform the functions involved in them. Additions and variations must be found which suit the individual problem. The patient still needs his own form of bed, chair, and toilet drill, even if he cannot manage the routine ones.

Adapted Equipment

Basic equipment can be provided to overcome a problem; for instance, a raised toilet seat for a patient who cannot rise from a standard pedestal. Alternatively, the basic equipment can be adapted to meet more specific needs. This subject is covered in some detail in Chapter 19.

Personal Help

In some cases the patient cannot be expected to function unaided, but informed help can change a difficult situation into a simple one. Instruction of relatives is an important aspect of this. Some simple 'tricks of the trade' can be invaluable in these cases and are given here as they apply to specific disabilities.

B. PARKINSON'S DISEASE

Introduction

The two major problems in retraining the patient with Parkinson's Disease are rigidity and tremor. His basic retraining methods are those for a patient with four functioning limbs (Chapter 15), but these two problems often inhibit his ability to perform the necessary movements. Modern medical treatments have helped many patients but there are still those who do not respond. The following methods have been found helpful for these people. Even those who do respond to medication will benefit from appropriate activity as well.

Relaxation

Tension in any form tends to increase both rigidity and tremor and so relaxation can do nothing but help. In order to help the patient to relax it is necessary that we ourselves should be calm and talk quietly and firmly. We must give him time to respond to what we say, and put him at his ease by letting him know we understand when he finds it difficult to do so. At all costs we should avoid pulling, pushing or lifting without relating our help to the patient's own efforts to move. Pulling against his rigid limbs demonstrates tension in ourselves and increases tension in the patient. It sometimes helps to ask him to try to relax consciously, but this should not be done to the point where the patient is irritated and frustrated by the very word 'relax!' We can hold his hand and shake it, saying 'now go all floppy' or something of the kind, or talk to him for a moment or two about something unrelated to the present task. When the patient reaches a point where he feels unable to move, it is pointless for us to press him to do so. This only increases his tension and the rigidity he is already suffering. A shared joke or thoughts on an unconnected subject may be helpful at such times. Specific relaxation exercises may be given by professional staff.

Initiation of Movement

Difficulty in initiating movement is one of the most disabling features of Parkinsonism. Once the patient starts a movement he can very often follow through, but in starting he tends to elicit the rigidity which puts him out of action. He is more likely to be able to respond to requests to perform complete movements which go with a swing than to the step by step instructions given to other patients in the retraining situation. If we give·him cue words such as '1, 2, 3 — up!' he is sometimes able to follow the movements through. We should always synchronise such cue words and the help we give him with his own effort. If we get ahead of the patient as we help him, we will inhibit the free flow of the movement.

Communication

Difficulties in communication are often added to the physical problems of the patient with Parkinson's Disease. His speech may be slurred, faint, or lacking in tonal variation. Busy people tend to avoid him because of the difficulty they have in hearing and understanding what he is trying to say. Writing is not generally the answer because this tends to be extremely small, and to fade away before the message has been completed. Even non-verbal communication by facial expression is not readily available to many of these people. The result is that other people tend to avoid them and consider them to be cold and unresponsive. It is no wonder that the patients themselves tend to withdraw and give up the effort to communicate with their fellows. It must be remembered that their need for human contact is the same as it was before they became ill. Their emotions, while lacking expression, are still as strong. If we understand this and see beyond the expressionless face to the feeling person behind it, we should not find it difficult to meet them a little more than half way in their effort to communicate. A natural, friendly approach and normal conversation on our part usually help the patient to relax in our company and so to speak more easily himself. It has been noticed that a sense of humour is usually well preserved and a light touch seems to help with this relaxation.

Suitable Activities

The abilities of patients with Parkinson's Disease vary widely between individuals, and in the same person at different times. Much of their job satisfaction depends upon the helper's skill in assessing their present capacities, and in choosing suitable activities. In his retraining the patient must be involved in all the usual moves to the full extent of his powers without feeling pressure from the staff. In creative activities his tasks should encourage smooth continuous movements without too many changes of pace or direction. Care should be taken that he is not placed at risk from sharp or pointed tools or hot liquids if tremor is one of his problems. A successful conclusion is essential to his satisfaction in the job. Social contacts in as many ways as possible should be encouraged by staff members. Careful seating arrangements in the group can help to promote participation in parties, sing songs, and games. Help from a protective fellow patient is often extremely valuable to these people. Many friendships have been formed as the result of such inter-patient care.

The Helping Hand

Helping the patient with Parkinson's Disease is a skill to be learnt and practised. Help should be given in response to the patient's needs and not automatically whether he needs it or not. The ability of these patients varies considerably from day to day and so does their need for help. Assistance should always be given calmly and in a matter of fact way, and any sense of haste or frustration should be avoided. The helping hand should have a light touch. Any move, to be successful, must involve team-work between the patient and the helper. The proposed move should be explained to the patient and he should be given time to respond. Then the helper and the patient should work together in a co-ordinated movement just as two dancers move to the same rhythm. Holding the patient tightly communicates tension from the helper to the patient. If possible it is better to let the patient do the holding. Rather than taking the patient's arm, we should offer him ours. Actual gripping by the helper is seldom, if ever, justified. If, as is common with these patients, a movement comes to a halt, the quickest way to restart is to stop trying to press on, to relax, and to start again. It is also the kindest way.

If the patient becomes completely rigid, and something must be done to move him, the best results are usually obtained by asking him not to try to help you, but to relax and let you position his limbs for him. A typical example of this is seen when a patient sits on the seat of a car, but is quite unable to bend his knees to move his legs into the cabin.

Relatives and patients together are usually surprised at the ease with which they can function once they learn this combination of relaxation and concerted movement.

Standing and Sitting

Difficulty in initiating movement, rigidity, and impaired sense of balance may all affect both rising and sitting. Step by step instructions do not help because they inhibit the free flow of motion. The following routines have been found useful when presented to the patient as smoothly and continuously as possible.

Standing Up

1. Make sure the feet are placed firmly on the floor.
2. Lean back in the chair and relax.
3. Rock forwards and backwards once or twice with a swinging movement and when ready continue the forward move until the weight of the body is over the feet.
4. Straighten up.

Note. The helper may encourage the movement with a light touch and the words 'one, two, three — up!' synchronised with the patient's rocking movements. For some patients a higher chair can be very helpful for rising.

Sitting Down

In sitting down the three main problems are a tendency to misjudge distance, a tendency to throw the body into the chair before a safe sitting position has been reached, and failure to bend the hips and knees in a co-ordinated way while lowering the body into the chair. All patients should be encouraged to touch the chair with their hands and to feel it with the back of their legs before sitting.

The patient who has difficulty lowering his body, and tends to get stuck half way down, may be helped by the following procedures.

1. Ask him to stand up again, and reassure him that the chair is in position. Move the chair forward to touch the back of his legs if he is unable to feel for it himself.
2. Stand in front of him and say 'let us go down together'.
3. Say 'one, two, three — down!' and go down slowly in time

with him in one continuous movement. The helper may find that he follows the movement more easily if she holds his hands lightly in hers, or places her hands on his shoulders.

Note. Some patients tend to fall back into a chair quite suddenly instead of bending their hips and knees and lowering themselves onto the seat. This can be dangerous as the average chair tends to topple backwards if used in this way. Wall bar exercises (see Chapter 16) are useful for patients with this problem.

Walking

Problems

The walk of a patient with Parkinson's Disease is usually easy to recognise because of these features.

1. The hands are held rigidly by the sides and do not swing in reciprocal movement with the lower limbs.
2. The head is thrust forward.
3. The gait tends towards a shuffle.
4. There may be a festinant gait in which the steps become faster and shorter until they cease altogether.
5. Having stopped, the patient may have difficulty in starting again. Hazards, turns and doorways may also lead to a full stop.
6. When one side is more badly affected than the other the patient will tend to lean, and possibly fall, to the weak side.
7. Some patients may overbalance forwards or backwards.

In advanced cases a walking stick is more of a hazard than a help. The two most satisfactory ways of improving the walking are the provision of personal help and the use of a walking frame.

Personal Help

Help in walking is given in the same co-operative way as has already been described for other movements. The method is applied as follows.

1. The patient takes the helper's arm or is held lightly, right hand to right and left hand to left.

2. The helper gives an appropriate cue word such as 'Quick March! left, right, left' etc.
3. The helper and the patient move off in step with the patient setting the pace. The helper should adjust her pace and her stride to his.

Note. If the patient tends to fall to one side the helper should stand on that side. The patient will feel more secure and it will be easier for the helper to control the balance if standing on the weaker side.

Initiation of the Movement

If we watch the feet of the patient who has had difficulty in resuming his walk after being brought to a standstill, we can usually see that an attempt is being made but that the foot, despite his effort, remains firmly on the ground. We will see that in fact he is trying to move without transferring his weight to the other foot. We can help him by 'rocking' him from side to side in the following way.

1. Ask him to start with the foot nearest to the helper.
2. Exert slight pressure against his rib cage, with the forearm, to encourage a swing to the opposite side just as he is seen to make an effort to move the foot. The helper's own foot should move forward in step with his.
3. Help him to swing back to the other side just as he attempts to take a step with the other foot.
4. By repeating steps in this way a gentle rocking movement from side to side should be encouraged.

Note. There must be no hard or sudden push or pull, because his reaction to such pushing or pulling will bring him down even more heavily on the leg he is trying to move.

Rocking

To continue walking after the first step has been taken a gentle rocking movement from side to side, with the two people moving in unison, will help the patient to raise his foot and lengthen his step. The principle is rather like that of walking a doll, where releasing the pressure on each foot alternately initiates a series of steps. It is essential for the rocking to coincide with the patient's voluntary effort and so the helper must watch the patient's feet and walk in step with him at his pace. The natural movement of the fit person from side to side helps to release the rigidity of the disabled one. If, as is more than likely, the patient should come to another halt, there is no point whatsoever in saying 'Come on, pick up your feet'. The patient is quite unable to do this, and that is why he has stopped. He should be asked to relax as before and to start again. Any sign that the helper is becoming impatient will only make him more tense and add to his difficulties.

The Walking Frame

Patients who are too heavy to be walked by one person, those who have no helper available at home, and those who have gross balance problems should be trained to use the walking frame. Ideally they should use this as described in Chapter 16, but to many this is not possible. Some common problems are as follows.

Inability to Master the Lifting of the Back of the Walker. Patients who do not lift the legs of the walker clear of the floor progress reasonably on a smooth surface, but can be immobilised on carpets, small steps, or rough ground. They are only made tense and irritable by constant reminders to 'pick up the walker'. A better plan is to take them for a walk over grass or to ask them to walk across a small mat. They then find it necessary to raise the back of the walker to progress. If neither a lawn nor a mat is available the same result can be achieved if the helper blocks progress by placing her foot in front of the leg of the walker to act as a stopper. The patient must then lift the back of the walker over her foot before proceeding. A patient who has learnt to lift the back of the walker over an obstruction in this way will not be immobilised by a similar hazard when he gets home, even if he has not learnt to lift the back of the walker at each step in the approved fashion.

A Tendency to Lean Backwards or to Pull up on the Walker as if it Were an Anchor. Patients who lean back in this way often believe that they are in fact standing upright. It may be very difficult to convince them that leaning slightly forward is necessary. In mild cases they may be helped by being asked to watch their toes as they walk until a safer posture is developed. In more serious cases it has been found that what we call a 'knee restrainer' can be of assistance. A metre of any material such as webbing, carpet, binding, unserviceable bandages or lengths of waste linen may be used.

This should be tied across the back of the walker, just below the level of the patient's knees. This makes it impossible for him to walk into the walker and ahead of his own hands. A forward lean is encouraged by placing the handgrips towards the front of the walker rather than at the back in the usual position. This, combined with the restrainer assures that the user must lean forward to hold them. Once the patient has learnt to lean forward onto the walker in this way, and feels safe doing so, he can usually return to a normal walking frame.

The Mat Class

The mat class (see Appendix C) has proved particularly helpful to patients with Parkinson's Disease. During retraining it allows exercise without the risk of a fall, thus encouraging confidence and wider movements. When continued regularly after discharge it helps to maintain the gains which have been made. Many patients are referred to the day centre for the continuation of social stimulation and for a regular visit to the mat class as part of their maintenance programme.

Steps and Stairs

Patients who find difficulty in initiating each step when walking, sometimes surprise their helpers by moving freely and quickly up a flight of stairs. The lifting of the feet comes quite spontaneously when there is something to step up to or over, although it is inhibited on flat ground. Some patients find great satisfaction in walking up steps, and they may even 'show off' by going too quickly. The helper needs to be aware of this because the steps do not improve the patient's balance or his awareness of his own safety needs. The ability to lift the feet over an object can be used to advantage for the patient who has initiating problems. If the rocking technique does not work for him he may be able to start if the helper places her foot in front of his and asks him to step over it. One patient with a stepping off problem solved it for himself by carrying with him a small block of wood on a string. He would drop this down in front of his leading foot and step over it to start walking. Once moving he would pull it up again by its string and tuck it into his belt until it was needed again. It is important that any patient who tries this method should be well aware of what he is doing so that there is no danger of his tripping over the block or failing to withdraw the string after the first step.

Out for a Drive

Helping a patient to get in and out of a car is just an adaptation of his chair drill. The same process of relaxation and continuous whole movements must be used. Some patients find it difficult to draw their feet into the car after sitting on the seat. If the knees are rigid, a conscious effort to try to bend them will only make them more so. Efforts to bend the knees passively will not succeed if the patient is trying to help the movement. When this difficulty is experienced the helper should ask the patient to relax and not to try to bend the knees himself. Supporting the limb under the thigh, just above the knee with one hand, the helper should exert gentle pressure on the front of the leg, just above the ankle with the other. In most cases the knee will bend quite easily and the legs can be moved into the car. In severe cases where these methods are not successful, the patient can be transferred from a wheelchair into the front seat by the use of a slide board. Care should be taken to fix the seat belt securely, and if necessary for safer balance, cushions should be packed around the patient.

Assistance to the Family

The problems of the families of these patients are usually physical, psychological and social in nature, reflecting those of the patient. Education concerning the disease itself, and their own patient's response to it can be very useful, helping the relatives to understand what previously seemed like 'difficult behaviour' on the patient's part.

Physical Problems

Physical help is usually more difficult than it needs to be if the relatives have not been made aware of the factors described above. The helper's task can be lightened considerably if she understands the problem of rigidity and the place of relaxation and good timing. Training sessions with a competent member of staff and the patient himself, in which the relative practises these skills can be invaluable.

Psychological Problems

Slowness, variable behaviour and apparent unresponsiveness of the patient can all be very frustrating to the relative when encountered day after day. Unless they have had sound, down to earth explanations of the disease it is easy for relatives to see these irritating symptoms as the patient's fault rather than his misfortune. Most relatives find it helpful to express these frustrations, to learn that the problem is a relatively common one, and to be given some practical hints on management. The patient who senses the frustration of his relative can only respond by becoming more tense, so increasing the very symptoms which are causing the trouble. This vicious circle can best be broken if we help the relative to understand and so accept the behaviour which has been disturbing her.

Social Problems

Frustrations can be increased if the relatives feel tied to the home because of the constant help needed by the patient. Their own social contacts may be affected or there may be difficulties in getting out of the house for shopping, entertainment or merely the short breaks we all need from our work. The various domiciliary services can be used to give relief. The day hospital or day centre may be particularly valuable (Chapter 9). Not only can the relatives look forward to some regular free time, but the patient can also enjoy an outing. If the day centre is attached to the hospital he can receive not only social stimulation but also such continued treatment as he may need.

Planned Readmission

In practice many patients improve markedly in their performance during retraining but drop back when the stimulus of the retraining programme is withdrawn. This fact combined with the family stresses already mentioned, has led to the concept of planned readmission. Arrangements are made in advance for the patient to be readmitted for a 'refresher course' after a certain period. The relative is encouraged to take a holiday at the same time for rest and relaxation. The timing is related to the needs of both the patient and the relative, and the two holidays can be mutually helpful. It is necessary for these admissions to come before the relative reaches breaking point and feels unable to carry on. With practical help of this kind the burden can be shared and so made bearable.

C. LOWER LIMB AMPUTATIONS

Introduction

The retraining needs of patients with lower limb amputations vary tremendously. They depend upon such factors as the site of the amputation, the general fitness of the patient, the condition of the remaining limb, the length and condition of the stump, the prospects for the use of a prosthesis, and perhaps most importantly, the spirit and resilience of the patient himself. It follows that each case must be assessed carefully so that the patient's real problems and assets can be known before retraining begins.

Factors Affecting Retraining

The Need for Retraining

All patients with amputations are likely to need retraining whether or not a prosthesis is to be supplied. There will be times when he must function without the prosthesis, because it is away being adjusted, because he is experiencing trouble with his stump, or because he can't wear it in the bath. The drills which teach transfers and mobility, should therefore be taught routinely to all. The choice of drills will depend upon what strengths and abilities the patient still has to build upon. There is usually waiting time between the operation and provision of a limb. This need not be wasted if it is used to make the patient independent and confident.

The Site of the Amputation

The site of the amputation is a crucial factor in selecting the appropriate drills. The needs of the single amputee approximate those of the hemiplegic, while the needs of the bilateral amputee are closer to those of the paraplegic. Because of these differences they are dealt with under separate headings in this chapter. In both cases the presence of one functioning knee joint can make the difference between successful use of a prosthesis and life in a wheelchair.

The General Fitness of the Patient

The majority of lower limb amputees who come to the retraining unit have lost their limbs as a result of vascular disease rather than trauma. There may be a history of a knock, a burn or even a badly cut toe nail but the underlying cause is the pre-existing condition of the patient. In retraining such patients we must remember that the remaining limb is probably still at risk from the same underlying condition. It is our responsibility to ensure that any drill we teach them, will not include the danger of further knocks or abrasions and that any equipment we supply is free from sharp corners or other dangerous features. If the patient has received even slight damage to his limbs, it should be reported at once to a responsible member of the team, such as the retraining sister or the physiotherapist. Many patients are weak after long periods of immobility resulting from illness, toxicity or pain in the pre-operative phase. Many have put off the operation long after the optimum time for it through fear or in the vain hope that an ulcer will heal. Others have co-existing or related chronic diseases such as diabetes, heart disease or bronchitis. All these things must be taken into account in the retraining programme. We must make haste slowly giving the patient time to build up his strength and so to improve his stamina and his work tolerance. In the beginning we should encourage short periods of activity at regular intervals and stop him working if we see signs of stress or fatigue. The amount of effort can be increased as the patient's state of fitness improves.

The Condition of the Limbs

The Condition of the Remaining Limb

What we can or cannot expect from these patients depends very much on the condition of the remaining limb. In some cases this is not at risk, and can be used fully as soon as the patient himself is ready. In others it is in little better condition than the one he has just lost and should be used with discretion. If there is any doubt the matter should be discussed by the team and referred if necessary to the surgeon concerned. The patient whose second limb is not at risk should use the routine retraining drills for those with one functioning lower limb. If weight bearing on the remaining limb is contra-indicated the patient should use the drills as outlined for the paraplegic. The patient who has lost one limb and whose other limb is at risk, is usually slow to adjust to his disability and frightened to attempt even those things which he can do. Pain is often a very real problem and should not be treated lightly by the helper. If weight bearing is to be attempted in the presence of an ulcerated or otherwise painful foot, the provision of a custom made felt boot with a sponge rubber sole is sometimes helpful. The use of such a boot should be a team decision and even so it should be used for short periods only on a trial basis until its safety is established. Patients who spend lengthy periods in a chair should be taught and encouraged to push up on the arms of the chair at regular intervals. This relieves the pressure on their buttocks and helps to strengthen the upper limbs for use in transfers and in walking with a frame. More specific exercise than this is outside the scope of retraining but may be given by the physiotherapist. Elevation of the foot is often prescribed. For this purpose a padded fracture board attached to a chair or a specifically designed sloping stool may be used. In both cases it is absolutely essential to ensure that the limb is evenly supported and that no part of the limb is at risk from undue pressure. Bunions, the outer edge of the foot, heels and ankles should be watched carefully. The ankle joints should be supported with the foot board if there is any tendency to plantar flexion. Morale tends to be very low when a patient is worried about the status of the remaining limb. Understanding and the encouragement of positive thinking are needed. Fear of losing the second limb is often well founded and a second amputation must be faced. This situation is discussed on p. 276.

The Condition of the Stump

The condition of the stump may have a deciding influence on questions concerning prostheses. It may determine whether a prosthesis is advisable at all, what form it should take and when the patient should start to use it. Healing, pain, and the length of the stump are important elements in such decisions.

Immediate Needs. Before healing can be expected, the patient must perform many activities of daily living. Routine retraining is designed to help him with these by concentrating on the strength of the functioning limbs. Transfers for the single amputee involve the hands and one lower limb. Walking means the use of a walking frame. Both are usually achieved without much difficulty. In these moves the unhealed wound must be protected from bumps and infections but it is in no danger from the actual retraining routines. In performing routine transfers the amputee moves towards the strong side. His strong foot should be kept under the mid-line of the body and the stump should be on the outside of each turn. In this way there is no danger of knocking the stump on the bed or the chair. The bilateral amputee should also lean to the strong side when moving (by pushing up on his hands) if he experiences better healing or less pain in one stump.

Pain. Pain often inhibits movement, sometimes because of its severity but often because there is fear associated with it. With a little encouragement most patients will be able to accept the pain they inflict upon themselves in voluntary movement and prefer it to the pain of unexpected jarring when they are being lifted. If the pain is too severe it should be discussed with the patient's doctor at the clinical meeting.

Phantom Pain and the 'Invisible Leg'. The patient may complain of 'phantom pains' which are pains he feels in the part of the limb which has been amputated. These are real to him and he needs reassurance that they are commonly experienced by people after an amputation, and that they will tend to improve with time. Another patient may forget that his limb is no longer there and step out of bed only to fall over. This applies particularly when he is not fully awake, as when rising at night to use the commode, or when he is not aware of his surroundings. Care should be taken that such patients are well supervised so that falls are prevented until the problem is overcome. Helpers should realise that such problems are to be expected in a certain number of patients and are natural and not the result of confusion or dementia. If the problem is causing too much stress or danger it should be reported to the patient's doctor at the team meeting. The patient's relatives should also have the problem explained to them if it is still causing him trouble when he is ready to go home or if they are worried about it during his stay in hospital.

The Length of the Stump. The length of the stump may determine whether a prosthesis can be fitted and whether the patient can control it adequately. If it is below the knee the patient will have the advantage of a knee joint to help him rise and sit, but he may be in more danger of difficult healing or subsequent breakdown. If it is above the knee, one-legged rising will be necessary. Most patients manage this quite easily so long as the remaining limb is sound. It can be difficult in the presence of circulatory or arthritic problems in the remaining limb. A very short above knee stump may make the use of a prosthesis impracticable. It is unlikely that an elderly patient with bilateral above knee amputations will learn to walk or rise from a chair with two prostheses, but most other drills are possible to him if he has the right spirit.

Bandaging

Correct bandaging of the stump is important to satisfactory fitting of the limb and to the patient's comfort even when a prosthesis is not envisaged. It is usually the responsibility of the physiotherapist, but nurses must apply bandages when no physiotherapist is available. They should know the correct procedure. Many patients can be taught to apply the bandage for themselves and all should be given the opportunity to learn. If possible this should be achieved before discharge, but if not the relatives should learn, or arrangements should be made for the community nurse to call.

The Waiting Game

It is common for waiting to be associated with healing or the shaping of the stump. There may also be times when fitting difficulties demand that the limb must be returned to the limb maker. The last contingency applies particularly to country areas where there is no local workshop. This time can be used to advantage in mobility training, but once the patient is independent and is no longer in need of specific treatment it may be possible for him to wait at home. For many patients this helps morale but it should not be encouraged unless the relatives have received instructions concerning management. Any domiciliary service which is needed should be made available. An unsatisfactory trial at home can upset both patient and relative and make the eventual discharge more difficult and frightening.

Flexion Contracture at the Hip or Knee

One of the dangers of non-weight bearing is contraction of the muscles involved. To the amputee who is not walking, and who sits for long periods in a wheelchair, flexion of the hip joint of the affected limb is a special risk. This can be minimised by ensuring that the patient lies prone for a prescribed time each day. One to two hours is usual. Flexion of the knee following a below knee amputation may be controlled by a night splint. The supply of such a splint must be under the supervision of a suitably qualified member of the team. Prone lying is not always well tolerated by the patients who find it uncomfortable, but they should be encouraged to persevere.

The Prospects for a Prosthesis

The criteria for recommending a prosthesis are the physical condition of the patient, his personality and psychological status, and social factors such as his home conditions, family support and usual life style.

Physical Condition

The physical condition will determine whether it is possible to fit a satisfactory limb, whether the patient is strong enough to tolerate the work involved in learning to use it, and what degree of independence he is likely to attain. For one patient the result may be an almost normal range of activities, while for another acceptable appearance and improved transfers are all that we may expect. Aims and possibilities of this kind should be considered when decisions are being made about the provision of a limb.

Psychological Considerations

Psychological considerations qualify the physical ones. The demented or agitated patient may be physically able to tolerate the prosthesis but still be at risk through inattention or hazards or a tendency to panic. The well-adjusted frail person may have enough motivation to achieve the success which will elude the stronger but less spirited one. Positive attitudes, courage, and the will to persevere can be developed as the person adjusts to his new conditions, but it is usually wiser not to order a prosthesis until the patient himself feels motivated towards wearing it. A temporary prosthesis helps informed decision making by the team as well as helping the patient to find out how he really feels. There is nothing more wasteful than an expensive limb which is kept in a cupboard.

Social Considerations

Social considerations also play an important part in this decision making. Home conditions, the support of relatives, and previous life style are all relevant. The social worker is a key member of the team and her insights are as necessary as those of the retraining personnel. For instance, if the patient is unable to apply his prosthesis and has no-one to help him to do so, it will not be of much use to him. Decisions may well differ between the patient who was a keen member of his club and another who rarely left his house before he became ill. As the limb is intended for use in the patient's own place of living it is common sense to ensure that it will be possible to use it in the conditions which apply there. The specialised and sheltered conditions of the hospital do not always demonstrate the difficulties which may be encountered at home.

The Dangers of 'Wishful Thinking'

When the subject of amputation is first mentioned there is usually great shock and distress. The comfort that we give should be encouraging and positive without becoming an exercise in 'wishful thinking'. Many well-meaning people try to give reassurance by pointing out how very good modern prostheses are. They may even go so far as to say, 'Cheer up, in a few months you'll be walking as if nothing had happened!' Such promises are meant in kindness, but it is not within the speaker's power to fulfil them. If at a later date it is clear that a prosthesis is not the best answer for that patient a second period of anxiety and distress must be faced. Discussion of the use of a prosthesis with the patient should be factual and unemotional. The need for perseverance and work should be mentioned as well as the obvious benefits. Analogies with new dentures or new shoes may help some patients to understand and accept their own difficulties. Later disappointments are avoided if the patient's expectations are kept within his grasp.

The Irrelevance of Age

Little has been said here about the influence of chronological age upon any decision to provide a prosthesis because it should never be a determining factor. Patients in their nineties can learn to use a prosthesis perfectly well if their general health and mental capacities are good, while patients in their thirties may fail if theirs are not. If the other factors point to an affirmative decision, age is irrelevant. The older person has just as much right as the younger one to be given the opportunity to try.

A Team Responsibility

The final decision is a team responsibility, remembering that the patient and his relatives are part of the team. Careful observation and accurate reporting are required from all those who express an opinion. They must be fully aware of the importance of this decision to the patient's well-being, and future way of life. Having heard the opinions of the team it is the doctor who must finally decide and sign the appropriate request forms if a prosthesis is to be ordered.

If the Answer is 'No'

The patient still has a life to live whatever the decision about a prosthesis may be. He needs to be well adjusted and independent if his life is to be a useful and cheerful one despite his loss. He should not be discharged just because his stump has healed if he has not yet accepted his condition or learnt to overcome his physical problems. Routine retraining, adapted to his special needs, can help his adjustment at both the psychological and physical levels.

Learning to Wear the Prosthesis

Many elderly folk find it difficult to apply their prosthesis themselves and to develop the habit of wearing it automatically day by day. Explanations, however clear, are not the answer. The skill in applying it must be learnt by practice, and the habit of wearing it must be built into the daily routine. Both these problems can be overcome by making the application of the prosthesis a part of regular dressing each morning, and not something which is done later in the day expressly for use in the Physiotherapy Department. This practice should begin as soon as the condition of the stump allows it. Until the patient becomes proficient he should be supervised by any member of the staff who has the necessary knowledge and ability to give adequate instruction. Daily application of the prosthesis, as part of the dressing routine, provides an opportunity for control of the length of time the prosthesis is worn in the early stages of retraining, and also teaches the patient a behaviour pattern which will help him to continue wearing it at home. This helps the staff to assess the patient's tolerance of the limb and gives the patient a yard stick by which to judge his own progress.

The Single Below Knee Amputee

Little special retraining is needed by the single below knee amputee who has no complicating factors. What he will need is usually of a routine nature, along the following lines:

(a) Training in applying and using his prosthesis (under the supervision of the physiotherapist).
(b) Help in accepting his loss and developing optimism about his future.
(c) Routine retraining and transfers (one-legged version) for use when not wearing a prosthesis.
(d) Routine retraining in one-legged use of a walking frame, for use without the prosthesis.
(e) Encouragement to wear and walk with his prosthesis if he shows reluctance.
(f) Walking on rough ground, and possibly a bus trip and a walk in a crowd, if he seems nervous of these.

If the patient cannot wear a prosthesis his retraining follows the course for those with only one leg as described on p. 235. Elderly patients usually become more confident on a walking frame than on crutches, and gain independence more quickly and more safely. Having mastered the walking frame, a few may progress to the use of crutches. These are more convenient out of doors, but indoors a walking frame fitted with a tray gives greater safety and independence.

The Single Above Knee Amputee

Loss of the knee joint is usually more disabling than loss of the ankle because of the importance of the knee in rising and sitting. Nevertheless, when wearing the prosthesis, the single above knee amputee can become completely independent if there are no complicating physical or mental problems. The aims for patients with differing degrees of disability are as follows.

If Mentally and Physically Agile

Patients who are mentally and physically agile should learn to use a free knee joint in the prosthesis and to walk with a walking cane.

If Aware and Able to Learn, but Physically Frail

The patient who is less physically able but who is aware of his surroundings and who can follow instructions and remember to carry them out should learn to walk with a locked knee joint in his prosthesis. He should learn to free it for rising and sitting. A pylon or walking frame may be safer than a cane for such patients. If a pylon is used it should be of a height to help him to stand upright and not to lean to the strong side as hemiplegic patients are taught to do.

If Able to Learn Only by Repetition

The patient who is unable to remember instructions and who must learn mainly through repetition should lock and unlock his prosthesis only while seated. He should use the one-legged 'drills' for rising and sitting, walk with a fixed knee, and use a walking frame for safety. Such patients are often safer and more independent without the complication of a prosthesis, and are in fact inclined to neglect to wear their prostheses after discharge.

If the Remaining Limb is at Risk

The patients whose remaining limb is at risk may be unable to use a prosthesis for walking, but may find it useful for transfers. It can help to protect the other limb by sharing the weight bearing and may even become the 'good' leg. Should the second limb eventually be lost the patient will already have learnt to make good use of the first one. This is particularly valuable if there is a functioning knee joint.

If Facing a Second Operation

Because of the systemic nature of some of the diseases which lead to amputation, a second amputation, though not inevitable, is not uncommon either. Patients facing such an operation are often in the hospital for some time while the decision is being made and the staff's attitudes are of great importance to the patient. Emotionalism will not help. The patient needs to discuss the problem calmly and factually with someone he can trust. The staff member should be a good listener and show empathy rather than sympathy (see Chapter 11, p. 160).

Some ideas which may be helpful are:

1. To understand that fear of losing the limb and the pain and danger involved in trying to save it often lead to the rejection of any activity. These fears and discomforts may also lead to irritable responses despite kindness and a caring approach. There may also be unhealthy concentration on every sign and symptom which might be connected with the limb.

2. To reassure the patient that his surgeon would not recommend an operation unless it were likely to make him safer or more comfortable.

3. To explain to the patient that the majority of people become much happier, healthier and more independent once the operation is over and they no longer have fear and pain dragging them down.

4. To put it to the patient that those who respond to the threat by ceasing to function have in effect already lost the limb and are in danger of losing their spirit as well.

5. To explain to any patient who appears to feel that loss of a limb makes him incomplete as a person, that wholeness is a way of thinking and feeling. If we can think clearly and relate well to other people our personality is intact and we are still ourselves. Limbs are the tools of the body, but we ourselves are the people inside.

6. To be quietly optimistic in talking to the patient, remembering that the bilateral above knee amputee is one of the easiest patients to bring to independence once he accepts his wheelchair as his legs. He can think and learn more easily than most patients with strokes, and he can accomplish his transfers more easily than the paraplegic. Seeing some of these other patients managing in spite of their disabilities is often helpful to the double amputee.

7. Patients who have been through a second amputation themselves and have adjusted to it can often help the newcomer to their ranks. There seems to be a sense of camaraderie among amputees which is less obvious among patients with other disabilities. This can be encouraged with good effect. There are many examples of close friendships and helpful exchanges between these patients. The following incident is one of them.

A patient facing his second operation and finding it hard to accept, was introduced to an old timer from the day centre. Towards the end of what had been a very helpful discussion, a pretty young nurse walked past. The old timer shot out his arm, spun her round and landed her on his lap, saying, 'You see, you can even have a girl on your knee'. The value to the new chum easily compensated for the nurse's embarrassment. Such spontaneous actions by another patient who has been through the ordeal can have much more meaning for the frightened new patient than the usual reassuring talk from a member of the staff.

The Bilateral Above Knee Amputee

At first sight the person who has lost both lower limbs above the knee may seem to be among the most gravely disabled of people. In fact he has a better chance of independence than others, including the single amputee with an unsound second limb. Unlike many other disabled persons he can use his arms and hands as before, and his brain is still capable of functioning at its usual level. He has lost his ability to walk, and so must become mobile on wheels, and he has lost his ability to stand, and so must transfer while seated. Given practical retraining in these areas his achievements will depend upon his courage and spirit rather than his physical condition. Living alone, going up and down stairs to a top flat, gardening, playing trains with grandchildren, driving a car or a motorised chair, riding in a bus, going shopping and doing full-time office work have all been accomplished by patients in this situation. The major factors are as follows.

Morale

The morale of these patients is usually remarkably high provided that the general management of the case has been good. Adequate pre-operative preparation of the patient himself as well as his limb is important. Practical measures such as teaching him to use his wheelchair, strengthening his upper limbs by teaching him to push up on the arms of his chair, and, if indicated, more specific exercises can give him a positive view of the future. It also gives him something to work on during the trying waiting period before surgery.

There should also be ample opportunity to talk and to bring his uncertainties and fears out into the open as mentioned earlier.

After the operation, if there is no complication and healing takes a natural course, there is usually a rapid increase in morale and in a feeling of physical well-being. At this stage the patient should be encouraged to do everything he can for himself and to be proud of his accomplishments. Enthusiasm and praise for his efforts are part of the staff's responsibility to him. It is difficult to keep trying if no-one seems to notice. There will be bad times for some when pain, the acute awareness of loss or some limitation experienced for the first time, will seem unbearable. There will follow the usual pattern of mourning which has received so much attention in recent years. The feeling should be expressed and worked through, not hushed up and repressed. Even the best surgical result is devalued if the patient remains dependent and unhappy.

Appropriate Equipment

Appropriate equipment is necessary for all patients undergoing retraining but for none more so than the bilateral amputee. It can be the deciding factor in his eventual independence. His wheelchair is the nucleus of his equipment and most other items are related to it.

The Wheelchair. The bilateral above knee amputee must learn to accept the wheels of his chair as an alternative to legs and the more thoroughly he can do this the fuller his life can be. A wheelchair life can be a full one as demonstrated by such people as Marjorie Lawrence as a singer, President Roosevelt of the United States, and even Ironside of TV fame. Some features to be considered when choosing a chair for a bilateral amputee are:

1. Comfort. The patient will sit in it for long periods at a time.
2. Removable arms. The patient will need to move sideways on to other surfaces.
3. Removable foot plates. It should be possible to bring the front of the seat up to the bed or toilet seat so that the patient can move forwards and backwards without crossing a gap.
4. Satisfactory brakes. These should be easy to apply and release and really secure when applied. The top of the level should be below the level of the seat so as not to interfere with the side transfers.
5. The seat belt. This is required if the patient has poor balance. Without the feet to brace the body, even a patient with good balance can tip out of the chair if he leans too far forward,

goes down a ramp frontwards or strikes an obstruction which brings the chair to a sudden stop. A seat belt is a precaution against such accidents.

Matched Equipment (Figure 17.1). The independence of the patient in self care depends upon his ability to move freely on and off such furniture as his bed, commode, toilet seat, bath seat and favourite chair. This becomes much easier if all are matched in height to the seat of his wheelchair which eliminates the 'steps' which must otherwise be negotiated. Most patients can learn to move on an even surface with safety and ease, and for this reason the matching of equipment for height is routine.

The Slide Board (Figure 17.2). The slide board is an ordinary fracture board with its ends planed down to form a wedge and its surface polished to minimise friction. The patient learns to use it to cross gaps as when entering and leaving a car. It can also be used to allow rests on the way when the patient needs fairly heavy assistance from another person, and to give a smoother surface to

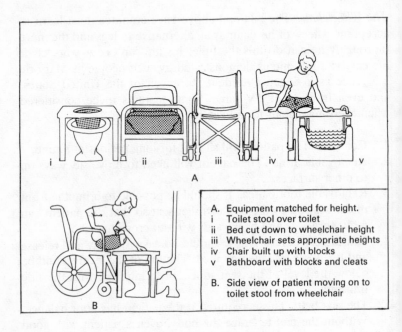

A. Equipment matched for height.
i   Toilet stool over toilet
ii Bed cut down to wheelchair height
iii Wheelchair sets appropriate heights
iv Chair built up with blocks
v   Bathboard with blocks and cleats

B. Side view of patient moving on to toilet stool from wheelchair

Figure 17.1: Equipment for Bilateral Amputee

move on when the patient has difficulty in lifting his body from the seat. In warm weather when moisture makes sliding difficult, it sometimes helps to sprinkle the board with talcum powder. Some patients prefer a smaller board in which case approximately 10in (25cm) can be cut from the end.

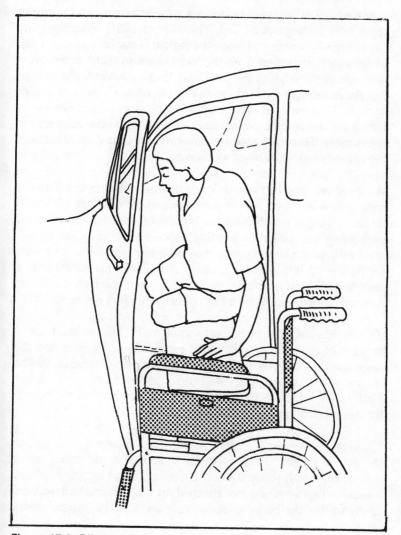

Figure 17.2: Bilateral Amputee Moves from Car Seat to Wheelchair

Hand Bats. Obese patients and patients with proportionally short arms sometimes find it difficult to lift themselves enough to move with ease. The lift can be increased by approximately 3in. with the use of these aids. They are not recommended for patients with poor concentration or poor balance.

Bed Rails. Bed rails may be necessary for some patients to prevent them from rolling out of bed. This is particularly so in the early days of readjustment and when the patient is not fully awake. Lack of sensory information from the feet can mean that the patient is unaware of the edge of the bed, while lack of lower limbs to control the movement may lead to rolling out of bed if he tries to turn over. Bed rails must always be offered with tact and suitable explanation for the patient, otherwise he is likely to be resentful and to reject them. This will happen almost certainly if he thinks that he is being treated like a baby or a prisoner.

A Bed Rope. The bed rope is made of plaited cotton to produce a rope approximately 1.5in. in diameter and 8ft in length (3.5cm × 275cm). This is attached to the bottom of the bed and used for supporting the patient in a sitting position until he learns to balance without the counter-weight of his lower limbs. It can be used for pulling up into a sitting position as well but this should not be encouraged as it prevents the patient from learning to sit up unaided. Its use should be a last rather than a first resort.

The Bathboard. The bathboard should be brought to the level of the seat of the chair as mentioned earlier. Some patients find the basic board too narrow and lack confidence when seated on it. The answer to this is to provide two boards side by side to give a wider platform on which to sit. Rails can also be attached to the boards for patients who appear to be at risk.

Cushions. Cushions are often helpful for building up the seat of the patient's chair. These cushions should be made rather like a sofa cushion with squared sides. Unevenness and lumps should be avoided. Tapes should be attached to all corners and secured firmly so that the cushion cannot slide away as the patient moves on it.

Wheelchair Steps (see Figure 17.3). Wheelchair steps are provided

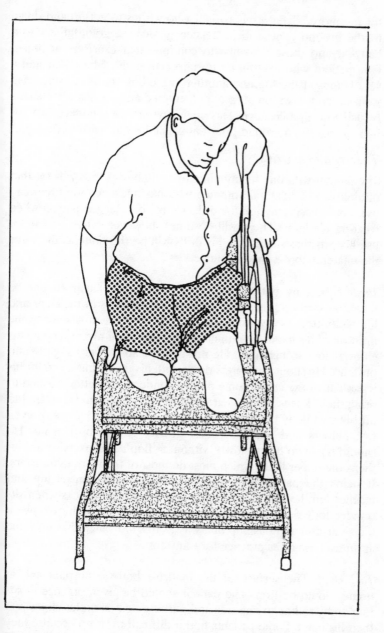

Figure 17.3: Bilateral Amputee Moves from Chair to the Ground and Back with the Aid of Steps

for the more adventurous patient who wishes to get up and down to the ground. These include keen gardeners, grandfathers who baby-sit and those who like to continue mat exercises at home. One patient who lived in an upstairs flat, had a wheelchair and a set of steps at the top and another at the bottom of the stairs. He went up and down on his seat and entered and left his wheelchairs by using his mobile steps. This manoeuvre made it unnecessary for him to move to a ground floor flat which he was loath to do.

The Retraining Drills

The patient with one functioning lower limb uses the drills for that disability. The bilateral amputee who has one knee joint and can use a prosthesis may use the drills for the one-legged person when wearing his limb. There will be times, however, when he cannot use his prosthesis and then his drills will be the same as those for the bilateral above knee amputee.

Push Ups. Any patient who must use a wheelchair should be taught as soon as possible to push up on the arms of the chair and lift his bottom away from the seat. To do this satisfactorily, he must place his hands near the middle of the chair arms, keeping his elbows close to his body. He must then lean forward slightly and push up. He should not press down with his thighs but try to lift his legs clear of the chair. Some patients understand better if asked to bring their 'knees' up to their chest. The patient who is too frail to lift his own body this way should be helped to rise by one or even two helpers and asked to resist gravity going down again. He should try to go down slowly without a 'flop'. This exercise strengthens the upper limbs which must do most of the work in transfers. It helps the patient to learn to balance when transferring and teaches him how to relieve the pressure on his buttocks when sitting for long periods. The patient should not lean on his elbow on the chair arm and push up that way as this movement has no value as an exercise or as practice for transfers.

Bed Drill. The surface of the mattress both in hospital and at home should be firm. The patient should be given practice in sitting up by rolling to one side and pushing up first on his elbow and then his hand. Some patients find it difficult to sit up because they feel top heavy without the weight of the legs to balance them. Practice usually solves this problem. Next the patient should learn to balance in this seated position by leaning forward from the hips. A rope may be used to get into position, but the patient should let go and try to stay up without it. Once he can sit, the patient should practice moving about on the surface of the bed by pushing up on his hands and moving his body. Walking on his buttocks should not be encouraged. It is not a useful movement and can be a painful one if the stump is not yet healed. If the patient's arms are not long enough to lift him, the hand bats may help. These are gripped in the hand and act as an extension to the arm giving him a slightly higher lift. If the patient has pain in the stump, he may find it difficult to move towards the weaker side. In this case he may enter the bed on one side and leave it on the other until the stump has healed and the pain has been resolved. Moving along the side of the bed is a useful exercise, but must be well supervised until the patient has achieved good balance. It accustoms him to the void in front of him and helps him to be more confident when seated on the bathboard, the toilet seat and other equipment. The other drills for the bilateral amputee all involve the use of the first two. If the patient can move from side to side and backwards and forwards by using his arms there are few situations in which he will be helpless.

Wheelchair Drill. If all the patient's other equipment has been matched to the height of the wheelchair, he can move back and forth between them by pushing up on his hands. The arms of the wheelchair can be removed if he wishes to go sideways. Care should be taken to instruct the patient in the use of brakes and to insist that he should use them at all appropriate times. To transfer without applying the brakes can be a very dangerous procedure. On rough or soft ground it is easier for the chair to go backwards, large wheels first. Patients who are alert and agile can master this if provided with a reversing mirror on the side of the chair. Correct use of a wheelchair should be taught to the patient and to his relatives before he goes home.

Commode Drill. The commode must be matched to the same height as the bed. It is placed with its front against the side of the bed so that the patient can go backwards into it and forwards onto the bed again. Alternatively one arm can be removed and that side can be placed against the side of the bed. In this case the patient will move on and off the commode sideways. Both of these methods are acceptable but some patients prefer one and some the other.

Toilet Drill. To give the patient a lavatory of the correct height, a built up toilet seat is used (see Figure 17.1). The wider part of the hole should be placed to the front. He is taught to bring his wheelchair right up to the seat, front to front and having applied his brakes, to move forward onto it. He can use it this way facing the wall without having to turn round. When ready, he just moves back again into the chair. Independence comes quickly by this method and nurses do not need to lift him on and off the seat.

Bath Drill. The bath should be fitted with a bath seat adjusted to the height of the wheelchair and a hose-type shower should be fitted to the taps. A double bathboard may be used if the patient is afraid of the narrow one. The chair can be placed either frontways or sideways against the board and the patient can move across in whichever way he finds easiest. The dimensions of his own bathroom often determine which way he must approach the bath. Once bathed he can move back to his chair for drying and dressing. A towel placed under him on the seat of the chair prevents it from getting wet and aids the patient in drying himself.

Shower Drill. The patient who uses a shower recess at home needs to practise its use during retraining. A waterproof chair or sturdy stool the same height as the wheelchair will be needed so that the patient can move on and off it using the front or side transfer as best suits his case.

Steps and Stairs. These can be negotiated by the more agile patient if he sits on the stairs and lets himself down one at a time. Most patients find it easier to have one hand on the step on which they are seated and one on the step below. Hand bats make the move easier for some by limiting the distance the patient must lean forwards and down to reach the lower step. Steps should not be tackled by those who are frail, frightened, or lacking in balance.

Car Drill. To get in and out of a car the bilateral amputee uses a slide board. The wheelchair is taken as close as possible to the car seat and the brakes are applied. The slide board is placed firmly to make a bridge from one seat to the other. The patient then moves across it and into the car by lifting up on his hands. A little help may be needed if the car seat is appreciably lower than the seat of the chair. A seat belt should be worn on every occasion, whether or not this is a legal requirement, because the patient has no way of bracing himself if the car comes to a sudden stop.

Leading a Full Life

The bilateral above knee amputee is at first sight one of the more badly disabled of patients. In practice he can live a very full life so long as he has good transport and reasonable health. As a rule he has not suffered brain damage with its associated problems, and he can use both hands to good advantage. Both intellectual and manual interests are therefore available to him so long as he is mobile in his chair. His greatest disabilities are caused by architectural barriers which pose similar difficulties for young mothers with prams and many younger disabled persons.

Acceptance of his loss and the determination to make the best of things are his greatest assets, and for this reason, morale building is just as important as the physical treatment he will receive.

D. FRACTURED FEMUR

Introduction

The combination of brittle bones with a tendency to stumble and fall, as is so often seen in the frail elderly, means that patients recovering from a fractured femur form a considerable group in the retraining unit. In earlier days these fractures were often seen as a death sentence, because pneumonia, pressure sores, and confusion followed long periods of bed-fastness while waiting for the bone to unite. Modern anaesthetics and surgical procedures combined with early mobilisation have changed this and the prospect is usually a hopeful one. The patient who is referred for retraining will probably have had one of the following procedures, and may or may not be ready for weight bearing.

(a) Traction with bony union. This will usually be a younger patient.
(b) A nail or pin for a fractured shaft of the femur so as to permit use of the limb before bony union is achieved.

(c) A three-flanged nail, driven up the neck and into the head for a fractured neck of the femur.
(d) A 'pin and plate' in which a nail is combined with a metal plate screwed to the shaft of the femur for extra strength.
(e) A prosthesis replacing the head and neck of the femur (and sometimes the acetabulum). These are usually seen when there is poor blood supply to the site, which may result in non-union.

Previous History

The previous history of a patient with a fractured femur is essential information when his aims of treatment are set down and his retraining programme is planned. The background to the fracture is almost as important as the condition of the limb. The aims for an active patient who is knocked over by a car, a confused and tottery patient who tripped over a mat, and a patient with Paget's Disease who suffered a spontaneous fracture, are likely to be very different from each other if the facts are known. The general health and life style of the patient and the degree of help available from his family are all relevant to his retraining and the goals which should be set.

Weight Bearing

The level at which retraining should begin, the equipment needed, and the actual 'drills' taught, will all depend in the first instance upon his weight-bearing status. Whether or not the patient is ready to bear weight must be the decision of his surgeon or the doctor who is now responsible for him.

Non-weight-bearing Procedures

If the patient is non-weight bearing he must use the drills appropriate for those with three functioning limbs. If he is unaware of his own safety (and many elderly folk are confused for a time after their fall and operation), he should be well supervised to ensure that he does not inadvertently put his weight on the damaged limb. Great care should also be taken that he should avoid any twisting of the limb when performing the drills as this can create problems at the site of the injury until healing is accomplished. The non-weight-bearing patient who is alert and careful can be quite independent in self care if he preserves sensible precautions. Walking is quite possible and safe if he walks with a walking frame, remembering not to put his foot to the ground. The process is as follows:

1. Stand on the strong limb, just behind the back feet of the walker, with hands placed on the walker towards the back.
2. Lean on the hands and raise the body by depressing the shoulder girdle.
3. In a controlled movement, without a swing or a hop, place the strong foot towards the front of the walker.
4. Transfer the weight from the hands to the strong limb.
5. Standing on the strong limb, raise the back of the walker about half an inch from the ground and push it forward on its wheels until its feet are in line with the toes of the strong foot.
6. This should bring the patient back to his starting point.
7. Repeat these moves as often as is necessary.

Partial Weight Bearing

Partial weight bearing is sometimes allowed in a transition period between non- and full weight bearing. This is possible with a walking frame or crutches, but not with a quadripod or walking cane. For an elderly patient the walking frame is the aid of choice (see p. 232). The process of walking with partial weight bearing is as follows:

1. Stand on the strong limb with the toes in line with the back legs of the walker, and with the hands placed comfortably towards the back of the frame.
2. Place the foot of the fractured limb lightly on the ground beneath an imaginary line drawn between the hands.
3. Taking most of the weight on the hands, but keeping the weak foot grounded, take a step with the strong limb towards the front of the walker.
4. Transfer the weight to the strong limb.
5. Standing on the strong limb, raise the back of the walker about half an inch from the ground, and push it forward on its wheels until its feet are in line with the toes of the strong foot.
6. Ground the walker and move the weak foot forward as in step 1 above.
7. Repeat the process as often as necessary.

Note. Partial weight bearing usually comes easily if there is some pain to remind the patient that he must take care, but if there is no pain, strict supervision should be maintained until the patient proves his reliability in remembering not to take full weight. This applies to all transfers as well as to walking practice.

Equipment

The equipment for a patient with a lower limb fracture should be stable, of good design and construction, and the correct height to suit his individual needs. It should also be suitable for use at home. We must remember that he has already had a fall leading to a fracture. As well as helping him to overcome his present problems and to get back on his feet, it is necessary to look to the future and to try to prevent it from happening again. Equipment should be chosen with this in mind.

Stability

Uneven legs, lost rubbers, poor brakes, strained joints and loose screws should all be attended to routinely. Each item should also be checked and made sound by the person who delivers it to the patient.

Sound Design and Construction

Simple well-made articles are preferred to elaborate ones which tend to go wrong or to lose detachable parts. However good the item, if it is not suitable for the individual it is not good design for him. A simple basic item can usually be adapted successfully to special needs, and so become 'custom made'.

Heights

The heights of his equipment are particularly important to the patient whose problems include stiffness or pain. The two main heights to be considered are the following:

Seating Surfaces. All seating surfaces used by the patient should be of a height to make it easy for him to rise and sit down again. His bed, toilet seat, and bath seat are involved as well as chairs and sofas. The patient with stiffness or pain usually requires a higher than average seat. The correct height can best be determined by trials with a series of firm cushions on a standard chair. All sitting surfaces used by the patient should then be adjusted to this height. Similar adjustments must be made at home if they are still useful to him at the time of discharge.

Walking Aids. The height of walking aids must also be suited to individual needs. A higher frame is needed for weight-bearing problems, and a lower one for balance. In the first case the patient lifts his body to reduce weight bearing, and in the second he leans down slightly to steady himself on the frame. This means that the required height does not depend upon the height of the patient so much as upon the reason he has for using it.

The height of a wooden quadripod should help him to stand straight, but it should not force him to walk with a sharply bent elbow, or push his weight over onto his damaged limb.

A walking cane should be short enough for him to swing it through with a slightly bent elbow, and to balance him comfortably when standing still. A good guide is the distance between his wrist and the ground when he stands straight with his arms by his sides.

Equipment at Home

The principle of teaching a patient on equipment he can use at home should always be remembered. Many elderly patients will continue to need aids to overcome a disability or as a preventive measure when the fracture is healed. A change to something different at the time of discharge will lead to the very dangers the equipment is supposed to eliminate. If a higher chair and toilet seat have been needed in the hospital, they will also be needed at home. If small scatter rugs create hazards they should be taken up. Adjustments of this kind are usually accepted readily at the time of discharge, but are less welcome at a later date.

Walking Frame or Crutches?

In the Newcastle Method of retraining the walking frame is almost invariably chosen instead of crutches, as being safer, more adaptable, and more practical for independent living. Elderly patients are unlikely to be using a walking aid on public transport where crutches would be an advantage, but they will be walking around their own homes and gardens, and perhaps down to the corner shop. In these places the walker is both safer and more useful. Some points in favour of the walking frame are:

1. It is stable and easy to control.
2. It gives confidence so that walking can begin early.
3. There is no danger of nerve damage by pressure in the axilla.
4. There are no parking and retrieval problems when sitting down.
5. It does not tend to slip on wet floors such as may be met in the bathroom or lavatory.
6. It demands less agility and sensory acuity than crutches.
7. It is safer in routine transfers.
8. It can be fitted with trays and bags to carry belongings and do the housework. This has particular importance for those patients who live alone.

For all these reasons the walking frame has become the aid of choice for elderly patients who are at risk.

Note. The wooden quadripod and two walking canes may help balance, but they do not reduce weight bearing, and they do not help to relieve pain as the walking frame can.

Footwear

Many frail elderly people wear unsuitable and even dangerous footwear because it is either smart or comfortable. The tight narrow shoes with a high heel and the lambswool slipper, twice the width of the patient's foot, can both lead to falls and fractures. It is surprisingly difficult to convince patients who lean towards either of these extremes that a low-heeled walking shoe would be better for them, but an attempt should be made. Many people tend to buy shoes with rubber soles in an effort to guard against slipping. It should be understood that in the older age groups tripping is more common, and so leather is safer and should be recommended. Leather is also safer in the presence of wet floors where rubber tends to slip and be dangerous.

Where swelling is present, particularly if only one foot is affected, it may not be possible to fit a suitable shoe. In such cases a felt boot may be the answer. These are made to open right down to the toe, and can be laced to fit almost any degree of swelling.

In some cases shortening may be present. A temporary build up can be made with cork or one of the new materials designed for the purpose if so ordered by the doctor. It should not be applied by a non-qualified person without authority and direction as to height. It is simple to apply if these requirements are met. If the temporary build up is successful, a simple permanent one can be applied by a bootmaker, but if there are complicated orthopaedic problems a surgical boot will be needed.

Pain and Fear

Pain is an almost inseparable part of beginning to walk again after a fractured femur. In many cases it is accentuated by tension and fear in the early days of retraining, and the patient's success in facing and overcoming it depends upon his own spirit. This makes it necessary for his helper to have skill in giving him confidence and encouragement. The intensity of the pain may vary from mild to severe, and the patient's tolerance of it will also vary widely. Whatever the patient's attitude to pain may be, some preparation for it will not go amiss. No patient should be encouraged to bear weight without a request from his doctor, but armed with such a request the helper can approach the patient with confidence, and provide the necessary encouragement.

The first effort should follow a pattern similar to the following.

The Helper's Approach

1. Ask the patient if he has much pain, and if so to tell you about it. (Let him put it in his own words.)
2. Tell him the doctor has said he can begin to take weight. (If the doctor has not given permission for weight bearing you should not be encouraging it in the first place.)
3. Explain that some pain is normal in the beginning.
4. Ask him to tell you if the pain becomes too severe, so that you can help him to sit down again. Let him feel that he is in control of this aspect, and do not push him to keep going once he asks to stop.
5. Give calm, definite directions, one at a time, and allow the patient plenty of time in which to follow them.
6. Give praise for a good try, even if results were not particularly good. The next try will almost certainly be better if this is done.

The First Try

It is important that the first attempt at standing and walking should be seen by the patient as a success, as this sets the pattern for subsequent efforts. Anything he is asked to do should be well within his capacity. At this stage assessment of his confidence and courage is as important as awareness of his physical capacity. If he is afraid or unreliable the helper should arrange for a second person to assist. A single helper should always stand on the side of the fracture, as any tendency to fall is likely to be towards that side. Helpers should give as little help as is consistent with safety, so that the patient will learn to rely upon his own efforts and not upon the helper's strength.

The first attempt at walking should proceed as follows.

1. Encourage the patient to stand up from his chair, pushing up with his strong leg and both hands.
2. Ask him to stand on his strong leg and to place both hands on the walking frame just in front of its back legs.
3. Let the patient feel his balance, leaning on his hands.
4. Ask him to push up on his hands and take his weight off his feet. He should try to clear the ground altogether, but some patients will be unable, either through fear or weakness, to do this on the first occasion. They should be encouraged but not forced.
5. Ask him to let himself down slowly onto his strong foot, controlling the downwards movement with his arms.
6. When he has mastered this, ask him to raise himself in the same way but to come down gently onto his weak foot. His arms will continue to take some weight if the pain becomes too severe.
7. If he complains of pain, and asks to sit down, allow him to do so. He will be more confident next time if he feels that he is in control of the situation.
8. If he manages well he should be taught to take a few steps as described on p. 287 (Partial Weight Bearing).

Note. Whether pain is present or not, the first session should be a short one. As in most retraining processes, little and often brings better results than too much too soon. Patients who become over-enthusiastic may have as many problems as the reluctant ones. They tend to 'crack hardy', and to bring upon themselves pain which they need not have. Pain has little value, except as a warning to go gently, or in severe cases, that all is not well. If pain is excessive, weight bearing should be discontinued until the problem has been discussed at the team meeting.

Pain on Rising and Sitting

After a fracture many patients find it difficult to lean forward and to push up with both legs when rising from a chair. If this is the result of stiffness alone, it may be useful to persevere with the movement as an exercise. If it is likely to remain a permanent disability, the patient's chair should be built up to a height from which he can rise unaided.

If temporary pain is the cause, it can be made less troublesome by the following procedures.

To Rise

1. Sit with the body turned slightly towards the strong side.
2. Place the weak foot slightly further forward than the strong foot.
3. Place the hand of the weak side on the strong knee.
4. Place the hand of the strong side on the arm of the chair.
5. Leaning slightly forward and to the strong side, push up with a steady movement until standing.
6. Place the hands on the walking frame, ready to move away.

To Sit Down

1. Turn the walking frame, and back up to the chair.
2. Feel the seat of the chair with the back of the legs.
3. Take a small step forward with the weak leg so that its foot is slightly ahead of the strong one.
4. Reach back for the arm of the chair on the strong side and transfer balance to that hand.
5. Reach back for the arm of the chair on the weak side.
6. Lean forwards and slightly to the strong side.
7. Lower the body slowly into the chair, controlling the downward movement with the strong leg and both arms.

Note 1. Patients who tend to flop backwards into their chair should be encouraged to watch their toes as they sit down. This ensures that the patient assumes the correct position. If permanent stiffness of the hip or knees makes this impossible, the patient probably needs a higher chair.

Note 2. As the fractured limb becomes stronger and less painful it should be brought progressively into the movement. This is achieved by sitting more squarely in the chair, and by bringing the weak foot back until it is level with the strong one.

Pain on Walking

Pain during walking with a walking frame can be controlled to some extent by the patient himself, if the method described on p. 287 (Partial Weight Bearing) is used. More or less weight can be taken by the painful limb, depending upon the extent to which the upper limbs are brought into use.

Aching at the site of the fracture after walking, particularly at night, is often a problem in the early stages. Patients should be warned of the possibility of this when training in walking is started so that they will not be afraid that some damage has been done. Most patients accept pain very well if reassured on this point. Medication may be requested if sleep is disturbed by the pain.

Analgesics

Control of medication is as always the responsibility of the doctor and the trained nurse. However, it is not always to these members of the team that the patient complains. Other team members who become aware of the problem (particularly if the patient is distressed, or is using it as an excuse for rejecting activity) should be careful to report the matter.

When analgesics are prescribed they should be given at a suitable time for the patient to gain full advantage from them in his walking practice, or when it is time for sleep. Much of the value is lost if the time does not relate to his programme.

Hazards and Steps

Because the patient has already suffered a serious fall it is not enough to ensure that he can walk on the uncluttered floors of the hospital. When he has learnt to do this he should be given practice over carpets, and taken outside for a trial on grass, gravel, and other rough ground.

Steps should also be practised, and a walk should be taken in a busy corridor amidst hurrying people. This applies whatever type of walking aid the patient will use on discharge. If a patient who has steps to negotiate does not progress beyond use of the walking frame, he may need to have two frames provided, one for use at the top and one at the bottom of the stairs. He would then ascend and descend sideways, holding a rail. Going down the weak side should go first, and going up the strong side should lead. Patients who need a walking frame on flat ground are unlikely to be safe enough to take it up and down the steps without help.

When possible, hazards should be removed for patients who do not achieve a reasonable degree of safety. These patients include the blind, those with residual balance problems or sensory disturbances such as those related to a stroke, and those who are confused or withdrawn, and unaware of their own safety. Badly placed furniture, electric cords, slippery surfaces, unsecured mats, children's toys, or even a demonstrative pet can all pose problems for such people. If they can be removed they should be. If not, both the patient and his relatives should be made aware of them. It is not good practice to clear the way for a patient who is walking with supervision, because he can gain experience by learning to cope with them in a safe situation.

Progress and Promotion

Most patients can become independent in the use of a walking frame. Some can progress further to a wooden quadrapod, a walking cane, or even to walking unaided. Whether they should be encouraged to do so depends upon home conditions and the reason for the original fall, just as much as it does upon the healing which has taken place in the limb. Patients should be made to feel safe and pleased with their efforts at each stage so that they will not feel they have failed if they cannot achieve the next. Safety should be the first consideration. It is far better to remain safely at home on a walking frame than to return to the hospital with a second fracture on a more advanced aid.

E. HEMIPLEGIA

Introduction

The treatment of hemiplegia has been the subject of many theories and many books. What is described here makes no claim to being another 'treatment'. *It is a method of managing the daily care of the patient in such a way that he learns from it.* By this method he is involved in his own progress, and becomes as independent as he can be at each stage of recovery.

Basic training in mobility and self care does not prevent those who can reach full independence from doing so, but it does help every patient to progress towards it without demonstrating failure along the way. At each stage the patient plays as active a part as he can in the activities of daily living, using the appropriate patterns of movement, and so becomes easier to help than he would have been without his 'drills'. This proves particularly useful when some residual disability is to be expected, and the patient is likely to need continued care. The high proportion of hemiplegic patients among the permanent residents of small hospitals and nursing homes is well known. Most of these people are there because no solutions have been found for practical problems posed by their residual disabilities. By considering the problems as well as the disease which produced them, retraining techniques give some hope to such people. They also contribute to the turnover of hospital beds without filling those of the nursing homes.

The Problems

The problems are usually practical ones related to the mental and physical ability of the patient to function in his former environment. The answers must include motivation and psychological support, training in the skills of self care, the supply of suitable equipment, and possibly alterations in the home. All these procedures should complement good medical care and are of little use without it.

In cases where full independence is not gained, the difficulties of the caring relative are as important as those of the patient.

Lifting, constant calls at night, and lack of time for shopping or relaxing are some of these problems. They are crucial to continuing support at home for the long period which may be involved. The patient's need for heavy help in daily care is more likely to prevent successful re-establishment at home than is a flaccid limb. What constitutes 'heavy help' differs with each patient depending upon the help available to him.

The programme described here takes account of these factors, accepting that the return of movement in a limb is of secondary value if it does not lead to useful function, if the patient is not motivated to use it, or if his relatives are over-protective and will not allow him to try to do things for himself. Routine retraining methods provide motivation, encouragement of self help, and the education of relatives in management of the case. Even minor gains by the patient are held to be worth while if they make this management easier or lead to further useful function.

Retraining Principles

The principles behind the retraining of hemiplegics are the same as those outlined for the general retraining programme (see Chapter 14).

The following concepts should be stressed:

(a) Emphasis is placed upon ability and not disability.
(b) Practical retraining begins where the patient is. It should not wait for the problematical return of useful function in damaged limbs.
(c) Each activity leads to the next so that there is no need for relearning at different stages of recovery.
(d) Routines are simple and direct. They can be learnt and applied by all grades of staff, and by the patient's own relatives.
(e) Lifting is minimised. The helper's job is to direct and guide the patient's own efforts and the patient's weight is distributed through his own limbs.
(f) Safety and good balance take precedence over postural considerations when there is conflict between the two.
(g) Training comes through performing everyday tasks using standardised movements.
(h) At each stage the patient is encouraged to do what he can for himself, however little that may be. He receives help with what he cannot yet manage.
(i) Pushing up is taught in preference to pulling up. Hand grips, rails, and overhead rings are not used.
(j) The patient is taught to lean slightly to the strong side in all his drills, and to rely upon his strong limbs whenever balance or safety are involved.
(k) The technique does not depend solely upon the patient's ability to understand instructions. Aphasia, hemianopia, or other perceptual disturbance may also be involved. Therefore

the technique is based on the principles of spherant conditioning.

Note. Some of these principles are controversial and cut across established practice. The test is 'Does it work?' rather than 'How has it always been done?' For example, the walking pattern is controversial because it is based upon early gait training and upon gaining balance by leaning sideways on the pylon instead of trying to maintain a perpendicular posture. The safety factor in leaning to the strong side gives confidence to the patient and leads to positive attitudes towards his programme. The psychological lift provided by such means more than compensates for any postural disadvantage. In more than two decades of use no spinal problems have been reported as a result of this posture. Patients progress towards an upright stance as recovery takes place and it becomes safe to do so. When recovery is incomplete many patients achieve a practical walk who would otherwise be confined to a wheelchair. The early and regular weight bearing helps to minimise the risks of flexion contractures associated with a bed- or chair-fast condition.

There is nothing to stop those patients who can progress to more sophisticated patterns from continuing treatment as outpatients as long as is required. Others continue to improve after discharge with help from relatives who have been taught retraining principles.

Method of Application

It has been the philosophy of the Royal Newcastle Hospital for many years that 'rehabilitation of the stroke patient should begin as soon as the patient is in physiological balance and his life is no longer at risk'. The therapeutics team begins the programme of mobilisation at this stage by applying the patterns of movement used in the techniques described below. The patient is helped through the movements and given the appropriate directions whether he appears to understand them or not. Most patients can follow the directions for the movements of their strong limbs unless there are communication or perceptual difficulties. If these are present visual clues should be given in conjunction with verbal instructions. As the patient's ability improves and he comes to understand what is required of him, the help is progressively withdrawn until he reaches his own maximum level of performance. In some cases continuing help will be necessary, but rarely will lifting remain a major part of the problem of caring for him at home.

Teaching is by repetition in real situations when motivation is at its best. Setting of immediate goals, within the patient's competence, and building upon success helps build confidence and motivation towards further effort. Association is provided by linking exercises with necessary activities and everyday equipment. There is no need to translate exercise into an activity in a different situation. Reinforcement is provided by consistent instructions from all who deal with the patient, and by recognition and praise for each advance, however small.

Equipment

General retraining equipment is discussed in Chapter 18. The principles outlined there apply to the hemiplegic patient as well as to those with other disabilities. Factors which relate particularly to the hemiplegic patient as described here should be read in conjunction with the general chapter. It must be stressed that any equipment used in the hospital must be available to the patient at home. If such equipment is still needed at the time of discharge, it should be provided, preferably on loan from the hospital. If necessary, the patient's own furniture should be modified to meet his new needs before he is discharged.

Factors to be considered are as follows.

Beds

1. The bed should be placed to allow the patient to enter and leave it on the appropriate side.

2. If there is sensory loss the weaker side should be nearer to the wall and the stronger to the side he uses to get in and out.

3. The bed should be stabilised so that it cannot slip if the patient leans against it.

4. Overhead rings should not be attached. If such a ring is part of the hospital bed it should be firmly tied up out of reach and nurses should be instructed not to use it.

5. The mattress should be firm, so as to assist controlled movements. A board base may be necessary on the patient's own bed.

6. The height should be such as to allow the patient to sit com-

fortably on the side with his feet placed firmly on the ground.

Chairs

1. A 'bridge' type chair is usually satisfactory. It is an advantage to have runners rather than legs. Runners make it safer and easier for the patient to move up to and back from a table independently — particularly if they must do this with only one functioning upper limb. It is easier for the helper to move a chair with runners for a seated patient.

2. The arms should be directly above, or inside the line of the legs to prevent the chair tipping sideways when the patient is getting in or out of the chair.

3. The seat should be straight, and wide enough for comfort. It should be high enough to permit easy standing, and well upholstered if the patient is likely to sit in it for extended periods.

4. The back should be almost straight, and well upholstered to give comfort and good support to the patient. The sloped seats and back of 'easy' chairs should be avoided because they discourage movement and independence.

5. The height should allow the patient to rise and sit easily. If this means that his feet cannot be placed firmly on the ground a stool should be provided. This will give support to the feet to prevent sliding, and will also guard against pressure from the edge of the seat on the back of the thighs.

Wheelchairs

Wheelchairs are used sparingly so that the patient will not come to rely upon them. Disability and invalidism are associated with wheelchairs in many minds, and there is positive psychological value to the patient in sitting in an ordinary chair. At the stage when a wheelchair is necessary for transport, the patient should transfer to an ordinary chair when he reaches his destination.

1. Good brakes are essential. They should be firmly applied whenever a patient attempts a transfer, and when the chair is not in motion.

2. The helper must be very aware of the danger of damage to the patient's lower limbs if they are knocked against the footplates. Patients with sensory disturbances or flaccid limbs are particularly at risk. It may be necessary to pad the plates or to apply a protective bandage to the patient's limbs. Footplates which can be moved aside are helpful, but they are not always available.

Baths and Showers

1. Traditional domestic baths, at a height of approximately 20 inches (50cm) from the ground are the most satisfactory. They are used in conjunction with a hand shower or suitably placed overhead shower, and a bathboard.

2. Adjustments must be made to the bathboard to fit the patient's own bath when necessary. A small hand grip is attached to the board to be used if balance remains a problem. It is not there to be used to pull the patient along the board. For this he should push up on his strong hand and move as in moving along the side of the bed. In fitting the bathboard the handle is placed near the wall.

3. If the patient normally uses a shower at home he should practise using a shower during retraining, and not waste time on 'bath drill' which he will not need.

4. A shower chair is used in the shower recess if there are no obstructions such as a hob at the entrance. If there should be such an obstruction a long stool can be placed with two of its legs inside, and two outside the wall. The patient sits on the outside part of the stool, and moves along, lifting his feet over the obstruction.

Toilet Facilities

1. Commodes with arms are used by the bedside, heights being adjusted to the needs of the individual. Each female patient should have her own commode.

2. Urinals are used at night by male patients who are taught to empty them directly after use into a bucket by the bed.

3. If the lavatory seat is too low for easy rising, a removable stool of the correct height is provided.

4. In the retraining unit toilet rolls are fitted on both sides of the lavatory. In the home it may be necessary to fit one within the patient's reach.

5. A device for one-handed tearing of paper may help.

Walking Aids

1. A wooden pylon is preferred to a metal quadripod because it gives more stability and a greater sense of security. As a result patients walk independently more quickly, and are less inclined to walk close to walls when left to go alone.

2. For cosmetic reasons some younger patients ask for a metal

stick. If they are safe with this they can usually progress to a walking cane, but each case is decided on its merits.

3. A tray and a handbag can be attached to the wooden pylon for carrying belongings.

4. Walking frames are only used if there is a complicating problem such as rheumatoid arthritis, a fracture, or an intractable balance problem. In such cases adaptations are usually needed (see Chapter 19).

Minor Personal Equipment

This may include:

1. A back slab to support a flaccid knee in the early stages of walking.

2. Special boots to accommodate oedematous feet or support an unstable ankle.

3. Bandaging over a shoe or boot to give extra support to a flaccid ankle.

4. A sling to support a hemiplegic arm, to minimise a tendency towards subluxation of the shoulder and stretching of the joint capsule. It also helps with the problem of oedema and pain, and facilitates balance.

5. A caliper may be prescribed for a few selected cases after other measures have proved inadequate. Apart from a certain amount of patient resistance for cosmetic reasons, a caliper is difficult to apply single handed, and so may inhibit independence.

Rails

Rails are rarely needed, because the methods taught rely upon the patient pushing up on the surface on which he lies or sits. Pulling up on additional equipment is discouraged because it limits the patient to places where such equipment is provided, encourages movements of flexion rather than extension, leads to unnecessary expensive alterations at home, and interferes with the patient's routine retraining drills.

The Drills for Hemiplegics

The following notes provide a 'job breakdown' of the various movements needed by the hemiplegic patient for independence through routine retraining.

Principles and Concepts

1. Concentration on maximum use of the strong limbs.
2. Distribution of body weight over the strong limbs.
3. Actual help to the patient kept to the minimum required for safety.
4. Gradual progression, building strength on strength. Literally 'one step at a time'.
5. Teaching of pushing up and leaning rather than pulling up and holding.
6. Constant repetition and habit forming as the basis of teaching.
7. Generous praise for a 'good try'.

Sitting in a Chair

Many hemiplegic patients are quite unable to support themselves when first allowed out of bed to sit in a chair. They tend to lean strongly to the weak side, and to be very restless. Eventually they are in danger of sliding to the ground. The natural reaction of most helpers is to prop them up with cushions on the weak side, most will agree that this brings only very short-term relief, and that these patients need almost constant supervision and repositioning. The

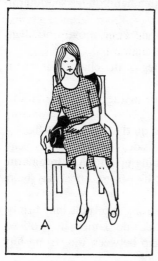 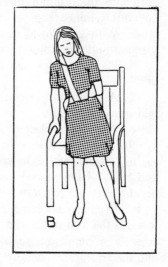

Figure 17.4: A. Hemiplegic patient sits in a chair supported by a low cushion on the strong side. B. Hemiplegic patient rises from a chair balanced over her strong limbs

following procedure, based upon retraining principles, has been found to be more comfortable for the patient, and less frustrating for the nurse (see Figure 17.4A and B).

1. Ensure that the patient is using a suitable chair. It should be low enough for his feet to be placed firmly on the ground. If they cannot be so placed, a stool should be provided. The seat of the chair should slope slightly backwards, but it should not be so deep that there is a space between the patient and the back of the chair. If such a space exists it should be eliminated by a firm cushion which should be attached to the chair by tapes so that it cannot slip. Two smaller cushions should be ready for supporting the patient when he is repositioned.

2. Whatever the patient's mental condition, stand on his strong side, gain his attention, and tell him what you are going to do.

3. If the patient can co-operate ask him to work with you in the moves as described. If he cannot, have a helper who will assist you in putting him through the same moves. In both cases, give a step by step explanation as you proceed.

4. Stand on the patient's weak side, and help him to sit upright. Support him in this position with a hand on his shoulder if he tends to fall back.

5. With your hand against his strong knee move both legs together until his hips are straight in the chair.

6. Place his weak foot against the leg of the chair, as in chair drill.

7. Ask him to place his strong foot in the centre under the mid-line of his body.

8. Ask him to place his strong hand on the arm of the chair.

9. Ask him to lean to the strong side, and to lift his seat slightly off the seat of the chair, by pushing up with his strong arm and leg. A hand placed firmly against his strong knee may help him to carry out this move.

10. Placing your hand against his strong hip, pull him firmly towards the arm of the chair on the weak side. Unless he is obese or of large build, this should leave a gap between the strong hip and the arm of the chair on the strong side.

11. Pack the larger of the two cushions in this gap so that he cannot move back into the space.

12. Check the position of his feet to make sure that the weak

one is placed widely, and the strong one is under the mid-line of his body.

13. Bring the weak shoulder forward and support it by placing the smaller cushion behind it in the corner of the chair.

14. If necessary attach this cushion to the back of the chair with tapes or a band of webbing.

15. Speak to the patient, standing on his strong side, and ask if he is more comfortable.

Note 1. The patient usually remains comfortable and safe in this position for extended periods. His strong limbs are placed so that he can use them to push himself back if he starts to slide. He can relieve the pressure and discomfort caused by long sitting by placing his strong elbow on the arm of the chair and pushing up with the strong limbs. In this way he feels more able to control his own position.

Note 2. The patient who has been restless because of discomfort can relax in this position, but a new patient who still has some degree of cerebral oedema must be expected to remain restless. It may be necessary to use some form of restraint for these patients, but they should not be subjected to the indignity of being tied in by a folded sheet. A lap/sash seat belt, as fitted to cars, is more efficient and more acceptable to the patient. It should be shown to him and explained as a safety measure such as we all wear in cars and aeroplanes. This should be done whether the patient appears to understand or not. Being less obtrusive and more comfortable than other forms of restraint it does not produce the same resentment and frantic efforts to remove it. Some special jackets are also available and have proved useful.

Chair Drill (Figure 17.5)

The ability to rise and sit is essential to independence. It is important that the patient be taught this drill as soon as possible rather than becoming accustomed to being lifted. The drill is done by placing two chairs facing each other and then encouraging the patient to rise from one, turn, and sit in the other. It is the basis of the other drills.

It should be used every time the patient is transferred from one seat to another (bed, chair, wheelchair, commode, bathboard, car seat etc.). Correct placement of the patient's feet and hands is essential, and except in the very early stages there should be no

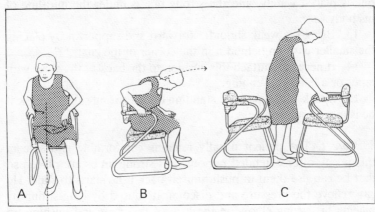

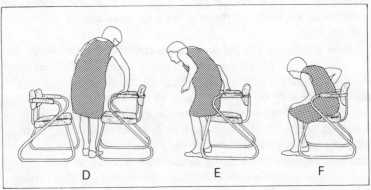

Figure 17.5: Chair Drill for Hemiplegic Patients. A. Hemiplegic patient positions herself in a chair when preparing to rise. B. Patient pushes herself forwards and upwards using her strong limbs. C. Patient stands and transfers her strong hand to opposite chair. D. Patient turns to weak side transferring her strong hand to the other arm of 2nd chair. E. Patient leans to her strong side and lowers herself slowly into chair avoiding a 'flop'. F. Patient moves back in the chair and makes herself comfortable

need for actual lifting by the helper if this is understood. On no account should the patient be dragged up by the helper's arm in the axilla, as this can lead to serious damage to the shoulder joint.

The movements are as follows.

1. Seat the patient in a suitable chair.

2. Place a similar chair opposite, approximately 5 inches (12cm) from his knees.

3. See that the patient can place his feet firmly on the ground. If necessary see that he moves forward in the chair to accomplish this.

4. Place the patient's weak foot so that the heel touches the leg of the chair. Make him aware of this move and gain his co-operation in attempting it.

5. Ask him to place his strong foot back in line with the chair legs, and under the mid-line of his body (see Figure 17.5A).

6. If the weak arm is not held in position by a sling, place it across the body to the strong side, thus bringing the weak shoulder forward.

7. Place the patient's strong hand forward on the arm of the chair in a comfortable position with the elbow held close to the side of his body.

8. Standing on his weak side, place your hand between his arm and his body, with the back of your hand pressing gently against his ribs. Do not grip his arm with your hand, or support the patient with your arm high under his axilla. The first of these procedures can lead to bruising or abrasions, and the second to structural damage to the shoulder joint if the patient should lose his balance.

9. Allow the upper part of your forearm to support the patient gently, just behind the shoulder, making your arm a firm bar which will give him confidence. The patient should not be dragged up by the hemiplegic arm.

10. Tell the patient to lean forwards and towards the strong side, and to push up with his strong leg and strong arm. Ideally, the strong leg should raise the body, while the strong arm acts as an auxiliary. If the effort made by the arm exceeds that of the leg the patient's weight will be pushed over to the weak side and balance will be lost (see Figure 17.5B).

11. If necessary, give just enough support to keep the weak side level with the work the patient is doing with his own strong limbs, but do not lift or allow the patient to lean back towards his weak side while you take his weight.

12. Encourage the patient to stand and balance his own weight. To do this his strong foot must be below the mid-line of his body. The weak limb should take progressively more weight as it becomes able to do so with safety.

13. Ask the patient to transfer his strong hand to the arm of the opposite chair, and to lean on it to help him balance (see Figure 17.5C).

14. Making sure that his weak foot clears the leg of the chair, ask him to pivot on his strong foot towards the other arm of the new chair. Some patients understand this move better if asked to stand on the ball of the foot and turn their heel towards the leg of the chair.

15. Ask the patient to place his strong hand on the far arm of the new chair, with his fingers pointing outwards. Balance again on to the strong hand (see Figure 17.5D).

16. Pivot again on the strong foot and in the same direction until facing the original chair. Throughout the movements the weight should be balanced over the strong limbs.

17. Ensure that the patient is straight with his new chair, and bending slightly forwards and to the strong side (see Figure 17.5E).

18. Ask him to lower himself slowly into the chair without a 'flop'. To do this he must bend his elbow and knee in unison. If the elbow is held too rigidly, his weight will be pushed over to the weak side leading to loss of balance. Patients who do not understand how to bend their hips and knees as they go down, sometimes do better if asked to watch their toes as long as they can.

19. The downwards movement is the reverse of the one used for rising (see Figure 17.5F).

The position of the body and the balance are the same, but in rising the patient pushes up against gravity, and in sitting he goes down resisting it enough to control the movement.

Note. Patients who have trouble in rising and sitting sometimes benefit from an exercise where they change direction half way up and down. Chair drill should be repeated as a lesson two or three times daily in the early stages until it is mastered. It should also be used every time a patient is moved from chair to bed, bed to commode, wheelchair to car seat, and in fact, whenever the patient changes one seating surface for another.

Bed Drill

Bed drill is divided into two actions — learning to get in and out safely, and learning to move in bed. The first is based very closely on chair drill. In both, the main principles involved are those of keeping the weight over the strong limbs, and of pushing rather than pulling. Bed drill is particularly important for resettlement as it teaches the patient how to avoid the need for lifting by a second person. It also teaches the independent use of a commode so that the family need not be disturbed if it is needed at night.

Before Getting into Bed

Placement of the patient's bed and bedside furniture should be considered in relationship to his needs and not to suit the symmetry of the ward. Access should be on the patient's strong side when he is actually in bed, and his locker and commode should also be on that side so that he can reach them safely. This is particularly important for patients who have diminished awareness on the hemiplegic side. Staff members and relatives should approach the patient on this side so that he can be aware of their presence.

The patient's bed at home should be placed so that he can use the same side as he has used in hospital. Occasionally such placement may not be possible, and only in such cases should the patient be retrained to use the weak side for access.

Getting into Bed — Adaptation of Basic Method to Hemiplegia

1. Turn the bedclothes right back so there is no need to pull them from under the patient's body once he is on the bed.
2. The patient should use that side of the bed which allows him to sit on the edge with his strong side near the pillows.
3. If the patient is in a wheelchair, place it so that he faces the bed just below the pillows with his weak side towards them.
4. If he walks with a pylon or cane, ask him to walk to the head of the bed and face across it with his weak side towards the pillows.
5. Teach the patient in the chair to rise as in chair drill.
6. In both cases ask the patient to proceed in the following way.
7. Place the strong hand on the bed, about 6 inches (15 cm) in from the edge, and lean on that hand.
8. Pivot towards the pillows on the strong foot as in chair drill.
9. Move the strong hand 10 inches (25 cm) closer to the pillows, lean on it, and complete the pivot, until he has turned far enough to sit safely on the bed. Throughout this manoeuvre he should be leaning to his strong side.
10. The patient should now be sitting close to the pillows, but if he is not well placed he should move up or down on the side of the bed, by leaning to his strong side and pushing up with his strong

limbs as if to rise, and at the same time moving himself in the required direction.

11. The patient should be sitting well back on the bed. This may be difficult if the patient's bed is too high.

12. Place the strong foot under the weak ankle, and with a rocking movement, swing both legs up on to the bed. At the same time the head should go back on to the pillows.

13. If the patient is unable to swing his legs up unaided, he may be assisted by the helper supporting his shoulders with one hand, and placing the other under his crossed legs. Saying 'One, two, three — up!' she should put him through the same movement he is intended eventually to manage himself. The patient should be involved at each step of the movement and try to assist the helper so that he will eventually learn the knack for himself.

Moving in Bed

Many hemiplegics find it difficult to move back in the bed, to turn over for comfort, and to sit up unaided. These patients should be taught to roll over on to the strong side, and then to move their bodies by pushing against the mattress. The movements involved should be taught to the patient by the night staff when he needs to be turned over so that he learns them in the conditions which apply when he is sleepy, and the ward is dimmed.

Turning Over to the Strong Side. The patient should bend the strong leg until the foot can be placed under the knee of the weak leg. The weak arm should be placed across the body to bring the weak shoulder as far forward as possible. By pressing the strong foot into the mattress, and pulling the strong shoulder back towards the body the patient should be able to learn to roll to the strong side in a controlled manner.

Turning Over to the Weak Side. The weak arm should be placed a little away from the body so that it will not be completely underneath the body when the movement is complete. The strong knee (and if possible, both knees) should be drawn up with the feet placed flat on the bed. The patient should reach directly across his body with his strong arm, placing his strong hand on the far edge of the bed. At the same time, his knees should be rocked over towards the weak side, so that the whole body turns in that direction.

Rolling Drill. These two turning movements can be combined in an exercise so that the patient moves alternately from one side to the other in a smooth rolling motion. They may be practised during the day in a mat class (see Appendix C) or on the patient's own bed. These exercises will reinforce the practice in real conditions at night time.

Moving up in Bed — Outside Method. This method can be used for patients who have not yet mastered the turn to the strong side. It makes it possible for one person to move the patient instead of the two who are needed for a shoulder lift. At the same time it gives the patient practice in self help. It is an important move for patients who are likely to need continued help at home, because it involves positioning rather than lifting.

The helper should ask the patient to proceed as follows.

1. Place the strong foot under the weak ankle so that it can support it during the move.
2. Sit up, pushing up on the strong elbow. If he needs help, the helper should place her hand behind his back and give light pressure behind the weak shoulder.
3. Raise the lower limbs slightly and, swivelling on the buttocks, place the legs over the side of the bed.
4. Sit up by pushing up with the strong arm, and make sure to place the feet safely on the floor.
5. Place the strong hand on the edge of the bed, about 7 inches (18 cm) away from the body.
6. Lean forwards, and slightly to the strong side, and begin to rise as in chair drill.
7. Move the hips towards the strong hand, and then sit again on the side of the bed.
8. Repeat steps 5 to 7 as often as necessary to reach the required position on the bed (see Figure 17.6A).
9. Place the strong foot under the weak one to support it.
10. Reverse the outwards movement and swing the feet back into the bed. If help is needed the helper should place one hand behind his shoulders and one arm under his knees, and work in concert with his efforts, using the words 'one, two, three — up!'
11. The helper should make the patient comfortable by ensuring that he is in a good position, and that pillows and bedclothes are appropriately arranged.

Note 1. Some patients find it easier to get right up in the bed if the pillows are removed before this manoeuvre, and are arranged when the patient is safely back in bed.

Note 2. Movement along the side of the bed is a natural movement, and is easily managed by the majority of patients. Moving to the weak side needs a little more practice than moving to the strong one, but does not usually cause much difficulty. The patient must still lean to the strong side to half-rise, but should push his hips away from his strong hand instead of moving towards it.

Note 3. As well as being useful for moving along the side of the bed, this drill is used in moving along a sofa to make room for someone else, in moving along a car seat after entering so that the door can be safely shut, and in moving along to the centre of a bathboard. Like chair drill, it is one of the basic movements of the Newcastle Method.

Moving up in Bed — Inside Method. Turning slightly to the strong side (see p. 310) the patient should bend the strong leg until it can be placed under the weak leg in such a way that its heel can press into the mattress. He should then press up with the strong elbow to raise his shoulders. By straightening his strong knee at the same time he should lift his body backwards, carrying the hemiplegic limbs. He should avoid throwing his head back on to the pillows, or letting his shoulders down on to the bed until the move is completed.

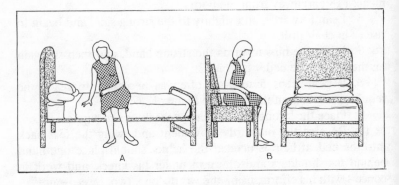

Figure 17.6: Bed Drill and Commode Drill. A. Moving along the edge of the bed to move closer to the pillows. B. Using chair drill to get out on to the commode and back again.

Note. This movement usually needs more practice than the previous one, but is more convenient for the patient who masters it. Obese patients, and those who are severely disabled or suffer from impaired body image do not learn it readily, and are probably better served by the outside method. Other complicating illness or disability must be taken into account when determining which method to employ.

Sitting up in Bed. The patient should turn on to his strong side as described on p. 310. He should then press his elbow into the mattress to raise his shoulders from the bed, leaning towards the strong side. By straightening his elbow he should then come up to a sitting position, supporting himself on his strong hand. In the early stages help may be given by helping him to keep his weak shoulder forward. Some patients find it easier to sit with their legs over the side of the bed rather than sitting straight up with their legs on the bed.

Getting out of Bed

Getting out of bed is a danger point for falls and the patient should be encouraged to pause at each part of the drill to make sure he has his balance before going on to the next step. Balance is often disturbed at night and when the patient first rises, so the patient should be made aware of the need for extra caution. The drill itself is very important for use at home because it is the first part of getting out to a commode. If independence is not reached in this, independent night care may present insuperable problems.

1. Teach the patient to use his strong hand to place his weak arm across his body, and so bring his shoulder forward. Help may be necessary at first, but the patient should make an attempt from the beginning, to help him become aware of his damaged limb.
2. Follow steps 1 to 4 as in 'Moving Up in Bed — Outside Method'. At the end of this the patient should be sitting safely on the side of the bed with his feet firmly on the ground. He should wriggle forward if necessary to achieve this.
3. If the transfer is to a wheelchair or a commode, the article should be placed facing the patient where he sits on the side of the bed. He should place his hand on the edge of the bed, and stand by leaning to the strong side and pushing up with his strong limbs. He should then complete chair drill by transferring his strong hand to

the chair arm, and pivoting as described on p. 305.

4. Care should be taken by the helper to ensure that the patient's feet are safely placed on the footplates, and that the flaccid arm is in his lap before the wheelchair is moved. The patient should be made conscious of this positioning of his limbs, and encouraged to take responsibility for them.

5. If the patient is rising to walk with a pylon stick, this should be placed 4 to 6 inches (10 to 15 cm) wide of the strong leg, and at right angles to the bed. The patient should place his strong hand on the edge of the bed, lean slightly to the strong side, and push up firmly with his strong limbs. A jerking or swinging movement should be avoided. When balance is achieved he should transfer his hand to the pylon, and lean on it before starting to walk. The whole movement should be controlled, and he should not grab for the pylon when half way up, as over-anxious patients tend to do.

6. Before starting to walk the patient should be reminded to take a breath and look about him. This helps to establish balance and minimises the danger of falls.

Commode Drill (Figure 17.6B)

Commode drill is simply a combination of chair drill and bed drill. It is most important for patients to become independent at this for their own self respect, and also for the sake of relatives, who find constant calls for attention at night an almost unbearable burden. Independence at night can mean the difference between going home and having to be placed in a nursing home.

1. The commode should be placed near the bed on the side that the patient uses to get in and out. It should face the bed, and be far enough away from it to give room for pivoting and for swinging the legs up again on the return to bed.

2. The patient should sit on the side of the bed, as explained in bed drill (follow steps 1 to 4 as in 'Moving up in Bed — Outside Method'). If necessary, he should wriggle forward to ensure that his feet are safely grounded (see p. 311).

3. The strong foot should be placed under the mid-line of the body, and the weak foot about 6 inches (15 cm) away from it to the weak side.

4. The patient should lean forwards and to the strong side, and push up with his strong leg as in chair drill.

5. When standing, he should transfer his strong hand to the arm

of the commode and complete the usual chair drill.

6. If his balance is good, the clothes can be arranged before he sits down. If not, this should be done when seated.

7. To return to bed the patient stands as in chair drill, places his strong hand on the bed and leans on it and uses the drill for getting into bed.

Use of a Urinal

Male patients usually use a urinal at night. So as to avoid spillage, or the need for someone else to empty it after use, a bucket is placed beside the bed on a plastic sheet, and the patient is taught to empty the urinal into it himself after each use.

Note. Close supervision of toilet drills is necessary at night until the patient is absolutely reliable because it is more difficult to act safely when half asleep and in semi-darkness than in a training situation during the day.

Bath Drill (Figure 17.7)

There is often a certain amount of fear of falling in the bathroom until patients become used to the routine, and it is necessary to give directions clearly and with confidence. If the patient needs support this should be given by placing the arm between the patient's arm and his body from the back, so as to provide firm support, at the same time this leaves the helper's other arm free to help when necessary in moving the weak leg.

The helping arm should not be used for lifting by pressing up in the axilla, but as a steadying agent, pressed gently against the rib cage, while the patient learns to use his own limbs.

The bath seat is placed at that end of the bath which allows the patient to enter with his strong side towards the wall. A chair without arms, and of equal height to the top of the bath seat, is placed beside the board so that there is no gap (see Figure 17.7).

During all movements the patient should lean towards his strong side while the helper gives light support, if necessary, on the weak side.

1. The patient sits on the chair to undress.

2. He places his hand on the board, and beginning to rise as in chair drill, swings himself to the strong side so as to sit on the end of the board.

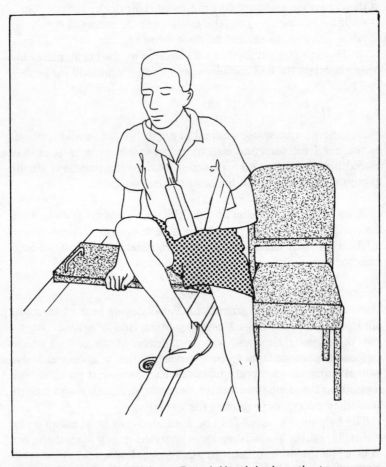

Figure 17.7: Bath Drill Using a Board. Hemiplegic patient moves on to a bathboard from a chair of appropriate height placed beside the bath

3. The patient puts his strong leg into the bath, and moves along a little way on the board.

4. He puts his weak leg into the bath. He may need help with this, but should try to achieve it unaided by lifting it with his strong hand. Some patients manage by placing the strong foot under the weak one, and lifting both in together as in bed drill.

5. He should move up to the middle of the bathboard, using the same movement as in Bed Drill ('Moving up in Bed — Outside

Method' p. 311). The patient sits on the board to wash or to be washed.

6. When washed the patient moves back to the outer end of the board and puts his weak leg over the edge of the bath — or is helped to do so if necessary.

7. He moves a little further and puts his strong foot out, grounding it safely on the floor.

8. With his strong hand on the board he half stands, moving his body across to sit safely on the chair. He should make sure he is sitting comfortably in a well-balanced position.

9. He dries himself, or is dried, seated on the chair. He should then stand, with help if necessary, to be dried underneath.

Note 1. A towel placed on the chair before use facilitates drying and adds to the patient's comfort.

Note 2. Heavy patients and those with sensory loss find bath drill easier if the chair is placed about six inches further back than the bathboard before they enter the bath, and six inches further forward before they move out again. This means that they sit further back on the bathboard going in, and further back in the chair when coming out. It also gives the patient with sensory loss more chance of seeing the chair and knowing it is there.

The manoeuvre is not recommended for the average patient who is expected to regain independence, because it demands the help of a second person to move the chair and thus works against the final aim.

Shower Drill

Some patients strongly prefer a shower to a bath, and others only have a shower at home. It is a waste of time to train them in bath drill, and a shower should be substituted. If possible, arrangements should be made for a hose-type shower to be fitted at home if only a fixed one is present. This makes it easier for the patient to direct the stream more selectively. It also makes it easier for any helper he may need to avoid being soaked at the same time as the patient.

A sturdy chair which cannot be damaged by water should be provided. The patient should approach it and sit down, using his ordinary chair drill. He washes himself while seated.

If a hob prevents him from walking into the recess, a long stool may be necessary. Two of the stool legs are placed inside the hob, and two outside. The patient sits on the stool outside the recess and moves along as in bath drill. He lifts his feet over the hob as he would lift them over the side of the bath.

Car Drill

Car drill is another extension of chair drill. It is important in that it makes outings possible for a patient whose family can arrange it, and also makes possible the use of voluntary or taxi transport instead of an ambulance for those who are to continue treatment as an out-patient.

For the walking patient the drill is as follows:

1. Open the car door as widely as possible.
2. Walk right up to the seat of the car, facing inwards, and standing as close as possible.
3. Place the strong hand on the car seat. Pivot on the strong leg as in chair drill.
4. Move the strong hand along the seat and complete the turn. The patient should now be facing outwards with his back to the driver's seat.
5. Sit down slowly on the seat, being careful not to bump the head on the way down.
6. If necessary, move backwards on the seat to leave more room for bringing the feet in.
7. Put the feet in the car. The patient may be able to do this unaided, using the method he uses to put his feet into the bath. He may need some help to bend his knee and ease in the foot.

Note 1. In cases where the patient cannot wriggle back far enough on the seat the following procedure may help:

1. Ask him to place his strong hand on the seat behind him to prop himself up, and to place his strong foot against the helper's cupped hands at the level of the surface of the seat. The knee should be straightened and remain so throughout the move.
2. At an agreed signal he should try to raise himself on his strong hand, leaning slightly to the strong side. At the same time the helper should push against the stiffened strong lower limb.
3. The patient should slide gently back along the seat. If the first push does not move the patient far enough, the process should be repeated.

4. When he has moved far enough his feet should be swung round into the car in the usual way.

Note 2. This method is much less strenuous for the helper, and much less uncomfortable for the patient than the usual one of pulling him in by the armpits from the other side of the car. If the patient's feet are safely in the car, but he is too close to the door, he should move along the seat by using the method for moving along the side of the bed as described in Bed Drill (p. 311).

Note 3. The patient must be securely balanced before the car moves, not only for his own comfort, but also to ensure that he does not fall towards the driver and hinder her movements. The patient's feet should be placed firmly on the floor, about 10 inches apart. The seat belt should be firmly adjusted, and packing pillows should be provided when necessary.

Standing Exercise

In order to feel confident in attempting to regain his mobility, the patient must learn to stand and balance himself, and to experience again the bearing of weight through his hemiplegic lower limb. This is begun at a wall bar, preferably near an open window, and is an adaptation of Dr Marjorie Warren's *Bed End Exercises.* The patient is encouraged to use his hand to balance himself, but not to pull himself up. The lower limbs should be used to push up, because the exercise is designed to strengthen the lower limbs and accustom the patient to standing and weight bearing.

In the early stages some positioning and physical help may be necessary. The exercise is usually done three or four times on the first occasion with whatever help may be necessary. It is then built up until it can be performed twenty or more times unaided. As the patient's strength and ability improve, the weak lower limb should be brought progressively into the movement. The procedure is as follows:

1. The patient is seated facing the wall bar in a chair with arms and a straight seat. He is given instructions, and if necessary helped to carry out the following movements.

2. Place the weak arm in the lap if it is not supported by a sling.

3. Place the strong hand on the bar, about six inches wide of the body on the strong side.

4. Bring the weak shoulder forward.

5. Lean the body towards the strong hand.

6. Push up with the strong leg doing most of the work until a standing position is reached. Look out the window and relax.

7. Stand so as to be as tall as possible. (It helps some patients if the helper places her hand on the top of his head and asks him to push it higher.)

8. Lean slightly forward and to the strong side, to get into position for sitting down again.

9. Lower yourself slowly into the chair by bending your hips and knees together, watching your toes as you go down.

10. Control the downwards movement with the strong limb. Do not allow yourself to 'flop'.

Note. Flopping down into the chair should be discouraged from the beginning because it develops a careless movement which when transferred to chair drill can lead to falls. The exercise provided by a controlled downwards movement is as important as the exercise provided by pushing up. Besides the part it plays in safe chair drill it encourages balance and security in the early stages of walking. If the patient tends to fall back into his chair he should practise half rising and sitting again with his gaze on his toes. If weak knees tend to let him down suddenly, or make him unable to start and finish the drill with proper control, it may be helpful to raise the height of the seat by providing a firm cushion until his strength improves.

Walking (see also Chapter 16)

Before any attempt is made to walk, the patient should have mastered one-legged standing at the wall bar. He should also be reasonably competent at chair drill. He should feel safe standing on his strong leg and leaning on his strong hand. If there has been no return of tone in the affected lower limb he may need a back slab (knee splint) at this stage but this is used only while he is actually being taught, and is removed at other times. Every attempt should be made to teach him to lock his knee before resorting to a splint.

The walking method is kept as simple as possible, and as with the other drills it is taught by positioning and repetition. As soon as possible, the wheelchair should be discarded, and each move should be seen as an opportunity to practise. When we first learnt to walk we found our feet by pulling up on furniture moving around stable objects, and then stepping out flat footed and stiff legged until balance was gained. Only then did we develop the refinements of raised knees and heel and toe co-ordination. Elderly patients who are relearning the art respond well to this simple natural programme. Alert patients learn more quickly, but one of the main strengths of the method is that even mentally deteriorated patients and those with sensory loss can learn the pattern.

Basic Principles

1. Ensure that the pylon is the correct height (see below).

2. Help the patient from his weak side.

3. Teach the patient to lean sideways and to take weight down through the pylon. He should not push up and away from it.

4. Teach him to relax, and not to grip the pylon too tightly. He should be leaning on the palm of his hand, not gripping with his fingers.

5. Teach him to see that all four legs of the pylon are safely grounded before he takes each step.

6. Teach accurate movements from the beginning to guard against bad habits and the need for relearning. Changes should come as a development of the original pattern, and not as a new technique.

7. Repeat instructions one at a time, and give the patient time to carry them out, until the pattern becomes automatic.

8. Hold the patient as lightly as possible consistent with safety.

9. Never hurry the patient. If he needs to get to his destination quickly (for example, the toilet or an appointment) use a wheelchair rather than letting standards drop or causing him stress.

10. Help the patient to be pleased with his progress, and with the pylon as an aid. Do not encourage the use of a cane unless you are sure that he has the capacity to use one. If necessary, explain the value of the pylon to relatives. Their expectations should not exceed the patient's grasp.

The Height of the Pylon

The height of the pylon should be such as to cause the user to lean slightly to the strong side when he stands with it beside him, and holds it with a straight elbow. This is achieved if the overall height of the pylon equals the distance between the patient's wrist and the ground when he stands upright.

Average heights are:

Small Women	28 inches or 70 cm
Average Women	30 inches or 76 cm
Small Men	30 inches or 76 cm
Average Men	32 inches or 81 cm

Very occasionally, a 34 inch pylon may be needed, but it should be remembered that tall people usually have long upper limbs as well as long lower ones, and the difference at the level of the hands is not very great between the tall and the short.

The technique is learnt more quickly if the height of the pylon enforces the appropriate lean. In the early stages a pylon that is too short is preferred to one that is too tall. This gives more confidence as well as teaching the patient to lean on his stick instead of his helper. A higher pylon may be given later as he gains in strength and confidence.

The Method of Support

Normally, the hemiplegic patient should be able to stand at the wall bar, taking his weight on his strong leg and balancing himself with his strong arm before attempting to walk. It is a small step from this achievement to standing on the strong leg and balancing by leaning on the pylon. Demented patients, and those with some sensory disturbances, may need to start their walking without first conquering the wall bar. These will be discussed on pp. 337–45.

The helper should see her task as positioning and teaching, and not as a supporting agent or auxiliary pylon. Her hold should be light, but her concentration on the patient and what he is doing should be intense. Patients do not usually feel secure if held tightly, because the helper's tension is transmitted through her grip. The patient who senses that there is help available if it is needed, but that effort is expected of him in the meantime, is more likely to feel confident and keen to do well. The safety of the light hold depends mainly upon correct placement of the helper's hand, and her watchfulness over the placement of the patient's feet.

1. The patient's pylon should be placed in readiness on his

strong side, with its back legs level with the front legs of the chair, and its front legs pointing directly ahead.

2. The helper should stand on the patient's weak side, and help him perform the standing part of chair drill (see p. 305).

3. When the patient is standing, the helper's forearm should be between his arm and his body, pressing lightly against the rib cage. It should not press up in the axilla to take his weight. Not only does the latter position lead to damage to the shoulder joint, but it also throws the patient off balance, and stops him from using his strong limbs to good advantage.

4. Having stood up, the patient should place his strong hand on the pylon, and lean on it.

5. The patient supports himself on his strong leg, leaning for balance on his strong arm. The strong foot should be under the mid-line of his body. This position is the natural foot placement for anyone standing on one leg. (Helpers should stand on one leg themselves and analyse their own position when learning this drill.)

6. By these methods the patient is supported on the strong side by his own strong limbs, and the helper is ready to give extra support on the weak side if it should be needed.

7. Patients whose weak knee is not yet able to lock when weight is applied may need a back slab in the early stages. This can usually be discarded when weight bearing is established, but if the problem is not resolved, a caliper may be indicated. As it is very difficult for a hemiplegic patient to apply a full length caliper to his own limb, every effort should be made to achieve safe weight bearing before such support is provided.

8. A flaccid ankle may lead to dragging of the toe, and an inability to clear the ground with the weak foot. In the early stages a supporting bandage may be used to hold the foot in a more satisfactory position, until returning tone helps the patient to overcome the problem. If the problem persists, a below knee caliper may be necessary. These are easier to apply, and to use successfully, than full length calipers, but there is a certain reluctance to wear them — particularly by female patients. In some cases, a moulded splint, worn inside the shoe, is equally effective, and more acceptable.

9. In most cases a sling is recommended, at least in the early stages, to protect the weak upper limb and shoulder joint, and to help with balance.

The Walking Pattern

The routine walking pattern for hemiplegics is the same as that described for 'Pylon Walking' in Chapter 16. In the early stages, however, there are variations determined by the degree of recovery in the weak lower limb. Whatever the degree of help may be at this stage, the helper should keep in mind the eventual pattern, and work towards it from the start. As the patient gains in confidence and ability she should be careful to withdraw the help which is no longer needed, until the patient can walk alone. The ability to do this successfully depends upon the helper's own skill and confidence, and should come with experience. The pattern is as follows.

1. Help the patient to stand and lean on his pylon as in step 4 above.
2. Ask him to proceed as follows:
3. Lift the pylon and place it forward so that the back feet of the pylon are level with his strong toes. The pylon should be about 4 inches (10 cm) away from the feet when grounded.
4. Lean on his strong hand and balance himself again.
5. Bring his weak foot forward so that it is placed opposite the centre of the pylon, and about 1 foot (30 cm) away from it.
6. Lean on his strong hand, and sharing the weight between the pylon and his weak lower limb, bring his strong foot 'up and over'. The toes of the strong foot should be placed level with the front of the pylon and about 4 inches (10 cm) away from it.
7. Take his weight on his strong lower limb, and lean on the pylon so as to return to position 1.
8. Repeat steps 3 to 7 as often as necessary.

Note 1. At first the patient may need help to bring his weak foot forward or to place it correctly. A gentle upwards pressure against his rib cage with the back of the supporting arm may be sufficient. This pressure should be co-ordinated with the patient's own effort to move the limb. If this is not enough, his feet may be brought through by the same pressure combined with a gentle push behind the heel by the foot of the helper. If the placement is faulty the helper can guide the feet into position with her own feet. It is usually a left hemiplegic with sensory loss who needs such help. In order to make him aware of the placement the helper should give clear instructions and draw his attention to what she is doing. The movement should not be allowed to become an automatic one, used as an easy way of getting along with the patient taking no part. In such conditions the patient has little chance of learning and so eventually taking responsibility for the movement. Directions may need to be given by a second helper, who stands on the strong side (see pp. 342–9).

Note 2. Many patients find it helpful in the early stages to repeat the words 'pylon, lean on it, left, right' or 'right, left' as the case may be. This assists memory and the establishment of a regular rhythm. It should not be encouraged if there is a speech problem, without discussion with the speech pathologist. It may lead to perseveration (meaningless repetition) on the oft repeated words. Counting should also be used with discretion for the same reason.

Some Common Mistakes in the Walking Pattern

Unhelpful variations to the walking pattern quickly become habitual if they are not checked in the early stages. Any person walking with the patient should notice poor technique and correct it as soon as it appears. If this is beyond the skill of the helper she should discontinue the walk and report the problem to a more senior member of the team. A long walk with an unsatisfactory pattern may leave the patient with a habit he is unable to break. Such patterns are much harder to discard than to pick up.

Some examples are as follows.

A Long Step with the Weak Foot, Followed by a Quick Short Step with the Strong One

This brings the two feet together instead of causing them to pass ahead of each other in turn. It is caused by a feeling of security while the weight is on the strong foot, and lack of confidence while it is on the weak one. Most hemiplegics tend to walk this way if not taught otherwise. It leads to an unnecessary limp which is particularly unfortunate in those who may graduate later to independent walking or a walking cane.

Placing the Weak Foot too Close to the Pylon

This may be caused by weakened abductors, over-active adductors, or lack of awareness of the correct position, bringing the body weight back over the weak limbs and upsetting the balance. A fall to the weak side is likely. With this placement of the feet relative to the pylon the patient tends to remain dependent upon a companion to hold him up. The patient must be encouraged to place his weak foot widely and to ground it safely before attempting to move his strong one. If over-active adductors are the cause he should ground the weak heel just behind the front of the strong foot, thus using it as a 'stopper'.

Raising the Pylon and the Weak Foot at the Same Time

In the early stages this is usually a sign that the patient is treating his pylon as an anchor rather than a leaning post. It is sometimes helped by giving him a pylon which is too short until he learns to lean on it. Other patients learn to lean by sitting on a long seat or the side of their bed and practising pushing up on the strong hand. On no account should the helper continue the walk with the patient leaning on her with his pylon in the air. Raising the pylon and the weak foot at the same time can lead to falls unless the patient has really good balance. In later stages it is a sign of returning confidence, and may indicate that the patient is ready to graduate to a walking cane, and a normal 1-2 gait.

Miscellaneous Precautions

Make the Patient Conscious of the Need to Feel Properly Balanced before he Takes the First Step in any Walk he Attempts. This is a common time for falls to occur. Some patients forget the instability of the paretic limb, and stand on it automatically, without proper positioning, and others may be affected by a temporary fall in blood pressure, or giddiness associated with ear disease. Rising slowly, and waiting consciously to ensure that all is well takes time which is very well spent.

Make sure that he is Conscious of the Placement of his Weak Leg at each Step. Do not add to his difficulties in this by telling him to look up if he feels like looking down. Most patients need to watch where they place their feet in the early stages, and will look up when they gain confidence. Those who have sensory disturbance may need to continue to watch their feet indefinitely.

Elderly patients do not usually move quickly so as to be at risk from distant objects. They do tend to over-balance as a result of poor foot placement or to trip over some obstruction they have not noticed. Looking down may not look as elegant as standing up straight, but for the patients under discussion it is safer.

Watch for Fatigue, and do not Push a Patient Beyond his Limits. If a patient who has been doing well loses concentration, forgets his walking pattern, staggers, becomes breathless or says he is tired, he should be allowed to sit down. It is advisable to have chairs in the walking area placed conveniently so that they can be reached quickly if necessary.

Be Conscious of the Patient's Problems apart from the Obvious Ones, and make Allowances for them. Watch for poor vision, hemianopia, loss of body image, disturbance of the understanding of space and direction, giddiness, distractability, loss of sensation, deafness, communication problems, and any other difficulties which may be present.

Never Hurry a Patient. Let him take as long over each movement as he needs to do it accurately. Speed will come with confidence but not with pressure. If the situation is such that speed is necessary, it is better to revert to a wheelchair than to risk hurried walking.

Give Plenty of Praise and Encouragement and Make sure the Patient Sits down with a Feeling of Accomplishment. Elderly people respond badly to scolding, but usually do their best when appreciation is shown.

Junior Staff should Report Difficulties to a Senior Member (Sister, physiotherapist, or occupational therapist). In this way the problem can be investigated. It is not helpful to battle on under difficulties which might be solved by someone with a little more experience. It should be remembered that the relative will have the same difficulties when the patient goes home unless they are reported and overcome.

Steps and Stairs

General Precepts

1. Patients are usually afraid of their first attempt to negotiate

steps, and so it is of great importance that the person helping should feel and appear confident. No attempt should be made until the patient is competent at pylon walking on the flat. At first the drill should be tackled early in the day when the patient is fresh. If the patient is very nervous he should have a helper on each side for his first attempt, and until he gains confidence.

2.   The primary helper should stand on the patient's weak side, and place her arm between his arm and his body as described for the early stages of walking (see Chapter 16). She should neither grip his arm, nor support him by pressing up in the axilla. A light but steady hold, with slight pressure against his rib cage gives confidence as do clear and definite instructions.

3.   The patient should be told that he will only be asked to do one small thing at a time, and that he may go as slowly as he likes. It may help to let him watch some more advanced patients have their lesson first. Working with a small group of patients who take turns is usually a satisfactory way of teaching because they tend to encourage each other when working together. The very nervous patient, however, should be taught alone until he becomes more relaxed.

Some patients learn to manage steps without stress by going for an outside walk, and being shown how to go up and down a pavement step as a matter of course. The same technique is then applied to a small flight, one step at a time. Going up is less frightening than going down, because the drop below is less apparent. If the available steps are suitably placed it sometimes helps to tackle the problems by going up first.

Going Up

1.   Walk as close as possible to the bottom step.
2.   Place the pylon sideways on the first step, well out to the strong side.
3.   Raise the strong foot and place it on the step beside the pylon. Make sure the heel is well grounded on the step.
4.   Leaning to the strong side, straighten the strong knee, helping it to raise the body by pushing up on the pylon with the strong arm at the same time.
5.   If necessary, raise the shoulder and hip on the weak side to help the toes clear the top of the step. At first it may be neces-

sary for the helper to assist the clearance of the toe by raising it with her own foot.
6. Make sure the weak foot is well grounded and completely on the step.
7. Repeat moves 2 to 6 for each step.

Going Down

1. Walk up to the edge of the top step, and place both feet so that the toes are just over the edge (about 1 inch — 2.5 cm).
2. Place the pylon sideways on the step below. It should be to the side of the body to leave plenty of room for the feet in the area in front of the patient.
3. Taking full weight on the strong leg, put the weak leg forward over the edge of the step.
4. Lean on the pylon. Bend the knee of the strong leg, and lower the weak foot carefully to the step below. This should be a steady, controlled movement.
5. Ensure that the weak foot is well placed, and leaves room for the strong foot between itself and the pylon.
6. Balancing between the weak leg and the pylon, lower the strong foot to the lower step.
7. See that the toes are slightly over the edge.
8. Repeat steps 2 to 6 as often as is necessary.

Note 1. The weak foot is placed first going down because the second limb must support the weight and resist gravity as the body is lowered. The strong limb is moved first going up because that limb must lift the body weight up on to the next step. This procedure must be reassessed for individual patients who have complicating disease or injury to the 'strong' limb, or who experience spastic adduction of the 'weak' hip joint.

Patients and relatives sometimes find it helps them to remember if they think of the 'good' going up to heaven and the 'bad' going down below. However, the best aid to memory is to understand the reason for using one limb rather than the other.

Note 2. A wise helper ensures that help is near until she is sure of her patient's reliability. It is very difficult for a single person to cope with a patient who panics half way down a flight of steps. No-one should feel too proud to ask for help to prevent such a situation developing.

Note 3. Rewards are an integral part of the retraining process.

In Newcastle a special reward is reserved for patients who successfully negotiate the steps. The flight which is used goes down to a garden, and a rose is chosen by the patient and pinned to his lapel as a badge of honour. This token produces still more reinforcement as other people see the rose and remark upon it. The simple ceremony has been found to have positive meaning for most patients who remember it long after they have overcome their fear.

Some Problems in Communication

If a speech pathologist is available, all patients with speech problems should be referred to her, and her suggestions for management should be followed by the rest of the team. If there is no speech pathologist the patient will still need understanding and help with his communication problems from those who are caring for him. In such a situation the following notes may prove helpful.

Emotional Lability and Diminished Control

When the patient weeps frequently and inappropriately this may be a sign that the patient is upset or depressed, and causes for distress should be investigated and dealt with. In most cases, however, it is the result of diminished emotional control, which is a common feature of a stroke. It is seen most commonly in the early stages of the illness, but may continue for lengthy periods in some cases. Patients with speech difficulties are often affected. This can cause difficulty in finding out their needs because the response to questioning is a flood of tears. Tears may come with happy associations, as when a relative pays a visit, a familiar song is played, or the patient is praised for a good effort during retraining procedures. They are often seen at the successful completion of a task almost as part of relaxation after effort.

Men are usually upset by this symptom more than women because in our society it is less acceptable for them to cry. Unfortunately, the more the patients try to control their emotions the more likely they are to continue to cry. Tension appears to play a role in this process. In most cases it is wise to tell the patient that this is a normal part of his stroke, that it usually passes as the condition improves, and that we understand it and will not make a fuss. The tears usually subside if the person dealing with the patient carries on in an unemotional way with whatever must be done. Superficial comforting words and gestures do not usually have the required effect, and may even increase the patient's difficulties.

Relatives often misunderstand these tears and can be helped to accept them better if a simple explanation is given. Patients are usually greatly relieved to know that they are not the only patient to experience this embarrassment. It is of course necessary to ensure that we are in fact dealing with emotional lability, and not sorrow or depression. If the latter is suspected the matter should be referred to a suitably qualified person for advice.

Expressive Speech Difficulties

If the Patient has no Speech, or Repeats a few Stereotyped Words.
Make the situation as relaxed as possible.
Avoid the appearance of impatience or haste.
Ask single questions which can be answered with a nod or a shake of the head.
Understand that some patients cannot differentiate between 'yes' and 'no', and may give an inappropriate answer. Watch for facial expression, and if in doubt ask the question another way.
Talk to the patient as normally as possible.
Avoid raising the voice, using 'baby talk', and discussing the patient in his presence as if he were absent or unable to hear or understand.
Talk to the patient as often as possible and make sure that he is not left without conversation or knowledge of what is happening because he himself cannot speak.
Talk to him while you work with him, giving the usual verbal directions whenever there is change of position or activity.
If you are unable to understand what he wants, try using a set of pictures of common objects, but remember that pictures and writing may have lost their meaning for him.
Consider giving a bell or a buzzer to a patient who is unable to attract attention by voice.

If Speech is Slurred and Difficult to Understand. The patient may be producing normal sentences, but pronouncing the words in a way that is difficult to understand.
Listen for key words and try to get the gist of the sentence.
Repeat the key word as a question to make sure you are on the right track. (Your daughter? A drink of water?) Once the subject

is established the words naturally become easier to follow.

Do not be afraid to tell the patient you are having difficulties in understanding. Ask him to try to speak a little more slowly or a little louder.

If the Patient is Speaking Clearly but the Words do not Make Sense. This is not necessarily the result of confusion. The patient knows what he wants to say, and thinks he is saying it, but the wrong words come out. Sometimes he knows they are wrong when he says them, but he cannot find the right ones. If he is not aware that they are wrong he may even think that you are confused because you do not understand what he is saying.

Try to imagine what the correct word is and put it to him in a question. (Patient — 'I want a bubble.' Helper — 'Do you want your glasses? a drink? a tissue?' etc.)

If the Patient is Becoming Distressed and You Still Cannot Understand. If you have eliminated all the usual needs of the hospital patient and are still unable to understand it may be better to postpone the discussion rather than to add to the patient's frustration. If possible take the blame, saying something like — 'I'm so sorry, I just don't seem to be very bright today. I'll think about it, and if I have a good idea I'll come back'.

Do not take the aphasic patient to the toilet automatically every time he makes an attempt to communicate. Remember that everyone who comes along may tend to do the same. One recovered patient stated that one of the most frustrating aspects of the early stage of his illness was being rushed to the toilet, even when he was only trying to say 'thank you'.

Receptive Speech Difficulties (Figure 17.8)

Some patients cannot understand the spoken word. They are neither deaf nor confused, but words have lost their meaning for them. Avoid shouting, speaking quickly, using long words and long sentences, and standing out of the patient's sight when you speak.

Remember that there is more to communication than words, and do not be afraid to use gestures. A pat on the back for praise, a hand movement for 'rise' or 'sit down', and a touch on the knee as you say 'move this leg', all help the patient to comprehend. 'Do you take sugar?' may be answered with a puzzled look which will

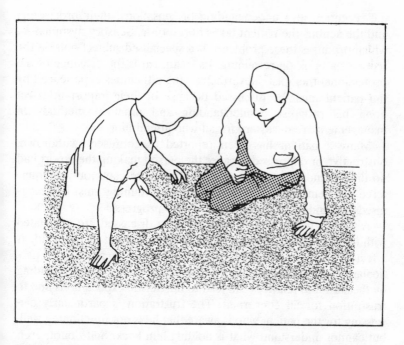

Figure 17.8: Receptive Speech Loss in Hemiplegia. Patient learns to get up from the floor and to move when down with the help of a mirror image demonstration

disappear if a finger is pointed to the sugar bowl as the words are said.

Just as a baby responds to the tone of its mother's voice before it has learnt to speak and a puppy understands the voice of its master without the knowledge of words, so the patient who has lost the meaning of words will understand the tone of voice and the attitude of his helpers. He should be given clear directions and be told what is happening in the same way as the other patients, even when he does not appear to comprehend.

Other Difficulties Associated with a Stroke

Apart from the obvious difficulties posed by loss of power in the affected limbs, and disorders of speech, many patients suffer more subtle problems associated with their specific lesion. These concern the reception and understanding of sensations, their processing, and the actions the patient takes in response. Sensory dysfunction, which produces these problems, is a specialised subject outside the scope of a book on retraining. Its treatment is the province of the professional therapist. Nevertheless, the difficulties experienced by the patient must be discussed because of their important effect upon his progress. Understanding and practical methods of management are necessary for all who attend him.

Many a patient has been reported as confused, withdrawn, obstructive or depressed because the person making the report had no understanding of these matters. The more commonly encountered problems and those which hinder retraining must be recognised and understood if the patient is to progress.

Although most of the problems to be discussed are associated with left hemiplegia they may also be present when the right side is affected. They can create great difficulties in retraining, particularly in the areas of safety and balance. Lack of understanding by the staff and relatives can lead to unrealistic expectations and to frustration for all concerned. The frustration is particularly distressing for the patient who is aware that he is not functioning well, but cannot understand what is holding him back. Self doubt, even concerning his own sanity, is sometimes encountered unless the patient has received confident reassurances that his problems are part of his stroke, and not unusual at his present stage of recovery. Natural recovery may take place, in which case the problem will resolve itself, but in many cases the disability persists, and it is necessary to help the patient adjust to it and compensate as well as he can.

The examples discussed below are likely to be encountered in retraining and will cause difficulties out of proportion to their incidence if they are not understood.

Disorders of Function Associated with Touch

Loss of Postural Sense (Figure 17.8)

Loss of postural sense is common in the early stages of hemiplegia but tends to improve by natural progression. In a minority of patients it persists and creates dangers associated with lack of awareness of body position and poor balance. The patient tends to fall to his hemiplegic side and lacks the ability to return to a safe position. If asked to try to sit up straight he may push himself further in the wrong direction, being unable to discriminate between the balanced and unbalanced states.

1. The method of supporting a patient in a chair, as described on page 304, is particularly helpful for these patients.
2. The use of visual cues, in the form of demonstration by the helper and the provision of a mirror will help some patients.
3. The patient should learn to stand by pushing up with his strong hand on the seat of the chair instead of using its arm. This encourages a lean to the strong side as he rises.
4. The patient should use a pylon which is shorter than would usually be chosen, to encourage him to lean to the strong side. This should be raised as his balance is regained.

Dulled Responses to Temperature and Pain

These patients have reduced awareness of feelings of heat, cold, pressure or pain on the affected side. This puts them at risk, particularly of sustaining burns. There is danger from such things as radiators, cooking equipment, showers and cigarettes. Staff and relatives need to be aware of this problem and to take protective measures. Adequate supervision should be provided in dangerous situations. Some patients can learn to compensate but many find it difficult to understand and accept that they have a problem. Each person's management must be considered individually to guard against the evils of exposure to risk, on the one hand, and to overprotection, on the other.

Tactile Inattention (Right/Left Rivalry)

The patient will not respond equally to bilateral stimuli. He will ignore the weaker message from the hemiplegic side when both sides are stimulated simultaneously. This makes bilateral activities difficult or impossible. A common example is eating with a knife and fork. Much frustration and waste of time can be avoided if the patient is taught to cut his food with a 'rocker knife', and to put the knife aside and feed himself one handed with the fork.

Reduced Span of Attention to Tactile Cues

The patient loses awareness of tactile stimulation more quickly on the affected side. This causes him to let go unexpectedly with that hand for no obvious reason. This can be dangerous when he is carrying an article without concentrating upon it, or if he uses his hemiplegic hand to support himself on a stair rail or to push up when rising from a chair.

1. The patient should learn to use visual cues rather than touch to remain aware of the hand's activity.
2. He should be encouraged to rely upon his strong limbs whenever his safety is at stake.
3. He should carry such items as cups of tea on a tray attached to his pylon, and not risk taking them in his hemiplegic hand, even if motor power is intact.
4. Handbags or purses should be attached to the pylon or money belt, because the patient is very likely to put them down without being conscious of the action.
5. If it is necessary to carry something in the weak hand it may help if he tightens and releases his grip consciously at fairly short intervals. This reinforces the feel of the article in his hands, but presupposes good insight and concentration, which he may not possess.

Retarded Response to Tactile Stimuli

The patient will respond more quickly and more strongly to stimuli on the unaffected side, tending to lag behind with the hemiplegic one. The patient is unaware that his movements are not synchronised, and believes that they have been carried out as he intended. This leads to the danger of falls if the hemiplegic limbs are expected to take an equal part with the unaffected ones in such movements as rising and sitting, or negotiating steps. It can also lead to danger in carrying a full tray or a hot baking dish.

A safety factor is built into the retraining drills in that they teach greater reliance on the strong limbs when safety factors are involved.

Unilateral Hemiplegia with Bilateral Sensory Changes

It is easy to take it for granted that the 'good' side will have normal sensation, but this is not always so. There can be disturbance of sensation on both sides. This makes it difficult for the patient to employ the usual compensatory measures with the 'unaffected' side. Repeated practice of the drills, and strong visual cues are necessary in this situation. The principle of using the patient's strengths still applies, but careful assessment of those strengths, and any deficits must be made.

Over Reaction to Sensory Stimuli

Some patients complain of pain or strange feelings which appear to be out of proportion to the mild stimuli which cause them. These patients are sometimes thought to be 'moaners' or attention seekers, but they really do experience the discomforts of which they complain. They may be upset by a sleeve brushing against their forearm, an attempt to help them move a hemiplegic limb, or a hand laid lightly on theirs in conversation. In some cases the unpleasant sensation is described as 'tingling', 'cold', 'heavy', or 'shooting'.

These patients need to be reassured that there is nothing dangerously wrong. Care should be taken not to expose them to unnecessary contacts with the affected parts unless this is required as part of a plan of treatment. Physical help consists mainly in good positioning when the patient is at rest, and minimal lifting and touching of the affected part during transfers and walking. Impatience should never be shown.

Disorders of Motor Function

Besides the obvious weakness and paralysis of hemiplegia some patients may suffer a variety of other disorders of motor function. Some may appear to be trying to co-operate, but will place their limbs without apparent reference to what they have been asked to do. Others will appear to oppose the directions of their helpers quite actively and strongly. Such behaviour must be seen as reflex action outside the patient's control and not as active rejection of treatment. If it is not so understood the patient's progress will be impeded by frustrations and cross purposes. Some of the more common problems, and those which most affect retraining will be discussed.

The Patient can Produce a Movement Spontaneously but not to Order

The patient is not being obstructive and refusing to act, but his attempts to act produce no movement, or a movement other than the one he intends. Tension appears to increase the problem, so it is useless to ask him to try harder. Better results can be obtained by asking him to stop trying. The primitive grasp reflex is an example. The patient opens his hand spontaneously to grasp a rail or the arm of his chair, but is unable to release that grip when required to do so. If he is asked to relax and not to try to let go it is usually possible to open the fingers quite gently. Rubbing the back of the hand may also help.

The patient should not be encouraged to use his hand in any situation where balance and safety are at stake. For example, it is dangerous for such patients to place the affected hand on the arm of a chair when rising or on a rail when negotiating steps. In both cases any forward movement will result in the patient being pulled backwards and to his weaker side, and a fall may result. The patient himself may be quite unaware that he is still holding on. The use of a sling may protect some patients from this danger, while others may always need supervision in mobility and ADL. It is neither wise nor kind to encourage such patients to use the hemiplegic hand.

Another example is the patient who bends his knee quite easily to sit on the seat of a car, but finds that the same knee extends strongly and cannot be flexed in order to put the foot into the car. If such a patient stops trying to help in the movement and relaxes instead, the helper can bend the knee passively, and help the leg into the car. Any help of this kind which is found to be necessary should be explained to the patient's relatives before he goes home.

'Counter-pull' in which the Patient Opposes Attempts to Position him by Pushing in the Opposite Direction

If the helper attempts to move a limb passively the patient pulls in the other direction and seems to be resisting the movement. If the helper attempts to push the patient's body to his strong side to improve his balance he will push back, sometimes very strongly. This is a reflex response outside the patient's control.

A good example may be encountered in chair drill. The patient is asked to lean forward to look at his toes so as to come into a balanced position for rising. It is natural at first for the helper to assist this forward movement, but as soon as the patient feels her hand pressing forward he leans back, pushing quite strongly in the opposite direction. If this is allowed to continue the patient may never learn to rise independently. The required movement can usually be elicited if the helper places her hand on the patient's forehead and asks him to push forward.

This reflex can be used to advantage if the helper places her hand and asks the patient to push against it instead of herself trying to push the patient in the required direction. Some common examples are listed.

In Standing Up Straight. A hand placed lightly on the top of the head and a request to 'be as tall as you can' brings much better results than lifting and supporting in an upright position.

In Balancing. A hand placed on the strong hip and a request to push it towards the pylon brings the patient's body back over the strong lower limb. A push against the weak hip only leads to the patient pushing back more strongly to the weak side.

In Early Walking. The patient should never be held up by the helper's arm around his waist or behind his shoulder as this teaches him to lean backwards and puts him at the risk of falling backwards when he attempts to walk alone.

Note. Many patients other than those suffering from 'counter-pull' respond well to this method of instruction. It is particularly helpful to the patient who does not understand verbal directions giving him visual and tactile ones as to the limb he is required to move and the direction it should take.

The Clenched Fist

Some patients who come for retraining with an old stroke present with flexed fingers which are difficult to open for hygiene and manicure. Pulling the fingers open usually leads to tighter clenching and in some cases to pain. The hand will be more easily opened if the wrist is flexed and the back of the hand and forearm are firmly rubbed to stimulate the extensors.

'As You Were' Movements, in which the Patient Carries out a Movement, but Returns to his Original Position before it can be Used

The patient achieves the first stage in a movement, but before the next instruction can be given he returns to his former state. This is seen in any drill when a series of moves must be made. For instance, in chair drill the patient may place his feet correctly for rising, but return them to their original position when asked to place his hands on the arms of the chair. Similarly, in walking the pylon may be placed forward and then brought back to its starting point before the first step is taken.

Constant practice is necessary, and the directions given by all staff members should be the same at each and every transfer. Most patients seem to overcome this difficulty if given this practice. Short cuts such as holding the limb in position have not proved helpful. The patient seems to have difficulty in remaining aware of the position of the first limb once his attention is redirected to the second. Examples are sometimes seen in dressing when the patient will begin to put on a garment, and then take it off again before proceeding to the next step. When recovery does not take place the patient will continue to need supervision after discharge, together with understanding and patience from those who help him.

Disorders of Constructional Ability

Some patients have difficulties in understanding structure and construction. They are unable to follow a pattern in two or three dimensions, or to perform tasks involving a logical sequence of moves. The patient knows what he wants to do, but cannot work out the processes necessary to achieve the required result. Writing, dressing, or making even a simple article may be impossible even for someone who was 'good with his hands'. Because these patients realise that they are are unable to manage tasks which others find easy, they are likely to be among those who reject crafts and creative activities. They will usually say that the task is too 'childish', or 'kindergarten stuff'. Unless the activity is being provided as part of treatment under the supervision of a qualified person it should be discontinued, and some more suitable task substituted. No patient should be made to appear stupid to his fellows, or to feel that this is happening.

In Dressing

The patient may have no idea of organising his clothes so that he can put them on. He may put both feet into the same trouser leg, put his shirt on back to front, or mismatch his buttons. He may sit and pick up a garment and handle it without making any obvious attempt to put it on at all. There are many degrees of deficit, but none should be seen as 'confusion'.

When a patient suffers disturbance of this kind it can be extremely frustrating, and long dressing sessions should be avoided. If the patient shows signs of fatigue or loss of interest in the task he should be helped tactfully to complete it. It is often better to start these patients with undressing than with dressing, because errors are less obvious. A simple part of the job done well will usually lead to more progress than an unsuccessful attempt at the whole.

Some patients overcome this problem, but some will always need help. The relatives of the latter group should receive instructions in easy dressing procedures, and an explanation of the patient's problems. This will make their task easier, and prevent them from seeing their patient as stupid or lazy.

In Drawing and Written Work

The patient may be quite unable to place lines on a page so that they have meaning. This can apply to drawing, writing, and written calculations. Both spontaneous and copied work may be affected. With a lesser degree of deficit the patient may approximate what is required, but the letters or shapes may be badly formed or badly placed on the page.

This difficulty may have great bearing upon the patient's prospects in returning to work. If possible a speech therapist should be consulted before any action is taken. If the patient wishes to practise writing he should do so, but he should not be made tense and unhappy about it.

In Crafts and Games

The majority of crafts involve construction in some form, and as would be expected, are beyond the compass of these patients. Because many of them know that they cannot produce work which they see others managing quite easily, they refuse to attend activity centres and work rooms. No patient should be asked to tackle something at which he must fail and feel inferior, but simple single-process jobs may prove the answer.

A patient who weaves the stakes of his basket into the working, takes the shuttle round and round the warp instead of through the shed of his weaving, or cuts a pot plant off at the main stem instead of trimming the dead leaves is more likely to be 'dyspraxic' than confused. Similar difficulties may be found with many games. For example, there may be difficulty in placing dominoes in the right way, although the game itself is well understood. The helper should be aware of such problems, and be ready to adjust the activity to suit the patient's abilities.

Disorders of Body Image

Disorders of body image are most frequently seen in patients with left hemiplegia. They concern the patient's feelings about his body rather than a picture that he has of himself. They take various forms and differ in degree from patient to patient. Retraining may be affected quite markedly because the patient's understanding of his body is different from ours. We may be asking him to use a part which he feels to be no longer there.

Some specific examples may illustrate this point.

The Patient Completely Disregards the Affected Side of his Body

When asked to move the weak foot to touch the leg of the chair at the beginning of chair drill he is unable to do so, because he does not feel that he has a left leg. If his weak arm falls over the arm of his chair he will make no attempt to bring it back, because he is unaware of its position.

This disregard for the affected side of the body leads to the danger of injury, and to difficulty in learning any process in which the hemiplegic limbs are involved. Movements in which balance and safety are the responsibility of the strong limbs are necessary for these patients. Some learning will take place by repetition, but supervision should be maintained while the problem persists.

The Patient is Unaware of his Paralysis, and may Deny it

Such a patient will make no attempt to take precautions against a fall. He will attempt to stand without leaning to the strong side, despite a flaccid knee, and fall heavily (and to himself, unexpectedly). In walking he may take two steps running with the strong limb without having moved the weak one, firmly believing that he has done so. Some patients with this problem will be unrealistic about their need for retraining, and in fact for any treatment. They may speak quite confidently about how they dress themselves, when what they are describing is what they did before their stroke. It is never wise to take a patient's word when completing an ADL assessment. Each section should be personally observed by the reporter.

The Patient Complains of Extreme Heaviness in the Weak Limbs

He may feel that he cannot rise because of the weight or that his hemiplegic arm is pulling him over. He may also feel unable to lift the hemiplegic lower limb when walking because it is 'too heavy'. There may be some substance in these complaints if the limbs are oedematous. They may also be the result of weakened muscles carrying the normal weight and feeling fatigue sooner and more strongly than those on the unaffected side. The patient's feeling, however, is of excessive weight, and he responds to it as such. Explanations, though they do not remove the feeling, can sometimes help the patient to accept it and to keep trying. A sling may help if the complaint concerns the upper limb. Some patients respond if they are reminded how a suitcase which seems dreadfully heavy to a frail old lady can be carried without effort by a fit young footballer, and this helps them to relate their problem to the strength of their muscles.

The Patient Complains of Pain 'Somewhere' but cannot Explain Where

He may even feel that the pain is outside his body. One patient admits to asking for an aspirin for a 'headache' because she did not want to seem stupid in explaining where the pain really was, and yet did want some relief.

The Patient Expresses Strange Ideas about the Shape or Size of his Limbs

This may be expressed as a worry, or as an excuse for not joining in activities. Sometimes the use of a mirror may help. At others the patient may be reassured by placing the two limbs side by side and having his attention drawn to the fact that they still match each other. This reassures him that it is only in feeling and not in fact that they have changed.

The Patient does not Recognise his own Limbs, and may Reject them

A dramatic example was the patient who picked up his hemiplegic hand and threw it from him saying 'whose hand is that? Get rid of it!' In this case the helper placed the patient's hands side by side within his area of vision and asked him if they matched. He agreed that they did. He was then asked if they could belong to the same person, which he agreed they could. When asked who owned the strong one he claimed it as his own, and finally agreed that the weak one could be his. He eventually accepted it as his own intellectually, but never reached the stage where he could 'look after it'. It can be imagined how difficult it is for such a patient to follow and remember instructions concerning his hemiplegic limbs when attempting his various drills.

The Patient does not Understand the Concept of 'Right' and 'Left'

Right and left may become meaningless to the patient, as may the words up, down, forwards and backwards. In teaching, this must be overcome by gestures, and by the use of alternative words such as 'this leg — that leg', or 'weak — strong'. Because of the negative ideas associated with calling a limb the weak one, the last of these alternatives is usually used only when more positive words have been tried without success. 'Good' and 'bad' should be avoided if possible, except on steps where patients and relatives find it easy to remember that the 'good' go up to heaven and the 'bad' go down below. In this way they work out how to start with the correct foot when rising and descending.

Some patients learn more easily if the helper demonstrates by standing in front of them and goes through the movement herself, back to front, so that he sees it as in a mirror (see Figure 17.8).

Disorders of Vision

Patients who have suffered a stroke may have pre-existing disorders of vision which will affect their retraining, but there are also disorders which result from the stroke itself. The latter differ from conventional blindness in many ways, and are not always so well understood, even by the patient himself. They have a strong influence on the patient's response to retraining, and so should be recognised and taken into account by the helpers. Those aspects which most commonly affect the patient's progress will be discussed.

The Patient Exhibits Poor Vision, but Blames it upon Conditions Outside Himself

The patient seems unaware that his sight is at fault, and so neglects

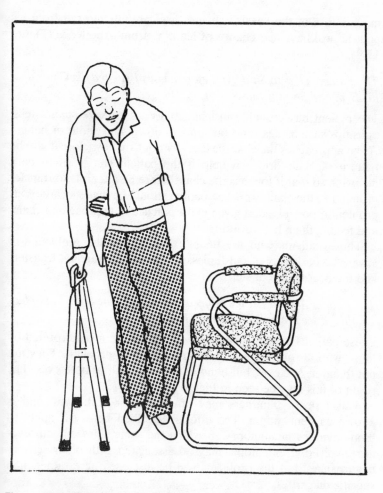

Figure 17.9: Patient with Left Sensory Neglect Practises Walking Past Objects Placed in his Path

to take precautions such as the use of a stick or the back of his hand to feel his way. He will blame poor light, glare, and other external causes for his blindness. This puts him at risk, as he will bump into obstructions, and be unaware of hazards such as steps and unevenness in his path. Even with good return of physical abilities the problem may persist, and he will need supervision in his walking and other activities.

Within reason he should be allowed to bump into things, and be made aware of the hazards. If they are carefully cleared from his path he will have less chance of learning from experience (Figure 17.9).

The Patient Tries to Sit down before he has Reached his Chair or his Bed, and Seems Unaware of the Danger

The patient has probably lost his ability to perceive spatial relationships such as near and far, up and down, and width or height. As he approaches the chair he is really not sure how close it is. The pattern of chair drill can help if the patient can learn to park his pylon so that it touches the chair before he attempts to transfer his hand to the chair arm. The patient should be made aware of his problem if possible, and given extra practice in approaching chairs and feeling them before sitting.

Those patients who are unable to adjust to the problem will always be in danger of falls unless supervised in walking, transfers and the negotiation of steps.

The Patient Appears to see Objects Clearly on One Side, but to be Unable to see them on the Other (Hemianopia)

These patients exhibit many signs which can be misinterpreted by those who are unaware of the nature of their problem. They are not 'blind in one eye', but blind in the same half of both eyes. The result of this may be seen in Figure 17.10.

This type of blindness may affect one or both eyes, and is known as hemianopia. The effects described here will apply to 'homonymous hemianopia' in which the same sides of both eyes are involved. Hemianopia may be associated with other sensory disturbances, but the problems will be discussed here rather than specific diagnoses.

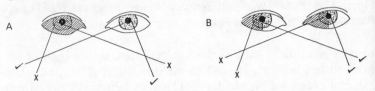

A. Blind in both sides of one eye. The patient can see both ways, but has difficulty in judging the position and distance of objects.

B. Blind in same side of both eyes. The patient can see normally to one side, but can see nothing on the other.

Figure 17.10: Hemianopia

The Patient Turns Away from the Speaker when Addressed from the Hemiplegic Side. Unless the speaker understands the patient's problem it will appear that the patient does not want to be spoken to. This is far from the truth. He is in fact looking for the speaker whom he cannot see on the weak side and so hopes to find on the strong one. This will be even more definite if the patient has hearing difficulty on the weak side, because he will actually hear the voice with the stronger ear. Nurses may report that the patient is withdrawn, and relatives feel that they are rejected unless they approach the patient on the side from which he can appreciate their presence.

There is one line of thinking which says that the patient should be approached from the weak side to help him to adjust to his disability and overcome it. In retraining it is taught that patients should be approached from the strong side so that their attention is gained, and that the helper should move gradually to the weak side so long as that attention can be held. This is good teaching practice, as we begin where the patient is, and gradually build up his ability without making him feel isolated or foolish. Many patients are reluctant to turn the head beyond the mid-line, which it is necessary for them to do in order to attend to stimuli on the weak side. They learn to do this with less fear if they follow the speaker into the unknown during conversation.

Patients who have otherwise made a good recovery may still feel uncomfortable conducting lengthy conversations with someone seated on the weak side. Short sessions for practice should be encouraged, but a change of position is indicated when fatigue, loss of concentration, or irritability are noted.

The Patient does not Follow Directions Given by the Helper on his Weak Side. The patient may not be aware of the helper for various reasons, including difficulties of receptive speech, touch, and body image. If hemianopia is added to these difficulties hand signals will only be effective if given within the patient's line of vision. A simple explanation of what is required, with a demonstration on the patient's strong side is often helpful. In badly disabled patients who must have full support on the weak side it is sometimes necessary for a second helper to give directions and hand signals on the strong side. The second helper should avoid giving unnecessary physical help, as this will delay the patient's relearning and encourage dependence.

The Patient Eats all the Food on One Side of his Plate and Leaves it on the Other Side. The line of demarcation down the centre of the plate may be so straight that it looks as if the patient is being obsessively tidy in his eating habits. Actually, the patient is unaware that there is another half plateful available to him. The patient should be taught consciously to turn his plate so as to bring the second half of his food into his line of vision. In the meantime, before he learns to do this, his food should not be removed by a nurse, wardsmaid or relative who says kindly, 'What's the matter? Aren't you hungry today?'

A similar problem exists if the patient's drinks and minor meals are placed on his weak side. Many a cup of tea has gone cold because the patient did not know it was there.

The Patient Completes One Half of his Craftwork and Leaves the Other Side Untouched. Crafts can be used to help the patient to adjust to his problem. The job should be made easy for him in the beginning by placement on his strong side. It can then be moved progressively into the area of difficulty. The patient should not be allowed to fail, or to look incompetent in front of the rest of his group. If this occurs he will probably reject further efforts as 'childish'.

The Patient has Difficulty in Finding his Way and Ignores Doors and Openings on the Weak Side. The patient has not seen the opening on his weak side and so continues straight ahead as if it were not there. This problem will mean that the patient will need a companion on all walks involving changes of direction unless he can learn to look for each turning well before he reaches it. Setting goals at intervals along the path has proved helpful to some. For instance, stopping at a door to see the next goal, before entering the room.

The Patient Goes through a Door without Leaving Room for his Helper, or even for his own Weak Side. The patient sees the door jamb on his strong side, but is unaware of the structure on the weak one. He keeps well clear of the one he can see, and in doing so collides with the one he cannot. He needs to practise walking close to articles on his strong side, and to become aware of obstacles well ahead while they are still in his line of vision.

The helper should encourage the patient to stop and look before entering any doorway or narrow passage. The patient will need constant supervision unless he can learn to make a conscious effort to look ahead.

Disorders of Symbolic Thought

The patient has difficulty in comprehending written symbols, which leads to problems with letters, numbers, and signs such as +, −, and =. Reading and writing will be involved if letters have lost their meaning. Calculations will be difficult or impossible if numbers are affected. Practice in these skills at a simple level may help if the defect is partial, and should be encouraged if the patient must manage his own shopping or business. Because it is usually a long and tedious process for the patient it is probably better not to stress the matter with those who will be living in a more protective situation. If a speech pathologist is available she should be consulted. Generally speaking, practice in reading, writing and calculating should not be introduced until more basic skills have been learnt.

Composite Problems

The foregoing problems have been discussed separately for the sake of convenience, but they will usually be found in combinations in the patient, depending upon the site and severity of his lesion. Allowance must be made for all the difficulties being experienced by the individual. For instance, the patient who suffers from sensory inattention, loss of vision, and lack of awareness of external space on his left side will receive no sensory stimuli from the general life of the ward if he is placed in a bed with his right side facing the wall. Far from helping him to become aware of such stimuli, this placement will lead to withdrawal and the danger of confusion related to sensory deprivation. An individual therapist may wish to treat the patient from the affected side for the short duration of her visit, but to isolate the patient from the normal life of the ward is counter-productive and verges upon cruelty.

Patients with these problems may have great difficulty in joining in activities, and so care must be taken to find something at which they can succeed if they are not to reject all activities or become depressed. Concern and ingenuity are the assets most needed by the helper in finding the right occupation.

Problem Solving for the Individual

The relative importance of the problems produced by these disorders of function will vary with the life to which the patient is to return. Treatment should be geared to the patient's real needs and his chance of achieving some success. Over-emphasis on an impossible goal usually leads to depression and withdrawal from even those things which the patient can accomplish. Some patients will recover spontaneously and overcome their problems. Others may have insight and be able to 'think through' an action quite consciously before attempting it. Unfortunately, there are some who are not able to understand what is happening, and so are unable to make the necessary adjustments for coping with it. Such patients will need continued supervision in the activities they are unable to master. This is particularly so if their safety is involved. In such cases the condition should be explained carefully to the relatives, who should work with their patient in the hospital before deciding to look after him at home. Because of the constant nature of their task the patient's attendance at day centre and planned periodical readmissions should be considered. Without continued support from the geriatrics service, the burden is likely to prove too much for them.

F. STIFF AND PAINFUL JOINTS
Introduction

Stiff and painful joints can result from many causes and treatment of the illness or injury behind the symptoms will vary accordingly. Any retraining, while not itself a 'treatment', must take such treatment into account, and should not conflict with it. Communication between all who handle the patient is necessary to ensure coordination of their efforts. There will also be patients in the retraining unit whose problems are residual ones and who are no longer receiving active treatment. Such patients will still have difficulties in performing daily tasks, but can usually be helped by the problem-solving aspects of retraining.

The Problems

The problems brought about by pain and stiffness are usually those of mobility and personal care. These problems are often increased because of accompanying weakness of muscles acting on the joints due to disease or disuse. In many cases there are also fixed deformities which have developed over a long period, and must be accepted as part of the problem. Many patients, despite severe signs and symptoms, will have found ways to do things for themselves, thus moderating their impact. Others will have given up, relying on their relatives for daily care. For this reason it is important to know what the patient has accomplished as well as his physical condition before assessing his problems.

Problems may be experienced in all the routine drills, and the answer is often found in adapted equipment and self-help aids rather than in working for any change in the patient's condition.

Retraining Principles

(a) Assess the patient's present strengths and weaknesses.
(b) Start with what he can do, and build upon his strengths.
(c) Involve the patient in all movements, but give help where it is needed.
(d) Avoid all jerky or sudden movements.
(e) Listen if the patient complains of pain or difficulty, even if the complaint is a regular one (see Chapter 13, 'Fear').
(f) Report all complaints of new or increased pain to a senior member of the staff.
(g) Watch for signs of fatigue, and give adequate rest periods.
(h) Allow the patient to decide when he has done enough in early sessions.
(i) Warn patients who are moving for the first time after a period of immobility that there may be increased pain and stiffness until they become used to the activity. This pain should not be confused with an acute 'flare up' of the condition.
(j) Avoid criticism and a suggestion that the patient could try harder. Praise for a good effort will encourage a better one next time.
(k) Ensure that all equipment is in good order, and adjusted to suit the individual.

(l) Try out self-help gadgets which reduce strain on the joints, and compensate for lost strengths. Adapt them as necessary.
(m) Ensure that relatives who will be helping the patient know how their help should be applied.
(n) Keep in touch with any new technical aids which may come on the market.

Some Precautions

(a) Follow the doctor's directions concerning activity, and if in doubt ask him for advice.
(b) Provide rest and not activity if there is active disease indicated by swelling, inflammation, pain or heat.
(c) Protect joints from further damage by reducing stress and energy requirements in essential tasks.
(d) Avoid activities which demand recurrent stress (hammering) or sustained tension (the holding hand in knitting).
(e) Encourage the patient to work within the limits of pain. Activity beyond that should be undertaken only after group discussion.
(f) Until the patient's abilities are established ensure that help is sufficient to prevent an accident.
(g) Avoid further damage to joints caused by unsuitable holding and lifting methods.
(h) See that patients lie or sit in positions which will protect and not damage their joints.

The Patient's Way

Many patients who present for retraining with stiff and painful joints have been subject to a slowly progressive deterioration over some years. They and their relatives have often adjusted to different problems as they occurred. They may have worked out a way to cope which serves their purpose, and of which they are proud. If such adjustments are functional they should be used in his retraining and not cast aside in favour of the routine method of the unit. If the patient does not continue to use his own method he may well lose it without learning to use the alternative one. The staff can in fact learn a new method, which may be useful to another patient at a future date.

If the patient's own method is unsatisfactory, or places too much strain on his helper, it should be adjusted or replaced by a more suitable method. This should be done tactfully because the patient's and the relative's pride may be involved. In most cases the change is readily accepted so long as the new method really is more practical than the old.

Attitudes to Pain

Attitudes to pain vary tremendously from person to person. Helpers should be aware of this, and allow for it when dealing with patients for whom pain is an inevitable part of treatment. Some will need encouragement to accept a certain amount of pain in order to increase their mobility, while others will need to be restrained from gritting their teeth and inflicting upon themselves more pain than is necessary or helpful.

Most patients find the middle way most comfortably if we discuss the subject of pain before starting their activity, and let them know what to expect. If we deny pain or ignore it when the patient complains we will almost certainly lose his confidence and co-operation. It is far better to accept the fact of pain and explain to the patient the necessity to put up with it as far as he can. It usually helps if we ask the patient to tell us when he has had enough, and to praise him for a brave attempt rather than to ask him to keep trying once he shows signs of distress. It helps the patient to do his best if he feels that you respect him for doing so.

A few patients may use exaggerated complaints of pain to avoid some activity they do not wish to attempt. This problem is never solved by a show of disbelief. In fact, such a response on the part of the helper is likely to elicit anger and further resistance. The real solution depends upon discovering why the activity is being rejected, and dealing with that problem in the most appropriate way that can be found.

If the helper is in any doubt as to the cause of pain or its severity she should refer the matter to the patient's doctor or a senior member of staff. No patient who complains of excessive pain should be written off as a 'winger'. If physical reasons have been eliminated by appropriate investigations, the patient will still need psychological support to help him overcome the problem.

The Routine Drills

The routine drills must usually be adapted for these patients to suit individual variations. The principles remain the same, with emphasis on protection of the weaker members. Some common variations are as follows.

In Chair Drill

If there is pain on rising as with a single arthritic hip or knee, this can sometimes be helped by teaching the patient to place the foot on the painful side ahead of the stronger one before he attempts to rise or sit down. Pain in both hips or knees may be eased by providing a higher seat or a seat with a forwards slope, thus reducing the angle through which the joint must be moved, and starting the upwards thrust in the easier range of the movement. A patient with a stiff hip fixed in extension, or with arthrodesed knees may be provided with a bicycle seat at an appropriate height so that he can back on to it without the need to raise or lower his body.

Painful shoulders, elbows, and hands can also make it difficult to rise and sit unaided. If the shoulders and elbows are involved the patient may find it easier to place the hands on the seat of the chair and to rock forwards rather than to push up on the arms of the chair. More height can be gained in doing this if the patient pushes up on the knuckles of a clenched fist and this is less painful for the wrists and fingers. This method should not be encouraged except as a last resort because it tends to increase ulnar deviation of the fingers. For some this may be a necessary risk, as when a patient lives alone, and independent rising from a chair is absolutely essential. In cases of doubt the matter should be discussed by the team. Some patients may learn to cup their hands over the edge of the seat, pushing up on their palms.

Pulling up is rarely helpful to these patients, but some manage by placing their forearms forward on a support such as their walking frame, and rocking forward over them, straightening up after their body weight is balanced over their lower limbs.

Some patients can benefit from one of the spring seats which are on the market if great care is taken to adjust the strength of the spring to the patient's own weight. However, these aids are relatively expensive, and tend to make the patient dependent upon them so that they become less able to manage if their own chair is not available.

Patients who are unable to balance or walk without the aid of a walking frame include that frame in their chair drill. They rise and stand in the frame, move it away from the chair, and then practise backing up to the chair and seating themselves again.

Note. Patients who sit in a high chair to make rising easier should be provided with a foot stool when seated. This should be a long stool and well padded if the knees are to be kept straight, or a stool to support the ankles in slight dorsiflexion if the knees are not at risk. A suitable stool should prevent pressure at the back of the thighs, assist sitting balance, and contribute to comfort.

Bed Drill

The patient's bed should be of the optimum height for rising and sitting. This will depend upon his stature, the degree of flexion in his joints, his strength, and the range of movement within which he can function. The chair from which he can rise most easily is a good guide. The mattress should be firm and flat providing for good posture, and greater support when moving on its surface. Other equipment may include a footboard or cradle to keep the bedclothes off the feet, a small neck pillow, a bed rope, and resting splints as recommended by the doctor or physiotherapist.

No pillow or folded blanket should be placed under the knees because this encourages flexion of hips and knees and can lead to disabling flexion deformities.

Getting into Bed. Bed drill is a modified form of chair drill, and so the variations suggested for chair drill will apply. The following aspects should be considered.

If one lower limb is more painful than the other some patients find it easier to enter the bed and leave it on opposite sides. The strong lower limb should lead both going in and getting out. This process may be useful in early days of retraining, but should not be continued unless the same move is possible in the patient's own bedroom.

Patients who cannot bear full weight should use their walking frame to transfer from commode, chair or wheelchair to the side of the bed. The chair is placed sideways beside the bed with the walking frame in front of it. The patient stands up in the frame, and completes a quarter turn to sit on the side of the bed.

When the patient is unable to use a walking frame and must receive help from another person, it is sometimes helpful to use a 'slide board'. This is usually a fracture board, polished and sprinkled with talcum powder to reduce friction. It is placed between the patient's chair and the bed, and the patient slides along it with whatever help he may need. This reduces heavy lifting for the helper, and stress for the person who is helped. It also permits both to take a rest half way through the move if this is needed.

Moving in Bed. The method used for moving in bed will depend upon which joints are stiff or painful. If the pain is unilateral the patient should roll to the strong side, and use the stronger limbs to their best advantage as described under hemiplegia.

The special problems of the rigidity of Parkinson's Disease are discussed on page 255. The 'rocking' movement described there can help some patients with stiffness from other causes.

The bed rope may also be of use. An overhead ring is not usually recommended because it places too much strain on hands and shoulders, and because it is not readily available at home. An occasional patient with strong arms but difficulties with their lower limbs may benefit from such an aid.

Getting Out of Bed. The movements for getting out of bed are usually a reversal of those used to get in. The exception to this is the patient who gets in one side and out the other in order to control pain. Slide boards, chairs with an arm removed, wheelchairs or walking frames will be needed as before, depending upon the method to be used.

Lying in Bed. If possible, the patient should lie flat in bed, with a small cushion under his neck to prevent neck flexion. The weight of the bedclothes should be supported on a footboard or cradle to protect the ankle, and to relieve pressure on other joints which may be painful. If night splints have been provided they should be worn to encourage relaxation in a good position.

When flexion is present in hips or knees, a certain amount of time should be spent by the patient in 'prone lying'. This should be discussed by the team, because it is not readily accepted by all patients, and there should be no doubt in the helper's mind as to whether it is necessary.

Sitting up in Bed. When sitting up in bed the patient should be as upright as possible and should have good support for his back. The knees should be kept straight, and the feet at right angles to the legs. The same general principles apply when seated in a chair. A stool will be needed to achieve them. 'Easy' chairs and a slouched position should be avoided as placing strain on the spine and the muscles of the back. If possible, patients with a tendency to flexion deformities of hips or knees should not sit for lengthy periods, but should stand, and preferably walk, at regular intervals. For this reason 'sitting up in bed' should not be encouraged as a way of life. It is much easier to move if sitting up in a chair.

Bath Drill

The patient with a stiff or painful hip may have difficulty in lifting his leg over the side of the bath when seated on the bathboard. He will be made more comfortable if the helper places a hand behind his shoulders and supports him as he leans back against it and raises the painful limb over the rim and into the bath. If he needs help to raise the limb and place it in the bath, this help should be given gently and smoothly. The leg should not be raised any higher than is necessary for the heel to clear the edge of the bath. The patient should be told what is happening, so as to be ready mentally as well as physically for each part of the move. Sudden or jerking movements should be avoided.

If the move is too painful for the patient, or the patient is too heavy for the helper, it is probably better to settle for a complete sponge in bed in the usual way, or the use of a mechanical hoist. The latter should not be used if the patient will not be able to use one at home.

There are many 'gadgets' for use in association with bathing, and more can be designed for specific problems. Some useful ones include a soap mit when the grip is weak, soap in a net bag tied to a shower fitting so as to be easily retrieved if it is dropped, a pad on the end of a dowel stick for washing the toes, a long-handled sponge for washing the back, and many more. Such gadgets should not be given to the patient for their own sake, but they can help in problem solving when no more natural way can be found.

Shower Drill

Shower drill is only chair drill carried out in a shower recess. If the patient is too disabled to move in this way, a shower chair on wheels may prove useful. Neither of these methods is possible if the shower has a hob. In this case, a long stool which crosses the hob, having two feet inside the recess and two outside, is a possible solution. The patient sits on it outside, and moves in as on a bathboard. A hose-type shower is easier to use when seated than a fixed one.

Toilet Drill

Rising and sitting can pose problems for patients with stiff or painful hips, and unstable or stiff and painful knees. A built up toilet seat provides an answer for many such patients (see Figure 17.1). The average height needed is 21 inches (53 cm) but this can be altered to suit the individual.

Patients with hips which have stiffened in some degree of extension find it helpful to have the seat raised higher at the back than at the front. Patients with stiff or unstable knees also find the sloping seat helpful. They should also be taught to sit and rise using the walking frame for extra support.

Commode Drill

This is a combination of the patient's chair drill and his bed drill. Many patients with stiff and painful limbs find it easier and safer to get out of bed onto their walking frame, do a quarter turn, and sit on their commode. They reverse the order to return to bed. This applies particularly to those with difficulties in weight bearing associated with their pain and stiffness. The commode should be built up to the optimum height for the patient, and a sloped seat is sometimes worth consideration.

A large patient with a stiff hip may find it impossible to sit far enough back in the chair to be in position over the hole in the commode. In such cases the back of the commode should be removed or sloped backwards, or a special commode should be constructed with an appropriately deep seat.

Car Drill

Getting into a car can prove difficult for patients with stiff hips or knees. This is particularly so with low seats and narrow doors. The former present difficulties in rising and sitting, and the latter make it impossible to bring a stiff leg into the car after the patient is seated. A specially constructed cushion which can be firmly attached to the car seat may help by raising the sitting surface. A firm seat belt and a firm cushion to support the feet will help with the balance problem of the higher seat.

Patients with knees in fixed extension can enter a car with a continuous front seat by using their chair drill. They should then move back towards the driver's seat until their feet clear the door, and forward again while turning to face the front. Cushions should be placed under the extended limbs for support.

This method is not possible with a bucket seat. In this case it is usually easier for the patient to enter from a wheelchair with the aid of a slide board. The chair is wheeled as close as possible to the car, facing inwards. The slide board is placed under the patient's legs, leading into the car and bridging the gap between the car seat and the seat of the wheelchair. The patient then moves forward along the board, turning his whole body towards the front as soon as his feet are well clear of the door. When he is in position the board is removed and the patient's extended legs are supported on a cushion. These moves are performed in reverse for getting out.

Adapted and Specially Designed Equipment

Because fixed deformities are so commonly associated with pain and stiffness, and because of the variety of disabilities which may result, patients with arthritic conditions require particular attention to their equipment.

Some General Principles

1. It should be light and easy to handle.
2. All moving parts should be in good order and well oiled so as not to cause strain to the operator.
3. Heights and angles should be suited to the individual.
4. The feet and back should be well supported, whatever the degree of deformity. Various shaped cushions, or specially designed ones should be used if standard ones do not solve the problem.
5. Hand grips should be built up, padded, or reangled to suit the individual.

6. Levers should be lengthened to decrease the effort required to use them.
7. Articles required by the patient should be placed within reach and not in cupboards which are too high, too low, or too deep.
8. For the patient with rheumatoid arthritis, methods of holding and working should be designed so that as little stress as possible is placed on the fingers. Methods which cause ulnar deviation (movement of the fingers away from the thumb towards the little finger) should be avoided with particular care.

Gadgets and Aids

Many gadgets and aids already on the market to help able people with common tasks can also help the person with arthritic joints. It is usually easier to adapt these by changing a handle, providing a method of support or lengthening a lever, than to make an item from scratch. The value of a gadget depends upon the patient's ability to understand and use it. Costly and elaborate gadgets tend to be left unused except by a few mechanically minded people. Patients should be given opportunities to use and learn about gadgets before taking them home, then any necessary alterations can be made to suit the individual, and the patient can build up confidence in the item's value to himself (see Chapter 19).

Aids for Recreation

Adaptations to equipment can be used in helping patients to participate in recreational activities which might otherwise be denied them. Such items as card holders, large housie cards with easy to handle cover pieces, remote control switches for television, built up knobs on radios, special handles on pens, pencils and paint brushes, clip boards to stop paper slipping, long-handled garden tools, and many other aids can extend the available range of activities. Stabilising the article on which the patient is to work, and providing equipment which will lighten the workload are the main considerations in bringing an activity within the patient's scope.

The Severely Disabled Patient

Patients with severe generalised disabilities as a result of long-standing and inadequately treated rheumatoid disease are not uncommonly referred to the retraining unit as the result of some change in their support system as opposed to a change in themselves. Typical is the almost helpless patient who has been cared for lovingly by a close relative. Only when this relative is no longer able to manage because of her own infirmity or illness does the original patient come to the retraining unit. In such cases the problems of both people must be recognised and dealt with. Lifting is usually one of the chief difficulties to be overcome and the need for constant attention may be another.

Every method for decreasing the demands on the helper needs to be considered, and implemented if it is practical. A slight increase in function in the patient, improved equipment, and better methods of managing by the relative may be enough when added together to help the situation; on the other hand, improvement in only one of these areas might be quite inadequate. Positive attitudes, practical measures, and good team-work are all required of the staff. Co-operation from the patient is essential as he must usually accept a certain amount of pain and discomfort in order to achieve the goal. Some patients come full of determination to do their best, but there are others who have long since accepted that their case is hopeless and that they must have everything done for them. Such patients need gentle handling in the early days, with small goals offered one at a time, and genuine interest from the staff in response to every small gain. Any suggestion that the patient 'isn't trying', should be avoided, because this usually leads to unhappiness and active resistance. The patient may even feel guilty if he finds that he can do something which he has allowed someone else to do for him for years, or he may treasure his helplessness as a means of getting help and sympathy. The psychological background should not be under-rated when helping such patients.

In the presence of severe multiple and permanent deformity and disability, no rule of thumb can be given for retraining. Each case must be taken on its merits, and gains should be sought wherever they seem possible. In no other patients are staff inventiveness and ingenuity of more importance. If these cannot produce enough answers the use of a mechanical hoist may be a necessary solution.

Domiciliary care is usually indicated for these patients, and the relative's needs are paramount. Help in the form of day centre attendance and planned readmissions may enable the relative to continue providing care as well as helping the patient to maintain his gains.

PART FIVE
Equipment and Materials

This section deals with the concept
of using simple basic equipment
and adapting it to individual needs.
Tools and materials used in the activity
programme are also discussed.

18 BASIC EQUIPMENT

The concept of 'Basic Equipment', standardised to suit the retraining programme. Its design, selection and delivery to patients are outlined and staff responsibilities are discussed.

Introduction

Equipment plays a significant part in the Newcastle retraining programme. It is one of many interconnected services, and all items have been chosen carefully to fit into the overall plan. It is used specifically as a problem-solving medium, attention being paid to everyday furniture as well as to specialised retraining aids.

The two main situations to which it must relate are the retraining programme in the hospital, and the residual needs of the patient after discharge. Basic equipment is chosen to suit both situations so as to ensure continuity for the patient when he goes home. This co-ordination has influenced the choice of items for the basic list. As in other aspects of the Newcastle Method, standardisation and simplification form a base from which to work, while adjustments are made in response to specific needs. The basic equipment consists of essential household furniture, selected standard aids for the disabled, and the tools necessary for making adjustments and additions.

Items on the basic list are used consistently during retraining, and are kept in stock for immediate delivery to the home when needed.

Principles in Selecting Basic Equipment

Over a period of more than 20 years, many items of equipment have been used and tested in practical situations. Some have been found to have general application, and to be in constant demand, while others have not lived up to initial expectations, and have been superseded or discarded in the light of experience. From this experience some principles have emerged which help the selection of new items to be more discriminating and practical, and incidentally, more economical, than the choice of isolated items which 'look promising'. These principles are:

(a) Equipment should be simple and practical, so as to be easily understood by the patient and all who help him.
(b) Safety in use should be a primary consideration.
(c) It should be suitable for use in the home as well as the hospital.
(d) It should be suitable for use with the retraining drills, and not chosen in isolation from the rest of the programme.
(e) Moving and detachable parts should be avoided or kept to a minimum.
(f) High quality should be demanded in construction and finish.
(g) New items should be well tested, and should prove themselves in a number of cases before being added to the basic list.
(h) Adaptability and a wide application should be considered.
(i) Economy should be considered so long as the patient's needs are met.
(j) False economies should be avoided. Poor workmanship, design, or materials usually lead to waste.
(k) 'Over' design is wasteful, and should be avoided.

The Economic Factors

Equipment can be a very expensive item if it is not selected and distributed with discretion. When it is selected with care, and used in problem solving, it can also lead to real savings in staff time and bed occupancy. The sidestepping of a physical problem by the provision of suitable equipment can shorten a patient's stay in hospital by days, or even weeks. For example, a patient with parietal lobe damage as a result of a stroke may find it impossible to place his pylon correctly so that it runs parallel to the line of his walk. Because of the natural angle of his hand as he grips the handle, he will tend to turn the front legs inwards in front of his strong foot. This leads to the danger of tripping or the production of an unsatisfactory gait.

Attempts to correct this problem by retraining are likely to take a long time for some patients and prove impossible for others. By using suitable equipment on the other hand, we can 'sidestep' the problem and produce the desired result almost immediately. In this case a special handle, placed at an angle to the pylon, ensures that the pylon comes down in the correct position when the patient holds his hand at the angle which comes naturally to him. It does not take many days of extra hospitalisation to counter any savings made by withholding the simple equipment usually needed for this problem-solving role.

When considering the economics of providing equipment the following considerations are relevant.

Standardisation

Even the simplest items of equipment are on the market in great variety. This applies to beds, chairs, wheelchairs, commodes, walking aids and most of the other items produced for hospital use. If any of these really solved all the problems the rest would not exist. It is therefore reasonable to choose a good average article and adhere to the decision unless real problems are found in its use. Some advantages of such a policy are:

1. The staff learns how to use the equipment more efficiently if unnecessary variety is eliminated.
2. Adjustments and adaptations become routine and do not need to be 'invented' for each new item.
3. The team will know exactly what is meant when equipment is ordered or discussed at clinical meetings.
4. Ward stock need not be so large, as standard equipment can be shared.
5. Storage for items on domiciliary care is easier because of reduced variety, and less need for reserve stocks.
6. Ordering is easier as it can be seen at a glance when individual items are getting low.

Simplicity

In choosing standard equipment, a simple, well-constructed article is usually cheaper and longer lasting than a complicated one with too many 'clever' ideas. Some modern equipment has become so specialised and complicated that elderly patients have difficulty in accepting it. They tend to react in one of two equally unsatisfactory ways. The first reaction is fear, particularly if the article looks difficult to manage or to apply. The second reaction is blind faith, which leads them to expect a machine-made miracle, and to put less effort into their retraining than they would otherwise do.

This unrealistic response applies particularly to items with numerous motors, leads, and moving parts. For these reasons, expensive equipment is not necessarily better than a simpler and cheaper article. Apart from this, expensive, elaborate equipment is more prone to breakage and loss of parts than the simple, more practical variety. The latter is easier for all staff members to understand and use correctly.

Over Design

Over design can add unnecessarily to the cost of equipment. It may be useful to have some adjustable articles in the retraining unit in order to assess the needs of individual patients. It is not necessary for the adjustable version to be provided for personal use. For instance, an adjustable walking stick may be used to determine the best height for each patient who needs one, but it is cheaper and safer to cut down an ordinary cane for training the individual and for his use after discharge. This eliminates accidental changes or alterations made by well-meaning but unskilled relatives and at the same time proves less expensive. Many of the clever ideas incorporated in an over-designed item may never be really needed, but they will certainly add to its cost.

Over-specialised Equipment

Highly specialised equipment may be necessary for an occasional individual, while the majority of patients can be retrained quite adequately by using the simple basic items. It is good practice to stock only the basic items, and to order more specialised equipment only in response to specific needs. This saves the expense of idle equipment in both capital outlay and in storage space. Deterioration is inevitable if equipment is stored for long periods.

Bulk Ordering

Standardisation leads to the use of fewer varieties, with larger quantities of the selected items. Savings can thus be made in ordering larger numbers with confidence that they will be used. This usually leads to a better price, and minimises transport and handling costs. It also helps in the accurate assessment of needs, so that mistakes in ordering are less likely to occur.

Re-use of Equipment

When standard equipment is used, it is freely interchangeable between treatment areas and between patients. When it is no longer needed by a patient it can be returned to stock for immediate reissue. Any adaptations can be removed, so that it returns to its original form, to be adapted again as necessary. The need for some of the adaptations has been regular enough for these adaptations to be added to the basic list, so as to be readily available when needed. These too, can be used and re-used as the occasion demands.

Organisation of Delivery to the Patient

The method of getting equipment to the patient is itself a matter of routine. There are three supply points, co-ordinated by discussion at the case conference. These are the ward, the retraining area, and domiciliary care. The staff members most likely to be involved are the ward sister, the retraining sister, the physiotherapist and the occupational therapist. The Social Work Department is responsible for delivery to the home of such equipment as is indicated by the patient's ADL assessment (see Chapter 8).

Ward Equipment

This covers the patient's bed, commode, bedside chair, method of bathing, and toilet facilities. The admitting nurse may see to these at the time of admission, but the responsibility belongs to the ward sister. If there is any problem which goes beyond routine, it should be referred to the retraining staff for special attention. Points to be considered are:

1. Suitable heights — All relevant equipment such as bed, chair, commode, toilet seat, bath seat, and stools should be checked to ensure that their heights match the patient's needs.
2. Placement of the bed in the ward — Such factors as medical status, need for companionship, side of bed to be used, sensory disturbance, mental capacity and ingrained habits need to be considered. It should be remembered that 'bed drill' is of key importance in a satisfactory return home, and all these factors may be involved in it.
3. Whether the patient will use a shower or bath at home — The patient should be retrained in the appropriate method from the beginning. The use of suitable equipment is a ward respon-

sibility. Information from the social worker or the relatives may be necessary, while practical problems should be discussed with the retraining staff.

4. Whether the patient has difficulty in using the standard toilet pedestal — The use of a raised toilet seat may be necessary if this is so. Lifting by the staff will only prolong the period of dependence, and so it is better to use equipment to solve the problem.

5. Whether a low commode poses similar problems to a low toilet pedestal — The legs of the commode should be built up to solve this problem. If the patient's bed drill demands a side transfer, the arm of the chair should be removed on the appropriate side.

Note. The ward staff is also responsible for seeing that the patient really uses all equipment supplied for his retraining and to ensure that he has it with him at appropriate times.

The importance of co-operation from the ward staff in the supply of appropriate equipment, and conscientious supervision of its regular use cannot be over-emphasised. Incorrect and badly used equipment is at best a waste of retraining time, and at worst a real danger to the patient concerned.

Retraining Equipment

Any equipment which the patient may need should be decided upon, ordered, and supplied in the retraining area if the problem has not been solved in the routine ward situation. This is particularly so in cases where the ward staff have asked for assistance. Some of the more specific items are usually the responsibility of the staff in the retraining area. Walking aids, feeding, cooking, and dressing appliances, and adaptations to basic equipment (see Chapter 19) are examples.

Some points to be considered are:

1. Equipment is a major tool in the problem-solving function of the special retraining staff — They should be aware at all times of the importance of correct size, fit, application and use. An inch cut off a walking stick, or added to a chair, may make all the difference between success or failure to the patient concerned. These finer points may not always be noted by the general staff, but should always be the concern of those speci-

fically concerned with retraining.

2. The retraining staff should make sure that any specific use of equipment is understood by the staff in the ward — There is no value in supplying equipment which is not used effectively in the patient's daily life. Routine methods will normally be followed by all staff members, so any variation for a specific patient must be made known to all who work with him and demonstrated if necessary.

3. A stock of basic equipment in all relevant sizes should be kept within easy reach of the retraining area — Appropriate individual equipment can then be assessed and supplied quickly and easily. In practice it has been found best to lend these items (walking aids, wheelchairs, slide boards, and stools) if the problem is solved by basic equipment, but to provide the article which will eventually go home with the patient if adjustments and additions are necessary.

4. It is desirable to have a fully equipped bathroom, toilet, bedroom and kitchen within easy reach of the retraining area — This ensures that items of equipment can be tested in that area with the patient concerned. If this is not possible, the ward facilities can be used, but this involves taking staff and patients out of the retraining area, and also causes some difficulties in the care and maintenance of demonstration equipment.

5. Care and maintenance of equipment is the responsibility of every staff member who uses it and finds it wanting — Because of their close association with the use and supply of equipment, the retraining staff should be specially concerned, and observant in this matter. This is particularly so at the point of issue to the patient, and any faults noted at this time should be attended to at once. Instability, loose parts, cracks, missing rubbers, poor brakes, and the like, can all lead to accidents. Cleanliness of reissued equipment should also be a matter of concern to all, but particularly to those who reissue it.

Domiciliary Equipment

The patient who has been helped towards independence by the use of equipment in the hospital will obviously need similar equipment if he is to maintain achievements at home. It is the responsibility of the retraining staff to list the patient's needs for equipment on his final ADL assessment, and give such details as to size, adjustment and adaptation as may be required. If required, they should also

see the relatives of the patient and instruct them in the proper use
of the equipment. It should be ensured that the patient's own bed,
chair, toilet and bath are suitable before he returns to his home,
and that adjustments are made as necessary.

Some points to be considered are:

1. Standard equipment, with standard adjustments as needed,
   can be delivered from the domiciliary care equipment store,
   but these adjustments must be made by a staff member, and
   not left to the relative or the patient.
2. If other than standard adjustments have been made, the item
   the patient has been using in the hospital should go home with
   him. The item should be replaced in retraining stock by standard equipment.
3. All items coming back into the store after use should be
   cleaned and serviced before being replaced in stock for reissue.
4. In the Newcastle Domiciliary Care Service, the equipment
   store is under the control of the Director of Geriatrics and
   administered by the Social Work Department. The staff of that
   department is responsible for delivery of equipment and for
   the accounting system.
5. The accounting system is similar to that of a library, where
   each item is numbered and has its own card, and each
   borrower has a card in his own name. Equipment cards are
   filed numerically under headings such as 'Commodes',
   'Pylons', 'Walking Frames', and the patients' cards are filed
   alphabetically. Two entries are thus made for each item as it
   leaves or re-enters the store.

Replacement and Exchange

If a patient's condition changes after discharge so that his equipment is no longer suitable, if he breaks it, or finds it unsatisfactory
for any reason, he (or the person looking after him) is encouraged
to refer the matter to the Domiciliary Care Service, so that the
team becomes aware of the problem. Simple replacement without
reassessment may lead to an underlying problem being missed. If
the fault is the patient's, he may need a refresher course. If the
fault lies in the equipment, it may need to be redesigned. Feedback
of this kind is of great value in developing sound, practical equipment for the basic equipment list. It is necessary for the patient,

who depends upon equipment for his independence, that such equipment should be in good condition and suited to his current needs. For this reason there must be provision for replacement and exchange after his discharge.

The Basic Equipment List

Items on the basic equipment list are those which are used routinely in the hospital, and most of them are kept in the equipment store, ready for distribution on domiciliary care. The list has been adjusted from time to time, in response to changing needs, or in the light of experience. This process will continue as needs arise. The present list includes beds, chairs, stools, commodes, built up toilet seats, bathboards, wheelchairs, walking frames, walking canes, and pylon walking aids. Adjustments, adaptations and additions to these will be discussed in Chapter 19.

Furniture

Standard Beds

1. The height should allow the patient to sit comfortably on the side with his feet placed firmly on the floor. In practice three heights are used. These can be further varied by providing a choice between inner spring and rubber mattresses. The relevant height is measured from the ground to the top of the mattress. Measurements should be taken without the patient's weight. The three basic heights are: 19 inches (48 cm) for short people and those with fixed flexion deformities of hips and knees; 21 inches (53 cm) for average people and those who use a wheelchair; 23 inches (58 cm) for tall people and those with stiff or painful hips.
2. A firm base is needed so that the patient can push up on it.
3. Bedclothes should not be too heavy, and neither should they be tucked in too tightly on the side used by the patient.
4. Overhead rings should only be provided in exceptional circumstances. Some paraplegics and patients who have already been trained to use this method are examples, but even they should be tested to see if the ring is really the best answer for them. If the patient can learn to push up instead of pulling up,

rings are unnecessary and lead to dependence upon a hospital-type bed.

5.   Placement of the bed is important to many patients. The bed should be so placed that when the patient sits on the edge his stronger limbs are nearest to the bed head. Patients with sensory problems should be placed so that they can make the best use of the senses which are still available to them. This applies to the blind and the deaf as well as to hemiplegics with sensory impairment.

6.   Lockers should be placed where the patient can reach them safely and easily.

The Importance of Bed Heights

Despite the recommendations of eminent geriatricians over many years, there is still opposition in many hospitals to cutting down the beds or replacing high ones with low. Frail and unstable elderly folks are expected to climb up on little sets of steps or to be lifted bodily by the nurses. The reasons which are most often given for such resistance are:

1.   Nurses will hurt their backs if low beds are provided.
2.   Varied bed heights will look untidy and inefficient.
3.   It will 'spoil' expensive equipment to cut it down.

Lack of understanding of the principles and aims of retraining, and basic conservatism underlie such thinking. Few units where some low beds have been introduced would willingly return to the exclusive use of high ones. Experience has shown that once a few beds have been cut down experimentally, a demand has grown for more to be similarly treated. Some of the answers to the points raised above are as follows.

The Nurse's Back. Serious injury to the nurse's back is usually sustained while lifting a heavy patient without concern for correct kinetic methods. Bed making may cause mild discomfort at first, until the nurse becomes used to the different height. It does not cause severe permanent damage as that which may result from heavy lifting. Dangerous lifting is kept to a minimum by the use of a low bed which permits the patient to transfer his weight through his own limbs instead of the nurse's back. The low bed protects the nurse's back at the same time that it helps the patient to become independent.

Lack of Uniformity. Military uniformity in bed heights may look efficient, but different patients actually need different heights for their well-being. True efficiency means being able to meet these various needs. Uniformity should not be seen as an end in itself, but should give place when it is incompatible with treatment requirements.

Damage to Equipment. As low beds are preferable to high ones for all but the sickest patients, cutting down some of the latter can be shown to improve them rather than to do them any damage. A few high beds should be left for specific nursing procedures and medical examinations, or a few 'HI-LO' beds may be provided. The relative numbers of such beds will depend upon the type of patient being treated. Where there is a problem of mobility a low bed should be considered.

Independence. Independent night care is one of the principal requirements for a satisfactory return home. Domiciliary care can break down as a result of neglect in this area, and yet independence cannot be practised nor assessed accurately from a high bed. Both the patient who lives alone and the patient who calls for help from a relative during the night are at risk. In a high bed the frail patient remains dependent upon another person to provide a bed pan or physical help until the day of his discharge. In a low bed the necessary degree of independence can usually be achieved.

Chairs

Chairs for the elderly disabled should be chosen for practical use as well as for comfort. They should be comfortable, but not 'easy'. Mistaken kindness often leads to elderly patients being placed in low, deep chairs, from which they have no chance of rising unaided. Not only do they miss the practice in rising from a chair, which is so important for their independence, but they also develop a habit of calling for help instead of trying to act for themselves. Easy chairs also encourage somnolence and a tendency to withdraw from the activity of the room. Some features to consider in choosing a patient's chair are:

1. The height of the seat. This should be suitable for sitting up to a table. A 'bridge' type chair is usually satisfactory for use at home if it is suitably upholstered.
2. Seats should be relatively flat, and firm but not hard. The width of the seat must also be considered if an obese patient is involved.
3, Backs should give support without the need for a cushion.
4. Arms should be firm, and directly over the legs to prevent tipping sideways when used for pushing up in order to stand.
5. Runners, if available, are preferable to legs. A chair with runners can be pushed back from the table or otherwise moved by the patient himself with greater safety than a chair with legs. It is also more easily moved by the staff with a patient seated in it.
6. The height may need to be adjusted for tall patients, those with stiff hips, and others who have difficulty in rising from a low seat. A stool should be provided for short patients so that their feet are well supported.
7. Strict attention should be paid to the stability of the chair in every direction.

Modern Chair Design

In recent years much work has been done on chair design and its relationship to anthropometrics. Principles which have emerged from this work will apply to seating for the elderly, just as they do for the population as a whole. Extra factors, however, must be considered when the furniture in question is to be used by the disabled whose bodies no longer comply with what can be expected of the 'average' person. Their chairs must be completely stable, easily adjustable, easy to move, easy to clean, and provided with well-designed arms. A chair which is quite satisfactory for a healthy young student or typist will not necessarily be suitable for someone with a physical disability. Each patient's specific needs should be considered when choosing or adapting a chair for him.

Stools

Two basic stool designs are used in the Newcastle programme. The larger one is long enough to support the lower limbs with the knees extended. The smaller one provides support for the feet.

1. The larger stool is used for patients with ankle oedema, plaster

casts, arthrodesis of the knees and other reasons for elevating the lower limbs. A small bolster cushion is placed at the back of the ankle to ensure that the heel clears the surface of the stool and is not endangered by pressure. Other cushions or sandbags are used in conjunction with the stool as may be necessary. The back of the stool should be of the same height as the front of the chair and it should slope gently to the front. Adjustments should be made if there is a 'step' between the two pieces of equipment.

2. The smaller stool is for supporting the patient's feet. It is intended for use by patients who find it difficult to make firm contact with the ground when seated in a chair. It is unsuitable for those who need to 'keep their feet up'. Very short patients, patients who need a high chair so as to be able to rise unaided, and patients who tend to slide forwards off their chair may all benefit from the use of this stool. It is also useful for supporting the feet while dealing with shoes and stockings. The stool is lower at the back than the front, to support the feet at right angles to the legs, and to help to prevent postural foot drop. The model used in the wards has adjustable legs so as to be adapted with ease to a variety of needs, but a simple, non-adjustable version is suited to most patients.

3. Stools, however stable, should never be used by elderly people for climbing into bed. The practice is dangerous, and teaches the patient nothing that will be of value to him on his return home.

Commodes

Adaptability is important in choosing a good basic commode for use in domiciliary care. Adjustment of height and the removal of one or both arms are such routine requirements that these are provided for with basic materials which are kept in stock. Standard 'build-ups' are stocked in four sizes, and can be attached quite simply. A screwdriver is all that is necessary to remove an arm. A wooden model commode has been chosen for its suitability for adjustment as well as its economy.

For many years the same model was used in the ward, but this necessitated removal by day, and replacement in the evening, causing unnecessary use of staff time. The chair which is now used in the ward is available in a fixed model, and one with adjustable legs, removable arms, and in its basic form has dimensions to match the wooden model the patient will use at home. It is aesthetically more acceptable than the more obvious wooden model, and so can be left beside the bed for day-time use as an armchair. For this purpose it was necessary to have cushions made, which do not come with the chair, because the commode was too deep to be comfortable and to give sufficient back support. In practice the proportion of one adjustable commode to every three fixed ones has proved satisfactory. If gross alterations are necessary the patient is provided with a wooden model from the domiciliary care store. This is adapted to suit his needs and taken home with him on discharge.

Toilets and Toilet Seats

1. Patients are taught to use a normal toilet pedestal if possible. Apart from being difficult and expensive to install in some homes, special bars, rails and chains limit the patient who relies upon them to places where they are provided. These are rare.
2. Rails for pulling up are not used, as the retraining drills are based on pushing up.
3. If a patient cannot rise from a normal seat, or if he needs a wider seat to push against, a special toilet stool of the height he needs is provided.
4. The basic toilet seat fits any toilet pedestal. The height is 22 inches (56 cm) to match the height of the basic wheelchair. A plastic bucket with the bottom removed is fixed beneath the hole, and fits into the toilet bowl to prevent splash. It also stabilises the stool so that it does not slip away from the pedestal.
5. The legs can be removed so that the seat is easily transported in the boot of a car. This gives the patient more flexibility as to where he can stay, and even makes a motel holiday possible for some.
6. The design suits the normal chair drill, providing space for the hands to be placed in the best position for pushing up.
7. The toilet roll may be mounted on the toilet build up on whichever side best suits the patient's needs.

Bath and Shower Equipment

In the Newcastle Method, patients are taught to use a bathboard (Figure 18.1) rather than to go right down into the bath. Most of them are relieved to find the latter process unnecessary, and those whose recovery is such that a plunge is possible will return to it spontaneously when they feel ready.

1. Both baths and showers are used in the hospital, depending upon the patient's situation at home, and not the convenience of the staff.
2. Shower equipment includes a plastic chair or a wide stool. Ordinary chair drill is carried out. A hose-type shower is preferred to a fixed one.
3. Bath equipment includes a chair of equal height to the bath. It may be without arms, or have the arm nearest to the bath removed.
4. A bathboard is used in conjunction with this chair. Patients do not go down into the bath, but use a hand shower or dipper.
5. The new, elaborate baths with cut away sides and built in handles are not necessary, and in fact create their own problems by being too shallow for easy rising, and unsuitable for easy fitting of a bathboard. Relatives should be warned against replacing an old bath before the patient's real needs have been assessed.
6. Rails are not used, but a handle is fitted to the basic bathboard for the patient who needs it for balance or confidence.

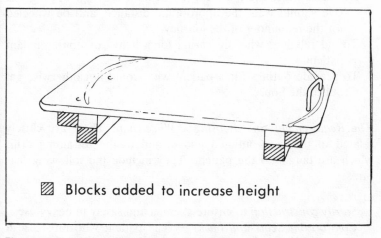

Blocks added to increase height

Figure 18.1: Adapted Bathboard. The height of the board has been raised by blocks to suit the specific needs of a patient

Wheelchairs

Surprisingly few patients who undergo retraining actually need a wheelchair when discharged. During retraining patients are encouraged to walk, with or without assistance, whenever it is possible for them to do so. The use of the wheelchair is kept to a minimum, and so the habit of walking is usually well developed by the time the patient goes home. Every walk is considered part of the patient's treatment, and the use of a wheelchair denies the patient that walking practice. When he goes home the unnecessary supply of a wheelchair can be dangerous. Unless used sparingly it encourages immobility and consequent deterioration. It can also lead to an attitude of dependence and invalidism.

Indications for the Use of a Wheelchair. These should be understood if the most suitable chair is to be chosen from the many to be found in the catalogue. The main uses are:

The early stages of retraining before walking is attempted.
Bilateral lower limb amputations.
Bilateral non-weight bearing or paralysis of lower limbs.
Quick transport to the toilet in cases of urgency. (The patient should walk back.)
Return to the ward of patients who become ill in other areas.
Distances which are too great for the patient's stage of progress. (He should walk the appropriate distance, and be wheeled for the remainder of the journey.)
To aid relatives who are caring for a heavy or non-ambulant patient.
To provide outings for a patient who would not otherwise get out of the house.

The Requirements in Choosing a Wheelchair. These are closely related to the uses outlined above, and to the retraining drills which are taught to the patient. They include the following features:

Sturdy construction to ensure stamina and safety in heavy use.
Comfortable seats and backs — The patient who must use a wheelchair for long periods is likely to be seriously disabled, and so may have difficulty in changing his own position or in main-

taining his posture. The basic chair must provide for this.

Removable arms — These are necessary for patients who must transfer sideways. Arms which are attached and swing behind the chair are useful because they cannot be mislaid or exchanged with those of another chair. Unfortunately, they are usually only supplied with rather expensive chairs.

Adjustable and removable foot plates — The patient's feet should be well supported at all times. The front of the foot plate should be higher than the back to help guard against foot drop. The foot plate should swing outwards as well as upwards, so as to be out of the way when the patient uses a standing transfer. It should also be removable for use by non-prosthetic bilateral amputees.

Long lever type brakes — The small 'modern' brakes are very vulnerable and a slight knock will render them useless. Forgetful and demented patients find the long lever type easier to apply because pulling on a brake comes more naturally than pushing it. The long lever is easy to adjust by attaching a removable extension handle for patients with weak hands. Brakes of both types need to be adjusted to maintain their strength as the rubber tyres wear down. The top of the brake lever without the extension handle should never extend above the seat level because this can cause obstruction in side transfers and may possibly lead to injury.

Solid tyres — For general use these are more practical than pneumatic tyres, which need more maintenance. Individual patients may need pneumatic tyres, but they are not recommended for the basic chair.

Wheel grips for self propulsion — This is an auxiliary ring attached to the large wheels. It protects the patient from soiling his hands, which is inevitable if he grips the rubber tyres to propel the chair.

A folding mechanism — This is particularly important for use in domiciliary care. Not only does it make it possible to take the chair in the boot of a car, but it also makes it easier to store in a restricted area. This is valuable in the base store and in the home.

Features over and above those listed here may be helpful for an individual patient, but they are not necessary in the basic chair, chosen for general use in the hospital or on domiciliary care.

Slide Boards

The slide or 'shuffle' board is the traditional fracture board with its ends planed down. Its main use is to form a bridge upon which bilateral amputees and paraplegics can move from wheelchairs to bed, car, or sofa, particularly if there is a gap to be negotiated. It is also used to reduce friction so that an obese patient can move more easily along a flat surface. It is particularly useful to help relatives manage a heavy patient, as it enables the move to be taken in stages, with rests in safe positions when necessary.

Walking Aids

There are three main walking aids used in the Newcastle Method of retraining. These are the Roberts Walking Frame, the Parbery Pylon Stick, and the traditional walking cane. The two former aids are stocked in a range of heights, and the canes are cut to the size needed by each patient. Generally speaking, the 'walker' is used by patients with two functioning hands, and either a balance or weight-bearing problem, and the 'pylon' by those with only one functioning hand, or the need for an intermediate support between the 'walker' and the cane.

It is rare indeed to find a patient whose needs are not covered by one of these basic walking aids, or modifications to them.

The Basic Walking Frame (see Figure 16.1)

The Roberts Walking Frame measures 27 in (69 cm) in its overall plan, and is stocked in two heights — 27 in (74 cm) and 31 in (77 cm). It has been refined through many stages, and the present model is stackable for economy of storage space. It stands upon two wheels in the front, and two rubbers at the back. The patient grasps the walker well back towards the rubber-shod legs, and leans on the walker before moving forward. This makes the rubbers act as a brake, and ensures that the frame does not slip. If the frame is held in the middle or even further forward its stability can be lost. Padded handles are placed in the correct position to prevent this from happening. Commercial walkers are available with four casters, or four rubbers, but the former have been found to be too mobile, and to undermine both confidence and safety, while the latter must be lifted completely from the ground, and so demand a greater degree of stability than is found in many of the patients concerned.

The advantages of the Roberts model are:

1. It is more adaptable for a variety of disabilities.
2. It is safer and gives more confidence to the patient.
3. It can be fitted with a tray for household use.
4. It is stackable.
5. It is better suited for the Newcastle drills, particularly for problems of weight bearing.

The Basic Four-pronged Stick (see Figure 16.1B)

The Parbery Pylon Stick is stocked in five sizes which cover all but the most exceptional needs. Special orders can be given for higher or lower sticks, but they are rarely needed. The basic heights are 28, 30, 31, 32, and 34 inches (71, 76, 79, 81, and 86 cm). These wooden 'pylons' are preferred to metal 'quadripods' because:

1. A larger ground base gives greater stability.
2. Weight is taken directly to the ground through the legs, so that 'whiplash' movement is eliminated.
3. The legs cannot be bent by rough ground or inaccurate placement, so there is little danger of them becoming uneven.
4. They are heavier, and so patients gain confidence in them more quickly.
5. They can be fitted with a tray or bag for carrying belongings.
6. They are cheaper. This would not influence the choice if they were in any way inferior, but is a bonus when they are preferred in their own right.

For these reasons the wooden pylon is considered essential to the efficient practice of the Newcastle Method of retraining in walking. When balance and confidence are gained some patients progress to a walking cane. A few younger patients sometimes buy themselves metal quadripods, and if it is safe, are taught to use them, but the practice is not encouraged. Any preference for them is for aesthetic rather than practical considerations, and they are not included in the basic equipment list.

Traditional Walking Canes

Walking canes are stocked in the simplest form, with the common hooked top. They are measured and cut to size for each patient. In most cases they are cut so that the top of the handle is approximately level with the wrist when the arm is allowed to hang loosely beside the body. For a patient progressing from a pylon stick the height is usually one inch (25 mm) greater than the height of the pylon.

Patients sometimes wish to use 'heirloom' sticks, or more attractive canes provided by relatives. These too should be cut to the correct size for the patient concerned. There is often resistance to cutting such sticks, but the problem can be overcome by lending a stick of the right height until the patient becomes used to it. Few patients wish to persevere with a stick of the wrong height once they have experienced the security and comfort of a suitable one.

Basic Additions and Adaptations

Those additions and adaptations which are in regular demand are added to the basic list, and stored ready for use. No item is added to the list or ordered in quantity until it has proved itself in actual use.

Items on the present list are as follows:

Alterations

1. Adjustments to the height of almost any article of furniture to make it suit the individual. Beds, chairs, commodes, bathboards, stools, toilet seats and walking aids may be cut down or built up as required. Some of the methods employed are described in Chapter 19.
2. Removal of parts as necessary. Arms from commodes, and foot plates from wheelchairs are the most common examples.

Additions

The following items are now included in the basic list because they solve recurring problems:

1. Trays for walking frames and pylons.
2. Elbow attachments for walking frames.
3. Eversion handle for pylons (see Case 4 p. 400).
4. Pull up ropes for beds.
5. Safety belts for wheelchairs.

6. Build-up blocks for beds and commodes.
7. Special build-up runners for 'diplomat' chairs.

Correlation of Basic Equipment and Basic Drills

The retraining drills, as described in Chapter 15, have been worked out to train the patient in the use of ordinary domestic furniture, so as to fit him for life at home. The equipment has also been selected or designed with this end in view. Some patients will need adjustments to their existing furniture in order to be independent, and others will need basic additions to it. It is usually possible to overcome these problems with the equipment described in this chapter. Special alterations are discussed in Chapter 19.

Heights are Important

The Newcastle drills are designed to help the patient to use his functioning limbs to the best advantage. This is obviously not possible if his equipment is too high or too low to permit the optimum movements. The double amputee who can be quite independent if all his equipment is matched for height, may be wholly dependent for his transfers if it is not. A patient with a stiff hip may be able to rise independently from a 23 inch (58 cm) chair, but need to be lifted by a nurse from a 16 inch (41 cm) one. The importance of correct height is stressed for any equipment used by a disabled person.

Pushing Up and Leaning Rather than Pulling Up and Holding On

The Newcastle drills encourage pushing up instead of pulling up. This affects the equipment in the following ways:

1. Overhead rings, bars, and rails are rarely used.
2. Firm surfaces are needed on beds, chairs, and anywhere the patient sits.
3. Stability is required in chairs, walking aids, and beds. Chair arms should be in the same vertical plane as their legs to prevent side tipping. Beds should have secure brakes or be wheel-less to prevent slipping if a patient leans against them. Wheelchairs must have reliable brakes.
4. Walking aids are somewhat shorter than those usually provided, to take the patient's weight directly to the ground through his own limbs and the aid.

Training in Real Situations

This aspect of the Newcastle Method means that artificial aids which are not generally available in the community, or which cannot be provided there are discouraged. Thus hand bars in corridors, overhead bed rings, island baths, and similar devices are rejected as leading to dependence except in the few situations in which they are provided. All equipment should be suitable for the average domestic situation.

Progress and Deterioration

In retraining, the patient's condition is unlikely to remain static. The performance of most patients will improve as they respond to treatment and become familiar with their equipment. The performance of others will tend to decline in the natural course of a progressive illness. Equipment must allow for such variations in ability, and be easily adapted to changing needs. This requirement is inherent in the use of the retraining drills.

Aesthetics and Acceptance

Few patients actively enjoy using equipment, but they accept it as the better of two evils. Acceptance is easier if the aid is well designed, well made, and well finished. Sometimes the most suitable aid may be rejected because the patient feels self-conscious about its use, and prefers something which 'looks better'. This may be an emotional decision, but it is very natural, particularly in younger patients. Compromise may be necessary, if familiarity with the article does not lead to a changed attitude. A patient who really dislikes a piece of equipment is unlikely to persevere with it once he leaves the hospital. A second choice, if he will accept it, may be the best choice for him. Some examples of this rejection of equipment include the refusal to carry a walking cane, to wear a caliper, or to use a commode in the bedroom.

Pride is usually the basis of this problem. We must see that the equipment is as good looking as we can make it. We can also try to help the patient to be proud of his skill in using the equipment instead of his ability to manage without it. Tact and understanding may bring results — compulsion will not.

Gadgetry

Gadgets and self-help aids could be the subject of a book in their own right. They are used to help patients perform tasks which would otherwise be difficult or impossible. They have been designed to cover every aspect of living, and are available in almost endless variety. Some have a very general application, and are included in the basic equipment for retraining. These fall into the following categories.

Dressing

1. A long-handled shoe horn.
2. Elastic bootlaces and a one-handed method for tying laces.
3. The use of 'Velcro' for fastenings instead of hooks and buttons.
4. Button-through dresses.
5. Elastic in pyjama trousers instead of cords, and in skirts instead of a placket.
6. A Velcro fastening for brassières and trouser tops.
7. A diagonal elastic brace to pull up trousers and skirts.
8. A stocking aid.

Hygiene and Grooming

1. A soap mitten.
2. Tap turner.
3. A suction-backed nail brush.
4. Bath plug stick.
5. A long-handled comb.
6. A toilet roll hook to facilitate one-handed tearing.
7. A long-handled sponge or back brush.
8. Electric razor.

Feeding and Drinking

1. A covered cup to prevent spillage.
2. A plastic straw.
3. A steep-sided plate.
4. Individually built up handles on cutlery.
5. Non-slip mats under plates.
6. Angled spoons and forks.
7. The 'Nelson' or Rocker knife.
8. A head hole serviette.

Cooking and Housework

Most elderly folk would rather use an old familiar knife than some modern alternative. The more closely any gadget resembles the old favourite, the more likely it is to prove successful. The two helpful features underlying kitchen aids are:

1. Steadying the item to be worked upon.
2. Providing an item which can be used despite the disability.

Steadying may be achieved by using suction cups, a damp wettex cloth, dycem mats, a ledge, or a clamp. Commonly used steadying gadgets are:

1. A vegetable board.
2. A bowl holder.
3. A hopper-type match box holder.

Items which are used normally with one hand, or make a task easier for weak hands include:

1. One-handed flour sifters.
2. Ratchet egg beaters.
3. Serrated jar openers.
4. Bar-type bottle openers.
5. Gas guns.
6. Tap turners.

Some items incorporate both these principles. Two of the most useful are the following.

The Electric Frypan. This can be placed conveniently for the patient to use sitting down, it can be stirred without the risk of tipping, it can be used with one hand, and the upright sides make it easy to pick up the cooked food and transfer it to a plate. Elderly men whose wives can no longer cook for them, find it much easier to understand the use of a frypan than the use of a stove, and people who live alone are more inclined to cook a balanced meal in a frypan than in multiple pots on the stove.

The Single-handed Drying up Apron. This is made of towelling, attached to a plastic band which can be put on one-handed and eliminates the need for a bow. The bottom of the towelling is turned up to make a pocket into which the washed articles are placed for drying. The apron is lined with plastic to prevent the patient's skirt from getting wet. The patient dries up while seated in a chair, so there is no danger for either the patient or the crockery. This apron has proved popular with elderly hemiplegics who wish to help in some way with household chores.

Gadgets, such as those mentioned here, are only provided when the patient really needs them, and will use them willingly. Younger patients, and those who live alone are the most common recipients. Many older patients find it difficult to adjust to a new way of performing old tasks, and others have already handed the tasks to someone else. The closer the new method is to normal the more likely it is to be used, and so simplicity in design is essential. Training in domestic activities and the use of 'gadgets' can be continued on an out-patient basis if the patient concerned is otherwise ready for discharge. Gadgetry can be of tremendous value to the right patient, but can prove time consuming and frustrating if persisted with unrealistically with the unwilling or confused.

Summary

Basic equipment is chosen to relate easily to the Newcastle retraining drills, and to be suitable for use in the patient's home. Care is taken that its dimensions suit the individual to whom it is supplied, and that he can use it efficiently. Any item which is found to be necessary in the hospital will be recommended for use at home, and if required, provided by the domiciliary care service.

19 THE USE OF EQUIPMENT IN PROBLEM SOLVING

The use, adjustment and design of equipment in the solution of problems which cannot readily be solved by treatment alone.

Introduction

The prevalence of multiple pathology and residual disability in patients who require retraining ensures that problem solving is an essential element in the programme. Suitable equipment can provide an answer when recovery is slow or incomplete. Problems which are common to many patients may be solved by the use of items from the basic list, but those which occur infrequently, or perhaps only once, need special attention and thought.

At this level, problem solving depends upon the inventiveness and positive attitudes of those who seek a solution. We can inhibit constructive ideas by saying 'he can't', or start them flowing by asking 'how can he?' Anyone who has driven through farmland, opening and shutting gates, will know that even a simple problem can have many solutions. The ingenuity of the farmer in devising ways to secure a gate is the kind we need when faced with a problem for which no immediate solution is apparent.

Attitudes and Ideas

Positive thinking and willingness to work with what is available are the main elements in this type of inventiveness. They produce original ideas, and make it possible to proceed at once, without long, frustrating delays. If an ideal item should turn up later, it is easily substituted, and no time has been lost in the patient's progress. Any equipment supplied is only successful if it is really used, and so the attitudes of the patient, the staff, and the relatives are as important as those of the inventor.

Attributes and Attitudes of the 'Inventor'

There is no monopoly on inventiveness. It is an attribute which all possess in varying degrees, but which some use more skilfully than others. Like most skills it can be developed with use and it is at its best when motivation is strong. Occasionally, solutions may present themselves in a flash of insight, but for most of us they are the result of thought, hard work, and conscious development of an idea. It is obvious that experience helps, but everyone must start somewhere, and it matters little to the patient who thinks of an idea, so long as it solves his problem. Some of the attributes which help in the problem-solving process are:

1. A positive approach — we must expect to find a solution, and seek it actively.
2. Imagination — we should be uninhibited in our preliminary thinking, letting our minds range over unlikely as well as likely answers. Extravagant ideas can help the flow of more practical ones.
3. A practical outlook — we should be practical in selecting which idea to pursue. Problems can only be solved with available material. The unattainable ideal should not blind us to the simpler possibilities.
4. Sensitivity — we need to understand how a patient may feel about using a special aid. In our design we should minimise any cause for embarrassment or inconvenience.
5. Perseverance — we should not give up too soon. If the original aid does not work, we should be prepared to adjust it and try again.
6. Open mindedness — we should be ready to listen to ideas from others. The patient, his relatives, or other members of staff may well see something we have missed. Hospital tradesmen such as carpenters and plumbers can be particularly helpful in advising on ways and means.

Attitudes of Staff Members

Staff members who have received their early lectures in retraining methods should be able to use basic equipment correctly, but new equipment or unusual ways of using the old should always be demonstrated and explained. The patient's acceptance of an article may well depend upon the staff's belief in it and the encouragement they give him to persevere. When staff members do not understand a piece of equipment or recognise the problem it is supposed to solve they will tend to place it out of sight and forget to encourage its use. No 'gadget' is better than the use that is made of it.

Once staff members become used to problem solving with equipment, they become interested in this aspect of retraining, and begin to initiate answers of their own. Positive attitudes are again the basis of success.

Attitudes of the Patient

Patients vary widely in their acceptance of special equipment to help solve their problems. Some are inventive by nature, and have already worked out useful ideas. Much can be learnt from them. Some are glad to use anything they can see as being helpful, and are proud of their skill in doing so. Some accept the aid quite passively, but forget to use it, or give up without really trying, while others are actively opposed to the use of any aid, either through pride, or because they would rather receive the attention of other people. These reactions have little to do with the degree of physical disability, but a great deal to do with the emotions and self image of the patient. We need to understand our patients in order to help them overcome these intangible barriers.

Many patients tend to take more interest in their equipment if it is fitted to their needs, and altered in their presence. Any suggestions from the patient should be incorporated if it is at all possible. A contribution from the patient himself is one of the surest indications that the article will be given a good trial.

The simpler and more normal a piece of equipment is, the less likely it is to be rejected by elderly patients. The pride which causes a deaf patient to reject a hearing aid, or a blind one to reject a cane, may have its counterpart in other forms of disability. Any form of aid should be presented with tact and understanding of the patient's likely attitude to its use.

Attitudes of Relatives

Once the patient goes home the attitude of relatives may well be the factor which decides whether his equipment will be used or not. Anything which is seen as damaging to the carpet or paint work, or as being ugly, bulky, or undignified, is likely to be put away and forgotten. Problems such as these should be avoided as far as possible in the design of equipment. If the patient's needs make a certain article necessary, and the relatives have some reason for rejecting it, a teaching session with these relatives is indicated. Most relatives will accept equipment if they are convinced of its value to the patient and understand the correct way to use it.

If the patient lacks understanding or motivation, or tends to forget instructions the relatives' co-operation in the use of equipment is essential. Much time can be wasted producing equipment for a patient who is allowed to retire to a chair to be waited upon because it is easier for the relative, physically, intellectually, or emotionally. It may be that this really is the best solution. If so, the choice should be planned for, and not left to chance. With the very dependent patient, the equipment needs and attitudes of the caring person must be taken into full account.

Identifying the Problem

Identifying the problem is much more than being aware that it exists. It involves understanding why it exists, its underlying causes, and the effects it will have on the patient's progress. An example of such identification might be as follows.

The Problem

Nocturnal incontinence.

Possible Causes

1. Slight urgency, investigated and treated; residual difficulty may not resolve.
2. Patient unable to transfer to commode unaided, dependent upon nurse arriving in time.
3. Obese and unable to sit up unaided.
4. Afraid, because once out on the commode she is unable to get back into bed.
5. Using ordinary low commode — unable to rise unaided.

Effects on Progress

1. Frail elderly sister unable to help at night — independent night care essential to going home.
2. Patient distressed by the problem and tending to let it over-

shadow other aspects of treatment.

The 'trigger questions' described in Chapter 5 can be helpful in bringing out relevant facts such as these, which might otherwise be overlooked. By bringing out individual aspects of the problem, they often point the way to the solution. The questions 'why?' and 'how?' are particularly helpful in this context. From answers such as those given above, it would appear, for instance, that the following solutions might be tried.

Treatment of the Patient

1. Check with dietitian.
2. Arrange extra bed drill.
3. Discuss at meeting — ? medication.

Help from Equipment

1. Pull up rope to aid sitting up in bed.
2. Lower bed so that feet are better supported on the floor when rising.
3. Build up commode to height from which patient can stand unaided.

When multiple pathology is involved it is particularly important to look for inter-related causes of difficulty. The presenting problem may be the tip of the proverbial iceberg.

Creative Thinking and Action

Once a problem has been identified, we should take any simple action which has been indicated as soon as we can. This will eliminate some of the minor difficulties, let the patient know that we are working on his problem, and perhaps most importantly, start us thinking about the larger aspects involved. If simple additions and alterations to equipment prove inadequate, original or 'creative' thinking is needed. We should not be afraid of it. Everything made by human hands was thought of by someone, and the process still goes on. The main thing is to make a start, and ideas will usually come. It is often helpful to follow a series of steps, quite consciously, if ideas are slow in presenting themselves.

The steps might be taken in some such order as this:

(a) Consider the aim of the venture — What are we trying to accomplish?

(b) Check the available assets — The patient's own strengths, existing aids or equipment, available tools and materials.

(c) Let the imagination run loose — Impossible ideas often point to something more practical. Try to see more than one solution.

(d) Select the most practical idea — Which idea is the most promising? the simplest? within present scope?

(e) Develop the article — Work out the details. Make a rough model or 'mock up'. Try it yourself or on another staff member. Refine it as necessary.

(f) Make a fair copy — You may understand your rough one, but the patient and others may be unable to accept your idea because of its presentation.

(g) Test and try — Take it to the patient and present it to be tried out. This gives both the patient and the 'inventor' a chance to retreat gracefully if all is not well. Make adjustments to suit the patient. Discuss these with him so that he feels involved.

(h) Supervise early use — This means ensuring that the article works satisfactorily before leaving it with the patient, and that other team members understand how it works. Regular enquiries as to the usefulness or problems of the article should be made.

Precautions

Ideas for problem solving may come from any member of the team, but should never be undertaken lightly. An article which could possibly involve risks to the patient should be passed by a professional person before being used. Some hazards of this kind are:

(a) Pressure to some area of the body which could cause ulceration.

(b) Friction leading to blisters or broken skin.

(c) Constriction of nerves or blood vessels.

(d) Injudicious splinting, putting joint function at risk.

(e) Use of materials to which the patient is allergic.

(f) Use of construction methods or materials which are not strong enough for the work required of them.

(g) Sharp points or edges which can cut or pierce if badly handled.

(h) Brittle plastic or glass components which create hazards if broken.

The safety of the patient and the 'inventor' are both served if new items of equipment are discussed with the team before they are finally put into use. The carpenter and the plumber and other tradesmen can give valuable help in this field as well as the medical and ancillary staff. Responsibility for the article and its results lies with the organiser unless team advice and acceptance has been sought.

Useful Materials and Tools

The materials and tools used in designing and making special aids are simple and easily acquired. Oddments and offcuts come into their own, because small quantities of a variety of materials are more helpful than larger quantities of a few. Some of the most useful items are regular hospital supplies, such as elastic bandages and adhesive tape. Others are available from various departments, e.g. unserviceable sheets from the linen room, offcuts from the maintenance department, and packaging material from the store. The tools which have proved most useful are listed in Appendix D.

The following materials have wide uses and may need to be ordered and kept in stock.

(a) A variety of sizes in nails, screws, tacks, staples and washers.
(b) A selection of padding and stuffing materials. Plastic foam in different thicknesses, foam plastic chips, cotton waste.
(c) A selection of threads, strings, twines and ropes, and wires.
(d) Adhesive materials for varied use. Paste for paper and cardboard, glue for wood, rubber solution for leather, and more specific adhesives if plastics or metal are to be used.
(e) Covering materials — head cloth, silk substitute, plastic sheeting, 'contact' adhesive plastic sheeting, leather.
(f) Supportive material — canvas, carpet binding, felt.
(g) Miscellaneous — cork sheets, plastic tubing, strawboard, plaster of Paris.

It may not be possible to order and store all these items, and the need for them will vary with the type of unit. In some units many of them will already be in use for patient activities. The list is included here only as a guide to the kinds of materials which may be helpful.

The Oddment Box

Whether or not there is access to new materials such as those mentioned above, a well-stocked oddment box should be organised. What it contains will depend upon local conditions, imagination and fate. Some more obvious items are empty cotton reels, old buttons and beads, jar lids, plastic food containers, disused belts and buckles, wooden and wire coat hangers, detached suspenders, hardware oddments, and similar flotsam and jetsam. Some less common items which have proved useful include suitcase fastenings, sample leather strips from a belt manufacturer, a handle from a dismantled door, broken broom handles, a variety of springs, bricks, burnt out kettle whistles, and lengths of pipe.

This list could be greatly expanded, but enough items have been listed to indicate the kind of thing which goes into the box. What comes out to be used will depend upon the need of the moment. Looking through the oddment box, and seeing strange or forgotten items can sometimes lead to a new and useful idea or a new twist to an old one. The oddment box is particularly useful in making the original 'mock up' before the item is finally produced with more orthodox materials. Its function is not primarily to reduce costs, but to provide a varied selection of materials and objects to start the ball rolling.

Some Specific Problems and Answers

In the following examples of problems which were solved by the use of equipment, it must be understood that thorough medical investigations, and treatment when it was indicated, preceded the decision to look for a mechanical solution to the problem. Problem solving with equipment is an addition to, and not a substitute for, medical care. It has its greatest value when there is residual disability which cannot be expected to resolve, or when the patient must function in the present, and cannot wait for some future return of function. Finding a solution to the problem by the use of suitable equipment is particularly helpful when the return of function is not assured. Some typical examples are given below.

Case 1. The Use of Basic Equipment

a. The Problem.
1. The patient needed a walking frame for all ambulation because of a painful osteoarthritic hip.
2. The patient needed to negotiate five steps to get out of the house and to get to her toilet which was outside.
3. The patient could not manage the steps with the walking frame, but could do so by turning sideways and holding the rail.

b. The Equipment. Solutions considered were a ramp, a chemical camping pot, and widening of the steps, and the provision of two walking frames. The last was decided upon as being practical, economical and immediate.

c. The Solution.
1. Two walking frames were provided, one for use in the house, and to the top of the steps, and one for use outside. The latter was parked within reach at the bottom of the steps.
2. The patient managed this arrangement well, and a side benefit was the ability to work in her garden with the outside walker and long-handled tools.

Case 2. The Use of Basic Equipment with Additions

a. The Problem.
1. The patient had been taught at another hospital to walk with the aid of two walking canes after a series of falls which led to a fractured femur. She was obese and clumsy, and still needed the support of both hands when walking.
2. The patient lived alone, and despite help from a housekeeper, Meals on Wheels, and a weekly visit to a day centre, there were many household tasks she needed to perform for herself. These were difficult and dangerous with two sticks to manage as well.

b. The Equipment (see Figure 19.1).
1. The patient was taught to use a walking frame instead of her two sticks.

2. A basic walker tray was fitted to a basic walking frame, and the patient was taught to use it in the retraining kitchens.

c. The Solution.

1. The patient was more secure in the walking frame than she had been with two sticks. She no longer tended to trip over her equipment, or drop it on the floor out of her reach.
2. The patient became independent with her lighter household tasks, but still had housekeeping help for the heavier ones.
3. She kept her two sticks for greater mobility when out and about, but used the walker and tray in the home.

Case 3. Adaptation of Basic Equipment

a. The Problem.

1. The patient was a bilateral above knee amputee with short stumps unsuitable for prostheses.
2. Her sitting balance was only fair, and she felt insecure on the basic bathboard.
3. The height of her own bath was 3 inches less than the level of the seat of her wheelchair.

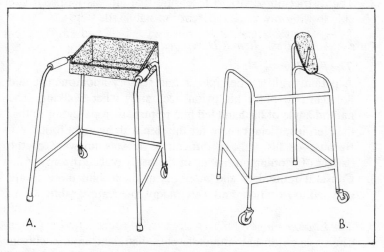

Figure 19.1: Adaptations to Walking Frames. A. A tray has been fitted to help a housewife carry necessary items from room to room and stove to table, etc. B. A splint is attached to help support a hemiplegic patient whose poor balance made a pylon stick unsuitable

4. She was blind.
5. Her frail, elderly husband could supervise and instruct, but could not give any help involving lifting.

b. *The Equipment.*
1. Two standard bathboards were joined longitudinally to give a wider surface.
2. Three-inch blocks were added under the boards to raise the height to match the wheelchair.
3. The cleats were lengthened to prevent the board from slipping on the bath.
4. A rail was attached to the back of the board to give the patient direction as she moved along it, and to support her back while she washed with a hose-type shower.

c. *The Solution.*
1. The patient practised the use of the board with staff members until she gained her confidence.
2. Her husband attended three sessions of training, after which both he and the patient could manage as a team.
3. The district nurse visited to ensure that all was well, but was able to withdraw once the situation stabilised.

Case 4. A New Basic Item is Developed

a. *The Problem.*
1. A patient with left hemiplegia and sensory impairment could not learn to place his pylon accurately when walking. The natural angle of his hand led him to turn its front legs in so that they left insufficient room for the step with his right foot.
2. Because of his sensory difficulties he was unaware of the danger of tripping on the leg of the badly placed pylon.
3. Constant reminders and attempts to make him more aware only led to irritation, and were in any case unprofitable.

b. *The Equipment.*
1. The basic pylon has its handle placed straight, in line with its base. Because of this a degree of external rotation is needed to place the walking aid parallel to the line of progress.
2. The patient could not make this adjustment because of his difficulties with body image and visuo-spatial relationships.
3. The patient's unsatisfactory placement of the stick was auto-

matic, and likely to remain so. The handle of the pylon was altered so that it was placed at an angle to the frame, in order to compensate for the natural angle of the hand. This allowed the patient to continue placing the stick automatically, while at the same time bringing the feet of the pylon down in the required line.

c. *The Solution.*
1. A rough model was made with a diagonal handle. This was turned inwards at the front and outwards at the back.
2. The model was tried with the patient and proved successful.
3. The patient was able to walk safely unsupported. Some supervision was still necessary pending his adjustment to left sensory neglect.
4. The difficulty is not an unusual one. Because the new handle proved effective for others the rough model was sent to the Rankin Park Work Training Centre where it was developed, refined, and put into production as the 'Fulton Handle'. The finished product has since been added to the basic equipment list.

Case 5. *Individual New Equipment*

a. *The Problem.*
1. A female patient with rheumatoid arthritis presented with her hips and knees fixed in extension. She was unable to rise or sit down again without being lifted onto her feet.
2. She lived with a relative who was away at work by day, but who could return to lunch at home.
3. They had worked out a programme whereby the relative put her on her feet in the morning, and left her to walk about until lunch time. Her only rest in this period was to lean on a verandah rail or the sink. When the relative became ill the patient was also admitted to hospital where the problem was fully investigated.
4. Surgery was not recommended, and it was essential for the relative to continue at work. Despite treatment, and some loosening of the joints the patient could not master the movement necessary to sit on a high stool.

b. *The Equipment.*
1. As the patient could only lie down or stand up, but could not

bend enough to sit, it was necessary to design a special seat.

2. The requirements of this seat were that the patient should be able to get on and off it unaided, and that she should be able to take her weight off her feet while her relative was away.

3. An old metal chair frame was used as a base, and a bar was welded across the centre of this from arm to arm. An adjustable bicycle seat was attached to this cross piece and fixed at a height which allowed the patient to shuffle backwards onto it. It was fixed at an angle which allowed her to sit on the wider part of the seat with the narrower front part between her legs. She could then relax on the seat and stand again using the small degree of mobility regained by exercise.

c.   The Solution.

1. When the relative was well again the patient was also able to return home with a much greater degree of comfort than she had known for some years.

2. Alteration to the height of the patient's bed, which had been too low for her needs, made the lifting done by her relative comparatively light, although some help was still needed.

Case 6. Gadgetry

a.   The Problem.

1. A patient with no return of function in his hemiplegic left hand found it difficult to tear off toilet paper, as the roll tended to run loosely as he pulled.

2. A container with folded sheets was considered, but the sheets could not be bought at his corner shop, and so this solution was discarded.

b.   The Equipment.

1. A gadget was made up consisting of a large rubber band, and a wire hook. The band was attached to one side of the toilet roll fitment; and the hook was clipped onto the other so that the rubber band held the roll in a stable position as the paper was torn. The hook could be released quite easily with one hand for the next sheet to be rolled off, and replaced for tearing.

c.   The Solution.

1. The patient mastered the use of this gadget at his first attempt,

and so a very simple idea overcame a small, but frustrating, difficulty.

2. The overcoming of small problems such as this is important for morale, and because it leaves the patient more energy to use in overcoming his many larger ones.

3. There are many gadgets on the market, and many more which have been developed in retraining programmes in different hospitals. This one is described as an example of how they can be developed if we ask 'how?' to overcome a problem, instead of accepting it as an inevitable nuisance.

Case 7. Adjustment of Clothing

a. The Problem.

1. A patient with Parkinsonism could not manage to pull up his own trousers, or to fasten them himself.

2. Pulling them up was beyond him because his balance was poor, and he needed to hold onto something when standing up. This left only one hand for pulling up the trousers, and when he let go to deal with the fastening, they dropped down again.

3. Fastening them was difficult, because of impaired dexterity as a result of his condition.

4. The patient was alone by day, and so help was not always available when needed. The patient was also embarrassed by his need for help with this function.

b. The Equipment.

1. A piece of ¾ inch elastic, long enough to be placed over his head was attached to the front and back of the trousers to act as a single brace.

2. A special fastening was attached to the top of the fly. This consisted of a leather 'keeper' on the right side, and a leather tongue on the right.

3. The leather tongue was long enough to pass through the 'keeper', and fold back upon itself, where it was secured with 'Velcro'.

c. The Solution.

1. The patient was taught to pull up his trousers while seated, and to place the elastic strap over his head.

2. He was then encouraged to stand up, holding his walker for

support. The elastic strap raised the trousers over the hips. They were then straightened if necessary with one hand.

3. The patient sat again, and used both hands for fixing the leather fastener. The leather tongue was placed through the keeper, and folded back to be pressed down on the 'Velcro' patch.

4. The patient then stood again, and pulled up the zipper with one hand. A small key ring attached to the tab of the zipper facilitated his grasp.

5. With a little practice the patient was able to be independent in managing his trousers, both at the time of dressing and in the toilet.

Case 8. Alterations at Home

a.   The Problem.

1. An elderly patient, with poor balance, and a minor degree of dementia, had been admitted because of a series of falls. She tended to be unaware of safety factors, and could not learn to avoid hazards. Her daughter, who lived with her, was anxious, and felt unable to leave the house.

2. A home visit led to the removal of numerous small mats, and attention to the placement of furniture to give less cluttered walking space.

3. The toilet was in a very small room added to the back verandah. It was realised that if the patient fell there it would be impossible to open the door to help her.

b.   The Equipment.

1. It was arranged that a son, who lived at some distance, but who was a 'handyman', should come and re-swing the door so that it opened out instead of inwards.

2. At the same time hand rails were placed in the toilet, as the patient was unable to learn how to turn her walker before entering the small room.

3. A sliding gate was placed at the top of the stairs which led off the verandah.

c.   The Solution.

1. Equipment helped in the solution of this problem, by eliminating some obvious risks, which were easily avoidable.

2. The daughter was further helped by attendance of the patient

one day per week at the day centre.
3. The practical help rendered by the son reassured the daughter that she was not as alone with the problem as she had felt, and she later remarked upon the value of this side benefit.

Case 9. Matched Equipment

This is not a description of one case, but of the procedure used in providing equipment for all bilateral lower limb amputees, and most paraplegics.

a. The Problem.
1. The patient who cannot bear weight on his lower limbs, even with the aid of a walking frame, must rely upon a wheelchair for his mobility.
2. Independence at this level means being able to move freely back and forth from other items of equipment such as his bed, commode, toilet pedestal, favourite chair, and car.
3. Elderly patients with this problem are usually neither very strong, nor very agile. Consequently, the fewer steps they must negotiate in these moves the easier their task will be.
4. The height of the basic wheelchair can be increased by a cushion, but it cannot be decreased.
5. For this reason it is the practice to match other equipment to the level of the seat of the wheelchair: 21 inches (53 cm) is the average height of the chairs used in the Newcastle Geriatrics Service, and the patients' equipment is adjusted accordingly.

b. The Equipment.
1. The patient is made comfortable in his wheelchair, with cushions if necessary.
2. His bed, commode, toilet seat, bath or shower seat, and easy chair are cut down or built up to match the level at which he sits in the wheelchair.
3. He is provided with a slide board for use when crossing a gap, or when a step cannot be avoided, as in his car.

c. The Solution.
1. The patient is taught to push up on his hands, until he can hold himself up off the seat of his wheelchair.
2. He is given practice in moving about on a flat surface, such as his bed, a sofa, or a wooden bench. The latter is useful if the

softer surfaces prove difficult. Moves should be made forwards, backwards, and to either side.

3. For the patient who is not to have a prosthesis it is helpful if the footplates are removed. This allows him to come right up to other furniture, and to use a smaller turning area than is otherwise necessary.

4. The simple expedient of matching the heights of his equipment usually leads to a dramatic improvement in the patient's independence, and consequently in his morale. It should be done as early as possible, whether or not he is to be fitted with prostheses. He can thus be independent long before he masters his prostheses, and at times when he must be without them for reason of repair, adjustment, or his own health.

Case 10. Equipment for Lifting

a.   The Problem.

1. A male patient of 25 was a virtual quadriplegic as a result of a myopathy developed in early childhood. In recent years he had become progressively obese, and his mother, who had done most things for him in the past, could no longer manage the lifting involved.

2. The patient's ability to help himself proved minimal, and little could be hoped for from treatment or retraining procedures.

3. His mother wanted to continue to look after him, whatever the cost to her own health.

b.   The Equipment.

1. Matched equipment and the use of a slide board were tried, but the task was still too heavy for a single helper.

2. It was decided that mechanical help was needed, and a small hoist, suitable for use in the home, was provided.

c.   The Solution.

1. The nursing staff were instructed to use the hoist in all the patient's transfers. In this way he became accustomed to the hoist, and learnt to trust it.

2. When the patient had gained his confidence, the mother was asked to attend the unit for instruction in its use.

3. Domiciliary services were offered to her so as to reduce the strain of her full-time task. Of these the day centre was particularly helpful, in giving her a free day, and giving the patient

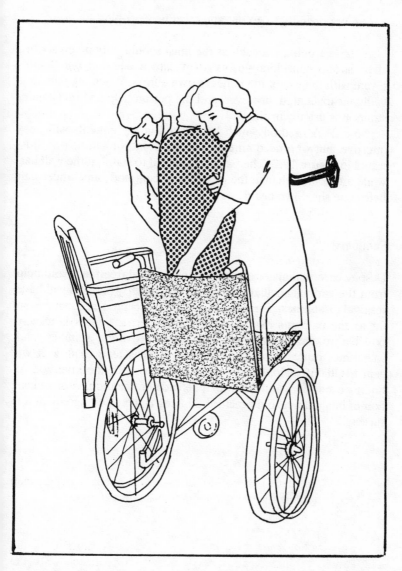

Figure 19.2: Early Commode Drill for Heavy Patient. Patient rises at the wall bar with help from two people. Chair and commode are changed and the patient sits again in the appropriate seat

an opportunity to go out and meet new people.

Note 1. Equipment such as the hoist should only be prescribed after careful consideration, as it involves a decision not to persevere with the use of the patient's own efforts. When the patient is badly incapacitated, however, and the person helping him is under strain, it is usually justified.

Note 2. A method which has helped heavy patients who may improve, but who need an easy starting point for self help is illustrated in Figure 19.2. The patient is helped to stand at the wall bar, while attendants change the positions of commode and wheelchair before he sits down again.

Summary

Despite careful diagnosis, medical and surgical treatment, and help from the various ancillary services, many elderly patients will have residual disabilities. These may have to be accepted as inevitable so far as the patient's own condition is concerned, but it is usually possible to ameliorate their effects by providing suitable, and sometimes quite individual equipment. Ideas tend to flow if we gain the habit of looking at such problems with the intention of finding a solution, and not with a defeatist resignation. A combination of imaginative and practical thinking is the chief ingredient for success.

20 TOOLS AND MATERIALS

The selection, storage and use of tools is important to the efficient running of a retraining unit. Safety measures are essential in their use and the staff should be aware of hazards with particular reference to individual disabilities among the patients.

Introduction

The tools and materials required in retraining are used by the staff in making and altering equipment as well as by the patient in creative activities. The balance between these two aspects of use determines the type and quantity of tools needed and the selection of materials which are likely to be used. A few good tools, well selected and well cared for, give better service than many cheaper ones which tend to bend, break and become blunt in even normal use. A wise choice of tools and materials can lead to savings both in money and in frustration and wasted time.

Tools

Basic tools for the major crafts have developed over many centuries and are ideally suited to the work they must do. 'Gimmicky' tools come and go as workers and others think of a new way to solve a problem, but they rarely do more than create a temporary fashion. It is wise when buying tools to choose the old familiar shape and a known manufacturer.

Before any tools are ordered it is wise to think out the aims of the programme, and to decide what activities are to be covered. Ordering should be directly related to those specific needs. Some institutions demand that a full list should be made, and all tools ordered when a new unit is being developed. This is wasteful and unnecessary. It is far more economical and practical to place a small basic order and make provision for acquiring more as the need for them is demonstrated. Many items which would be placed on a definitive list 'just in case', may never be needed if a more informal method of ordering is accepted. Basic tools which have proven value in retraining are listed in Appendix D. If the first method of ordering is insisted upon, a much fuller list will be required to cover future needs.

Preparing the List

In preparing the list, all the required activities should be set down as headings. Special requirements for each activity should then be listed under these headings. Tools which appear on more than one of these specific lists should be transferred to a general list to avoid duplication. The general list should also contain all the items needed for staff use in working on equipment.

In making these individual lists it should be remembered that only the simpler processes of any craft are likely to be attempted by the patients, and that it is not necessary to buy all the tools that would be needed by a professional craftsman. The basic list of general tools should be ordered first, and then as each new activity is added the list of required tools can be checked against this original list, and only those tools which are not already available need to be ordered.

Storing Tools

Storage space is usually at a minimum in retraining units and activity centres, and thought should be given to using it to its best advantage. Tools tend to be borrowed and not returned, put into work bags and otherwise mislaid if no adequate storage space is provided. This applies particularly to small items such as scissors, pliers and awls. The answer does not lie in throwing the tools together in one box. Firstly, they will blunt and bend each other by careless contact, and secondly, there is no way of telling at a glance that any individual tool is missing.

The Shadow Board. The most satisfactory way to protect and keep track of tools is to make a shadow board. This can be done by painting the outline of each tool on a firm board, or by cutting it out of adhesive plastic sheeting and sticking it on. Suitable nails or hooks are then inserted to support each tool over its shadow. Shadows may be placed upright on a wall board or on the back wall of a cupboard, or flat on a shelf, depending upon the type of tool and the space available. Some may be placed on the inside of a cupboard door, but it is necessary to ensure that moving the door will not dislodge the tools. Spring clips are usually needed in this situation rather than nails and hooks.

The shadow board has the advantage of making checking easy at the end of activity sessions, and of making it easy to find tools in a hurry, because each has its special place. If the supporting nails are correctly placed it also protects them from damage to their weaker parts and their cutting edges.

The Cutlery Drawer. Smaller tools which are not suitable for a place on the shadow board can be effectively housed in a partitioned cutlery drawer or container. If tools are kept in drawers partitions should be placed to separate them into categories, and to diminish the amount of friction between the tools. Even cardboard boxes placed in drawers can serve this purpose until more permanent fittings can be made or obtained.

A mass of mixed tools thrown haphazardly into a box is dangerous to the users, wastes time in endless searches for the right tool, leads to breakages and damage to cutting edges, and gives no indication that a tool is missing. For all these reasons the shadow board and the partitioned drawer are recommended.

Caring for Tools

The method of storage described above goes a long way towards caring for tools and preventing loss. The following factors should also be considered:

1. Have tools sharpened regularly by a competent person.
2. Ensure that all parts which need oil receive it regularly.
3. Clean tools after use whenever necessary.
4. Put tools away carefully after use.
5. Ensure that metal cutting edges do not contact hard or abrasive surfaces.
6. Have damage repaired as soon as possible after it occurs.
7. Teach staff members, and through them the patients, the correct care and use of tools.
8. Use the correct tools for the job, and discourage inappropriate usage.
9. Let the tool do the work. If correctly used, there should be no need to use great force.

Note. In the training course provided by the Newcastle Hospital for occupational therapy technical assistants' time has been allotted for a lecture and demonstration from a member of the maintenance staff on the care and use of tools. This has proved valuable not only to the individual assistants, but also to the hospital and the department concerned.

Some Precautions with Tools

Tools have made innumerable tasks possible for man which he could not have performed without them, but they can prove dangerous when used carelessly or incorrectly. This is particularly so with disabled people who may find difficulty in controlling or understanding them. The staff are responsible for ensuring that patients are not put at risk by the tools supplied to them or left within their reach.

Problems Caused by the Disability. Patients suffering from 'blackouts' or fits need special care. They should not be left unsupervised with piercing or cutting tools, nor placed where they may come into contact with heated surfaces or dangerous machinery.

Patients with only one serviceable hand will have difficulty with almost any tool if their work is not anchored securely. Weights, clamps, and non-slip surfaces can help to compensate for the absence of a holding hand. If the patient's dominant hand is affected there may be danger of tools slipping or going out of control until greater dexterity has been achieved in the remaining one.

Patients who have suffered loss of feeling in a limb, or who have poor recognition of their own limbs, should be protected from cuts, abrasions and burns which they may not be conscious of sustaining.

Acuity of vision should be considered when asking a patient to use a potentially dangerous tool.

Thought should be given to the safety of any tool given to a depressed or unstable patient, and care should be taken that no such tools are taken from the workroom.

Problems Inherent in the Tools. Power tools are not generally suitable for the elderly disabled person unless he has some previous knowledge of them and is still able to control them. The dangers may result from the speed being too fast for the physically disabled, the action being too strong for the frail, the concept being too difficult for the confused or demented patient, and electricity itself being too dangerous in the hands of those who may not treat it with due care and attention.

The previous paragraph is not to say that power tools should not be used by these patients, but that responsibility for ensuring that the tools are in safe hands rests with the staff.

Tools which employ heat have obvious dangers and should be treated with the same care as power tools.

Blunt tools should not be used. They should be sharpened as soon as possible after their condition is noted. The extra force needed to work them is beyond the power of some disabled people, and even if the power is there, a blunt tool is difficult to control and tends to cause accidents and injury if it slips.

When using sharp tools patients should be well seated and balanced. If possible, cutting should be done in a direction away from the body. Almost any tool can be dangerous if used in too confined a space, and sharp or pointed tools, particularly, should only be used if the worker has reasonable elbow room.

Staff Responsibilities. All staff members should be aware of their patients' needs and the dangers inherent in the tools they supply. Forethought and good supervision are necessary in every workshop. If despite these, an injury does occur it should be reported immediately to a senior member of the staff. Even minor injuries can prove troublesome if neglected, and what may seem minor to a younger person may have serious results for the old and frail. In the activity group as elsewhere, prevention is better than cure.

Materials

Tools are non-expendable items which are included in the inventory as permanent equipment. Materials, on the other hand, are expendable, being used up and replaced in the course of the work. They may come from many sources, and will vary from time to time depending upon current activities. Some may already be available to the group concerned, some may be used material for recycling, and some may have to be bought. At first, attempts should be made to discover what is readily available. Activities can then be built around such materials and there is no need to wait until an order has been passed by authority and filled by a business firm. It should not be necessary to purchase everything at high cost from a craft supplier.

As with tools, some materials serve basic needs for both equipment needs and crafts. Others only need to be ordered when a particular activity is to be introduced into the programme.

Ordering Materials

Most institutions have their ordering system well developed, and it is wise to find out what it is, and to comply with its rules. There will be items however, which are wanted in small quantities or at short notice which do not fit easily into the prevailing system. If it can be arranged, a small petty cash allowance is invaluable for these items. If the institution is unwilling to provide this, it is sometimes possible to approach a service club or auxiliary, or to hold a sale of work and raise money for the purpose. What course should be taken will depend upon the policy of the institution concerned, but some arrangement for small immediate purchases is needed.

If materials are to be bought from a commercial source it is usually cheaper to buy in large quantities. This is worthwhile with items which are in constant use and those which do not deteriorate with age. The savings are illusory if only part of the order will be used within a reasonable period. Losses will arise from deterioration, shop soiling, misplacement, and the prolonged use of valuable storage space.

Interest is usually fairly constant for major crafts such as woodwork, needlework, pottery, weaving, basketry, and potting plants, depending more upon the skill and enthusiasm of the helper than the interests of the group. Minor crafts on the other hand, seem to be subject to fashion, and what may be a craze at one time may be quite unwanted at another. Some examples are stuffed clowns, plastic lampshades, cut wool balls and shell-encrusted flower pots. Minimal quantities only should be ordered of materials for activities which are unlikely to have a lasting place in the programme, unless that material can be used for something else when the craze passes.

Salvage and Recycling

Much can be done to limit costs by using offcuts, disposable packaging, and recycled materials. One army hospital kept an average of 100 patients occupied with no official supply of materials for a period of nine months. This was accomplished by recourse to the salvage dump, the good will of local businesses and the ingenuity of interested people, both patients and staff. Some of the materials used were:

1. *From Salvage* — Wooden packing cases, lengths of string and cord, hessian bags, flour bags, various kinds of wire, nails, screws, and other hardware, cotton waste, and various shapes and sizes of discarded metal.
2. *From Local Businesses* — Leather offcuts, dressing and curtain material samples, wall paper books, parquet flooring blocks, broken lines in tiles, torn ends of newspaper from the local press, odd buttons and buckles, remnants of material, braids, and laces, tangled and damaged skeins of wool, good cardboard from photographic packaging and many others.

Using items such as these reduces costs for both the institution and the patients, and sorting, pressing, straightening, cleaning and polishing provide useful jobs for those patients who do not wish to make articles for themselves.

The art of using salvaged materials is to put them into good order before offering them to the worker. There can be pride in successful 'mend and make do' projects, so long as the finished article can bear comparison with a similar one made from new material.

Recycling materials are obtained by letting needs be known rather than by ordering in the usual way. Relatives, friends, service groups and hospital auxiliaries are fruitful sources of such materials as are some well-disposed shops and businesses. In some areas a service known as 'Reverse Garbage' may function, and recycled materials may be bought very cheaply. The possibilities of this kind of material are limited mainly by the inventiveness of the users.

The Choice of Materials

The Importance of Good Quality. When choosing materials to purchase it is not economical to take the cheapest without regard to quality or suitability for the job it is to do. It is wasteful and disheartening to do good work on poor material and to see it come to nothing. The quality should always be sufficient for its purpose. Cheap thin cord may make a reasonable looking landing net, but this is not an economy over a more expensive cord if the cheaper one breaks while holding a large fish. However good the knitting, a garment made from harsh, hairy wool will give little comfort to the wearer, and cheap hairy cane will not produce a smooth professional-looking basket.

There is usually some waste when poor quality materials are used, as the worst parts must be discarded. The usable part which is left may then prove very nearly as expensive as a better grade. If ordering must be done through an agent such as a purchasing officer, he should be made aware of the quality needs as well as being asked for a quantity. Tenders can only be compared if they relate to items of the same quality, and it is finally the patient who suffers if care is not taken at the time of ordering.

Choosing Colour Schemes. It is never wise to order 'assorted colours'. Such an order tends to be filled with those colours which are least popular with other buyers. Colour can be a stimulating part of craftwork, and it is well to have pleasant, cheerful colours available. If colours are bought to mix and match much better results will be achieved than from a collection of isolated colours which do not relate to each other. Ranges from dark to light in a few standard colours allows for more variety than many colours all of the same depth. The pattern we see depends more upon the arrangement of darks, mediums and lights than upon the actual colour used.

Suppliers should be asked for a colour chart for all materials where there is a choice, and the colours should be ordered to a considered scheme.

Gauges and Dimensions. When deciding which gauge or thickness of a material should be ordered, the main considerations are the durability of the finished article, and the ease of management by the user. Materials which are heavy need strong hands to work them, and materials which are fine usually demand good eyesight. These factors must be balanced against each other, and a compromise may be necessary in the middle range. Sturdy, reliable material is essential for materials to be used in making or altering equipment because accidents can result from materials which cannot bear the strains put upon them. Materials used by the patients should be chosen with their disabilities in mind. For instance, tapestry on coarse canvas will be more suitable than fine embroidery, and a shopping basket in medium cane better than a laundry basket in heavier grades.

Storing Materials

Many activity groups start with little more than a cupboard for storage, and it would be a rare unit indeed that had too much space for this purpose. The most can only be made of available space by care and organisation. It only takes one careless member in a team to spoil the best storage system, and in the process to damage many dollars' worth of material. For this reason responsibilities for storage should be carefully defined. In a large store separate areas can be allotted to different members of staff, and in a small one those who use it can take it in turn to be responsible for its care.

Some storage rules which have proved useful are:

1. Have a definite place for each item.
2. Have a box of suitable size for each item.
3. Do not place two different items in the same box without a partition between them.
4. Have a set of trays to carry boxes of small items. For instance, all nails, screws, cup hooks and other small hardware items on one tray, all 'Housie Housie' equipment and prizes on another, and all sewing requirements on a third.
5. Place all items which are rarely used in the inaccessible places, on the highest shelves, at the back of deep cupboards, and in corners. Christmas decorations are a prime example.
6. Place items which will have constant use at or just below eye level at the front of the cupboard.
7. Place large and heavy boxes at lower levels to overcome lifting problems.
8. Try to keep all the items which will be used together close to each other on the shelves. Woodwork in one area, games in another, needlework in another.
9. Mark each shelf with a distinctive colour, and each box which goes on that shelf with the same colour, so that misplacements can be seen at a glance.
10. Provide a place for people who are in a hurry to place things to be stored carefully later.
11. Have a regular place in the time table for cleaning out and tidying cupboards and boxes.

Certain kinds of material need special methods of storage. Some need to be stored away from heat, some are more vulnerable than others to dampness, some must be hung, and others must lie flat.

Poor storage methods can waste more material than the patients' use. Some of the more common special needs are:

1. Cardboard and thick paper should lie flat. If there is nowhere else they may be placed on top of the cupboard, or standing between the cupboard and the wall. They can rarely be used if left in a roll.
2. Almost anything that comes on a cardboard roll should be left on that roll to be stored. Thin papers, rug canvas, dress materials, adhesive plastic sheets, and book binding linen are examples. Rolls are easier to manage if placed upright in a tall box than flat on a shelf, and this also saves space on the shelf.
3. Materials bought on large reels store well if the reels are threaded onto a dowel rod supported on the wall or the end of the cupboard. Examples include 1 mm plastic tubing, some brands of string and twine, braids, and cords.
4. Items which might damage other materials should, if possible, be stored in a different cupboard, or at least on a separate shelf. These include all the 'wet' materials, such as glues, paints, polishes, putties and liquids, and 'dry' materials in powder form, such as plaster of Paris, powder colours, grout, chalk and whiting.
5. Always comply with storage instructions on the label of goods.
6. Sides of leather should be stored flat, or carefully rolled around a cardboard tube or roll of newspaper. This is to prevent damage from creasing. The surface can be protected by rolling the skin with the surfaced side turned inwards.

Much more could be written about the storage of individual materials, but these few examples have been given to demonstrate the need for thought in the method of storage which will lead to easy handling and to the protection of the item being stored.

Accounting and Disposal

Accounting Procedures

When activities are being introduced into an existing organisation the accounting system of that organisation will be established, and the new department will be expected to use it. Early discussions with the purchasing officer and storeman are recommended. More latitude is usually possible in a smaller independent organisation, but there will be more responsibility too. Storemen and auditors require exact and detailed records, but when a few people are responsible for all aspects of a complicated retraining programme, minute records of every item can bring the work with patients to a halt. Some people in authority may even see the activity part of the programme as a chance to make a profit. This is to misunderstand the very nature and purpose of the activities, and at its worst can lead to a form of exploitation.

The following points should be considered when deciding upon a reasonable accounting system.

1. Activities are provided to stimulate and motivate the disabled patient, and to this extent are part of 'treatment'. No patient should be excluded from the programme because he can't afford it.
2. Part of the stimulus to the patient comes from being able to decide for himself what he will do with the article he has made.
3. Some of the patients will have problems in learning ability and performance, and some wastage is inevitable if all are given a chance to participate.
4. Materials will be used in making and adapting equipment for treatment, and to this extent are in the same category as bandages, plaster of Paris, and prostheses.
5. Materials will be used in making gadgets to help disabled patients to perform independently tasks which would otherwise require help.
6. Materials will be used to make equipment for use in the department. Some examples are testing equipment, storage partitions, hand class items, games, percussion instruments and many others.
7. Materials will be used in group activities. Some examples are Christmas and table decorations, party hats, cooking ingredients, stage props for various entertainments, and materials for posters and notices of various kinds.

To keep accurate accounts for all the materials used in these different ways as well as for each individual patient is impractical and wasteful in itself. A compromise is for the hospital store to order and keep the main body of material and for small quantities in the workrooms to be supplemented as necessary by weekly orders on the main store. Accounting at the level of use is less detailed and stringent than in the base store, and depends upon the use made of the material.

In smaller and independent units materials are likely to go directly into the workrooms, and to attract the second form of accounting. The guidelines for this are:

1. Materials used mainly for departmental and retraining purposes are not costed individually unless an estimate is required by the administration. They are considered as part of the cost of the department. Some examples are pieces of equipment made for hospital use, standard aids for helping patients towards independence, adaptations and additions to basic equipment, material used in group activities, and material damaged in the course of use by a patient.

2. Materials used for the following purposes are costed: completed individual crafts; some individual aids which are outside the basic list; ADL equipment bought by visitors to the unit; items of equipment made for and supplied to other departments or institutions; and articles produced for sale through group projects.

3. The method used for costing the items in the second group is the cost of actual material in the item, plus 10 per cent of that cost to cover wastage and offcuts.

Disposal of Articles at the William Lyne Unit

1. The finished articles are not free to the patients, but are sold to them at the cost of materials plus 10 per cent as described above. Standard prices have been worked out for standard articles, but original articles are priced individually. Patients are encouraged to make articles which they want themselves, or which they wish to give as presents, to increase their involvement with the work, and so many articles are sold to the patients themselves.

2. So long as the standards of work are high there is a constant demand from members of staff and the public for hand made articles. If there is a patient for whom it would be good to fill an order, or if there is a suitable article not wanted by its maker, such sales are made. Orders are not taken as a business

to pose problems for both patients and staff. Articles sold to outsiders are priced at double the cost to the patient. Half the cost is returned to the hospital to cover the material, and the 'profit' is divided between the patient and a general patients' fund. The money in this fund is used to buy prizes for games, and other small comforts for patients.

3. Articles not wanted by their makers, and others made specially for the purpose can be sold at a sale of work. In this case the articles are listed, and the total cost is worked out before the sale. Price tickets are added, the price being the original cost plus whatever is thought reasonable in view of the standard of workmanship. At the end of the sale the cost of all items is returned to the hospital, and the 'profit' given to whatever cause the patients were working for. Unsold items are usually given to the hospital's auxiliary, who sell them for their own funds. These are presented as a contribution from the patients. This process has been described in detail, because disposal of 'unwanted' items can be difficult unless there is some regular channel for moving them on.

4. Sub-standard and damaged work provides a different problem. The patient concerned should not be distressed by seeing it discarded, but sales of work only keep the interest of buyers over the years if they gain a name for good articles and fair prices. It is best therefore, to unpick and recycle sub-standard work if this is possible without the patient's knowledge. If the material is unsuitable for recycling or if this will take more time than it is worth, the rubbish bin is the best place. It is useless to keep such items indefinitely, taking up shelf space to no purpose.

5. Particularly good work may sometimes be kept as a 'sample'. This gives a feeling of achievement to the maker, and is useful in encouraging and teaching others. Staff members may also make samples for demonstration purposes from time to time. These items can be costed in the usual way, and added to the department's inventory.

Conclusion

Whatever the attitude of the administration to accounting and the care of tools and equipment, it is the responsibility of the staff to

look after them and to use them carefully and economically. Ease
of workmanship, safety, and satisfaction in a good result depend
upon it, as well as the actual cost to the institution and the patient.

It is hoped that some of the concepts and procedures outlined in
this chapter will help newcomers to the activity aspects of retraining to avoid some of the more common problems encountered
even by 'old hands'.

APPENDICES

APPENDICES

APPENDIX A

GUIDELINES FOR ACTIVITIES OFFICERS CONDUCTING ACTIVITY GROUP PROGRAMMES FOR LONG-TERM AND GERIATRIC PATIENTS IN SMALL HOSPITALS AND NURSING HOMES

These programmes are conducted to serve the psychological needs of the patients. The activities undertaken must not be regarded as treatment, but as a means of stimulating and maintaining the patients' interest in the world around them.

If the programmes are to fulfil this function and make their full contribution to patient welfare, there are certain questions which must be asked and, if possible, answered, before patients are involved. Such questions are posed below, together with recommendations where appropriate.

Who Should be Involved?

(a) Who will have administrative responsibility for the scheme?
RECOMMENDATION: The Senior Executive Officer.
(b) Who will have responsibility for the medical aspects of the scheme?
RECOMMENDATION: The Matron.
(c) Who will be responsible for choosing patients to attend the group?
RECOMMENDATION: The Sister in charge of the ward.
(d) Who will be responsible for liaison between the Activities Officer and Nursing and Domestic staffs?
RECOMMENDATION: The Matron.
(e) Who will be responsible for liaison between the Activities Officer and outside agencies?
RECOMMENDATION: The Senior Executive Officer.
(f) Who will transport patients to and from the group?
RECOMMENDATION: Wardsmen or nursing staff.
(g) Who will plan and carry out programmes?
RECOMMENDATION: The Activities Officer.

(h) Who will be responsible for toileting and patient care?

RECOMMENDATION: A nurse allocated to the Activities Room during the time patients are there.

(j) Who will be responsible for submitting orders for equipment and material and finding sources of supply?

RECOMMENDATION: The Activities Officer with the cooperation of the Purchasing Officer.

(j) Who should be responsible for the actual ordering?

RECOMMENDATION: The Chief Executive Officer through usual stores organisation.

(k) Who will be chosen from the patients to attend the Activity Group?

RECOMMENDATION: Long-term patients whose morale can be maintained or improved by activity. At first, only willing and co-operative patients should be involved until the group is established. Then it should be possible to introduce a few difficult or withdrawn patients into an active situation with success.

(l) Who should decide if a patient is too difficult and is upsetting the group?

RECOMMENDATION: The Activities Officer after consultation with the Ward Sister.

What?

(a) What activities should be introduced?

RECOMMENDATION: Very simple crafts, social activities and group projects as suggested in Chapters 5–8.

(b) What equipment will be needed in the beginning?

RECOMMENDATION: Equipment as outlined in Appendix D.

(c) What expendable materials will be needed?

RECOMMENDATION: 1. *Bought through commercial suppliers*

Cane supplies, plastic, sewing supplies, stationery and art supplies, wool and knitting supplies, and materials for new crafts as they are introduced.

2. *May possibly be donated*
Offcuts or discontinued lines in masonite, tiles, parquetry floor fingers, dressmaking materials, vinyl tiles, wood veneer, old but good magazines, beads, Christmas cards, samples of wallpaper, ribbons, laces and other similar items.

3. *Prizes for games*
These should not be large, but some source of supply is needed. Handkerchiefs, soap, combs, stamped envelopes and similar items are used.

(d) What system of accounting should be followed?

RECOMMENDATION: This must depend upon local conditions but it should be kept as simple as possible so that time is spent with patients and their work rather than at book keeping. Patients should be allowed to keep any article made by them in the activity programme and pay for cost of material plus 10 per cent for wastage only. If the patient cannot afford to pay for the article but wishes to retain it, then some special arrangement should be made to allow the patient to keep the article.

If the patient does not want to retain the article, it may be sold to staff or visitors at the suggested price of twice the cost to the patient, as an encouragement to him. The patient should receive 50 per cent of the profit and 50 per cent should go to a fund from which all the group can benefit. Of necessity, these amounts are always small.

At no time should stress be put upon a patient by staff or visitors to make articles for sale as this can be detrimental to a patient and is quite contrary to the aims of the programme for patient welfare.

At no time can it be expected that the return from sales of materials will cover the costs of supplies.

(e) What procedure is to be followed in placing orders for:
  1. Expendable materials?
  2. Equipment and tools?
  3. Books of reference and ideas?
  4. Petty cash for small emergency purchases?

(f) What help will be available from:
  1. Nursing staff?
  2. Cleaners?
  3. Orderlies or wardsmen?
  4. Voluntary helpers?
  5. Local organisations, Service Clubs, concert parties, pianists, business houses, etc.?

(g) What furniture will be available?

RECOMMENDATION: If possible, patients should sit in chairs and not remain in wheelchairs. Chairs with steel-lined frames have been found most suitable. Arms are necessary for safety. Upholstered seats are advisable.

Tables to seat four patients are most satisfactory, as they can be arranged to suit a large or small group. Tables should be steady, but not too heavy to be moved with ease.

A trolley will be necessary to hold a tub of water for cane work and other activities if no sink is available.

Plenty of cupboard space is essential with storage capacity for both large and small items. Tidiness and elimination of waste through over-crowding both depend upon adequate storage facilities.

A solid table with good working top is necessary for preparation of work by the Activities Officer.

A shadow board for tools, a small notice board, and display cabinet for finished work and samples are all of value.

(h) What hours will be worked by the Activities Officer?
(i) What will be her rate of payment?
(j) What provision is there for increments?
(k) What are her other conditions of service?
(l) What are the local fire drill procedures?

Where?

(a) Where will the person appointed as Activities Officer be trained in the additional skills required to conduct the activity programme?

RECOMMENDATION: At the institution where the Supervisory Occupational Therapist is based or at an alternative venue acceptable to the occupational therapist.

(b) Where will the activities group programme be conducted?
(c) Where will materials, equipment and patients' work be stored?
(d) Where will the Activities Officer work with patients?

RECOMMENDATION: Only in the rooms provided to begin with. Work in the wards with bed-fast patients should not be attempted until the groups are a success. Both projects could fail if too much is expected in the early stages.

(e) Where can materials be obtained?

RECOMMENDATION: Some suppliers are listed in Appendix D, but these may be supplemented by local firms and by donations from friends of the hospital.

(f) Where is preparation to be done?

RECOMMENDATION: If two rooms are available, it would seem best to use one for patient activities and the other as an office, preparation room and store. Preparation and correction of patients' work should be done at the hospital in time provided and not in private time at home. This is mentioned as it is an occupational hazard.

When?

(a) When should the activity groups programme commence?

RECOMMENDATION: When orders have been placed and enough materials received to make it practicable. When the rooms and storage facilities are ready, when the Activities Officer has had time to prepare enough work in advance to make a good start, and when all the other people involved have been briefed on their role in the scheme.

(b) When should the patients be occupied in the groups?

RECOMMENDATION: This will depend upon local conditions — doctors' rounds, visiting hours, meals, etc. — but a pro-

visional time table is attached as
Appendix B.

(c) When can the Activities Officer see the Chief Executive Officer and/or Matron to discuss progress, problems and plans?

(d) When will there be time for shopping, preparation, looking for ideas, making up samples, etc.

(e) When can the Activities Officer return to a Geriatric Unit for follow-up training?

How?

(a) How are the activities to be supervised?

RECOMMENDATION: An occupational therapist should be present to give some supervision and consultation and be available to discuss problems and ideas both with regard to the activities and the method of introducing them.

(b) How can the activities be increased and varied in response to need and experience of local conditions?

RECOMMENDATION: In one month of training, it is only possible to absorb some basic principles and slight proficiency at a few simple activities.

It is strongly recommended that provision be made for the Activities Officer to return for further training when she has had a chance to put some of these into practice and to discover what her own needs and difficulties are.

(c) How many patients should form the groups?

RECOMMENDATION: For crafts and individual work, the maximum number at any one time should be 10. For singing, quizzes, housie and such group activities, the number will be limited by the size of the room. Over-crowding should be avoided, as elderly folk are difficult to move in and out of crowded rows, but the activity itself places little restriction on the size of the group.

(d) How will patients be allocated to the different groups?

RECOMMENDATION: By consultation between the Activities Officer and the Ward Sister. Withdrawn and reluctant patients usually do best if started in the social activities, only moving to the craft groups when their interest and co-operation has been gained. It should be remembered that the social group demands less of them than the individual work, and progress can be made from one to the other.

(e) How should the day be planned?

RECOMMENDATION: See the provisional time tables attached as Appendix D.

APPENDIX B

SOME TYPICAL TIME TABLES FOR RETRAINING PROGRAMMES OF VARIED INTENSITY

Some General Guidelines

(a) These programmes are offered for guidance only. They can and should be adjusted to suit the needs and abilities of each separate group.
(b) The activity programme should be seen as part of the retraining programme and not as an end in itself. It should provide interest and motivation to complement the physical aspects of retraining which are linked to all daily tasks.
(c) The retraining drills should be used every time the patient moves from one place to another. The Activities Officer should be as aware of this as other members of staff, and should be trained in the same procedures.
(d) The fact that there is an activities programme should never be seen as an excuse for neglecting the drills and other retraining procedures in the patient's daily life. Physical retraining in real situations is the basis of the programme.

Sample Time Tables

(a) One Half Day Weekly. For example, in a nursing home with a visiting Activities Officer coming one morning per week.

Time	Activity	
Up to 9.30 a.m.	Permanent staff ensure that patients are dressed and ready. They should attend to toilet needs and walk patients to the activity room, taking the opportunity to check walking patterns and chair drills. The visitor prepares the room and receives the patients.	
9.30 a.m.	Morning song	Sing a few songs well known to the patients. Add variety with rounds or action songs.
9.45 a.m.	Keep fit session	Choose suitable exercises from Appendix C. Vary them each week.

10.00 a.m.	Morning tea	Make use of this time to celebrate birthdays or other suitable occasions if there is an opportunity to do so.
10.15 a.m.	Individual activities	Provide a selection to suit many tastes and levels of ability. Crafts, games, hobbies, letter writing and simple cooking are all suitable. Involvement of the patient is the main aim.
12.00 md	Lunch	The Activities Officer says goodbye to the patients and proceeds with tidying up. Nurses take the opportunity for supervised chair drills, walking and feeding as necessary.

(b) Five Mornings per Week. For example, in a nursing home or small hospital with a part-time Activities Officer. A daily programme similar to the one above can be implemented, offering more variety over the five days.

Time	Mon	Tues	Wed	Thurs	Fri
Up to 9.30 a.m.	As in above				
9.30 a.m.	Morning song	Recorded music and discussion	Rounds and action songs	'Skiffle' band	Morning song
9.45 a.m.	Keep fit session — vary the choice of exercises each day.				
10.00 a.m.	Morning tea — Celebrate appropriate birthdays and special days. Encourage patients to help serve and collect cups if any are able.				
10.15 a.m.	Crafts and hobbies	Group games	Discussions and quizzes	Crafts and hobbies	Social activities (party, group entertainment, etc.)
12.00 md	Lunch as in (a) above				

Patients' Time Table in a Residential Retraining Unit

Time	Monday	Tuesday	Wednesday	Thursday	Friday	Saturday	Sunday
Up to	Preparation for the day — Rising, washing, toileting and dressing, receiving help as necessary, and instructions in methods which will lead towards independence. Supervised walk to dining area and breakfast. Walk to activities area, receiving help and instructions as necessary. Some patients may need a wheelchair, or may only manage to walk part of the way.						
9.00 a.m.	Morning Activities — Each patient is given an individual activity suited to his interests and abilities. These may be crafts, hobbies, games, puzzles, reading or writing. Patients will be taken singly from the group for medical or nursing procedures, baths, exercises.		Doctor's Round Patients move to the activity room when the doctor has seen them. Individual activities are provided.	Morning Activities — Individual activities as on Monday and Tuesday. Treatment changes will be made in the light of Wednesday's clinical meetings. Work will be finished for those going home, and new patients will be welcomed and introduced to the programme.		Grooming Day Nurses attend to hair, nails, pedicure, etc. Exercises and games are provided in the wards.	Church Service Or hymn singing for those who wish to attend. Exercises and games are also provided in the wards.
10.00 a.m.	Morning Tea						
10.15 a.m.	Continuation of Morning Activities					Unstructured period. Patient's choice, including television.	
11.30 a.m.	Return to the ward dining area. Supervised walking practice and chair drill. Lunch followed by a rest on the bed or unstructured activities of the patient's choice.						
1.40 p.m.	Patients move back to the activity room, receiving walking and chair drill instruction as before.						

Time Table Contd

2.00 p.m.	Group Exercises	Prepare for Visitors	Group Exercises	Prepare for Visitors
2.30 p.m.	Afternoon Tea			
2.45 p.m.	Group and Social Activities — These may include games, quizzes, parties, discussions, sing songs, etc.	Visitors	Group and Social Activities — as on Monday and Tuesday. The choice of activity varies daily.	Visitors
After 3.30 p.m.	Return to the Ward — Chair drill and walking practice. Frail patients are helped to undress. Tea. Prepare for visitors and bed. Television for those who want it. Supper and lights out. Night staff continue retraining procedures for patients who need attention for toilet or positioning in bed.			

Activities of Daily Living Assessment Form

THE ROYAL NEWCASTLE HOSPITAL
ACTIVITIES OF DAILY LIVING ASSESSMENT
(Functional Evaluation for Independent Living)

....
SIGNATURE
OCCUPATIONAL THERAPIST

U.R. ....

SURNAME MR. MRS. MISS
.... PLEASE PRINT NAMES .... GIVEN NAMES .... PLEASE PRINT NAMES .... SEX ...... AGE ......

ADDRESS ....

DIAGNOSIS: ....

KEY
{
+ + + + CAN DO UNAIDED
+ + + SUPERVISION FOR SAFETY
+ + NEEDS VERY LIGHT ASSISTANCE
+ NEEDS HEAVY ASSISTANCE
0 CANNOT DO
}

ACTIVITY	FIRST TEST	PROGRESS REPORT
	DATE	DATE
1. FEEDING		
USE CUTLERY		
CUT MEAT		
BUTTER BREAD		
DRINK		
CLEANLINESS OF EATING		
FOOD INTAKE		
MANAGEMENT OF MEDICATION		
2. BED		
GET INTO BED		
FROM LYING TO SITTING		
MOVE UP IN BED		
TURN OVER IN BED		
REACH BESIDE TABLE		
FROM BED TO STANDING		
3. DRESSING		
PULL CLOTHES OVER HEAD		
PULL UP PANTS		
SHIRT OR DRESS		
FOUNDATION GARMENTS		
FOOTWEAR: PUT ON/TAKE OFF		
FASTEN		
STOCKINGS/SOCKS		
DO UP AND UNDO BUTTONS		
FASTENERS		
CALIPERS, PROSTHESES, ETC.		
4. HYGIENE		
TURN TAPS ON AND OFF		
BATH/SHOWER		
WASH SELF AND DRY		
CLEAN TEETH/DO HAIR		
SHAVE/MAKE-UP		
ON AND OFF TOILET		
USE TOILET PAPER		
CONTINENCE		
NIGHT CARE		
SLEEP PATTERN		

078717

NAME ....   ACTIVITIES OF DAILY LIVING ASSESSMENT   U.R. No. ....

ACTIVITY	FIRST TEST DATE	PROGRESS REPORT DATE
5. MOBILITY		
WALKING — BRIEF OUTLINE		
FROM CHAIR TO STANDING		
SELF-PROPELLED CHAIR		
UP AND DOWN STAIRS/RAMP		
IN AND OUT OF CAR		
CROSSING ROAD		
USE PUBLIC TRANSPORT		
GET UP FROM GROUND		
6. COMMUNICATION		
SPEECH		
COMPREHENSION		
FOLLOW DIRECTIONS		
HEARING		
VISION/READING		
WRITING		
USE OF TELEPHONE		
7. DOMESTIC		
REACH HIGH/LOW CUPBOARDS		
COLLECT INGREDIENTS		
TRANSFER/KETTLE/SAUCEPAN		
SCREW TOPS		
TAPS, SWITCHES, ETC.		
LIGHT STOVE — GAS/ELECTRIC		
PREPARE VEGETABLES		
PREPARE AND SERVE SIMPLE MEAL		
WASH AND DRY DISHES		
TIDY UP		
DUST/SWEEP		
WASH CLOTHES		
IRON		
MAKE BED		
HANDLING MONEY		
GO SHOPPING		
8. GENERAL		
MOTIVATION		
SELF-ORGANISATION		
ORIENTATION — TIME AND PLACE		
ADJUSTMENT		
CONCENTRATION		
TEMPERAMENT		
9. ANY DIFFICULTY NOT NOTED ABOVE AND GENERAL REMARKS		
10. EQUIPMENT SUGGESTED		

078717

APPENDIX C

EXERCISE PROGRAMMES

General Exercises or 'Keep Fit' Group

These exercises are not presented as specific treatment, and there should be no pressure upon patients to hurry or try to do more than they can manage with comfort. They should be used in conjunction with the instructions given in Chapter 6, page 61. Some typical exercises are described here, but many others can be introduced from time to time to provide variety.

The Shoulder

1. Reach for the sky. Place your hands on your shoulders. Circle your elbows forwards and then backwards.
2. Place your arm outside the arm of your chair, and swing it loosely forwards and backwards like the pendulum of a clock. Repeat with the other arm.
3. Shrug your shoulders.

The Elbow

1. Reach out as far as you can in front of you.
2. Bend your elbow and place your hands on your shoulders. If one arm needs help, hold both hands together and bring them up under your chin.

Supination and Pronation

1. Tuck your elbows into your sides.
2. Hold your hands out with the palms turned up.
3. Turn your hands over until your palms face the floor. Turn the palms up again, and repeat.

Wrists

1. Move your hands as if you are having a really good wash under a running tap, and then shake the water off with loose wrists because you have no towel.
2. Rotate your wrists like the propellor of an aeroplane.

Hands

1. Open your hands as far as you can. Now make a fist and pretend to have a 'box on'. Open your hands again as far as you can.
2. Spread your fingers like a fan. Close them and open them. If one hand can't do this, place the fingers of the strong hand between the fingers of the weak one.
3. Pinch hard with your thumb and first finger, and then with your thumb and middle finger.
4. Twiddle your thumbs.

The Hips

1. Sit well back in your chair, and sit up as straight as you can.
2. Raise your feet from the ground, and place them well apart on the floor. Raise them again and put them back together. If necessary, help the weak leg with the strong hand.
3. Raise the right knee as far as possible, and then the left. Continue alternately 'marching on the spot'. (If the group is suitable, singing 'Pack up your Troubles', 'Tipperary', or some other marching song adds variety.)

Knees

1. Ask those patients who can stand safely to place their feet firmly on the floor, and their hands on the arms of their chair. Now lean forward, look at your toes, and stand up. Sit down slowly.
2. The staff should then go to those patients who cannot yet stand, and help and encourage them to do the same.
3. When seated again, raise first the right foot and then the left foot by straightening the knees. Hold the foot up for a few seconds before putting it back on the floor. If necessary, place the strong foot under the weak one and raise both feet together.

Ankles

1. Place the feet firmly on the floor. Raise the heels from the ground as if standing on the toes. Now place the feet flat again and raise the toes as if standing on the heels.
2. Cross the legs and rotate the ankles taking each leg in turn. Rotate in both directions.

Toes

Move your toes inside your shoes as if you are trying to wrinkle up the insoles.

The Trunk

1. Place your hands over the arms of your chair. Lean over as if you are trying to reach something on the floor. Go to one side and then the other.
2. Place your hands on your knees and run them down the front of your legs. Try to touch your feet. Patients with poor balance should not attempt this exercise without supervision.
3. Turn round to see what is behind you. If it is a person, give them a smile. First turn to one side and then the other.

The Neck

Patients who complain of dizziness or neck pain should not do this exercise.

1. Look up to the ceiling and then back. Look down to the floor, and then back.
2. Sit up, looking straight ahead. Turn your head as far as you can, first to one side and then to the other.

Grand Finale

If there is time and the patients are not too tired it is good practice to finish with 'Simon Says', an action song, or a seated version of the 'Hokey Pokey'.

The Mat Class

There are many movements besides those listed here which can be introduced into the mat class, but the ones given are those which link most closely with the retraining process. The bed drills are particularly suitable for practice at ground level. General strengthening exercises can be added if approved by a suitably qualified person.

Getting down to the floor and up again is itself one of the exercises, and patients should be taught a safe method for doing this. See Chapter 15 for method based on retraining principles.

Once the patient is down on the floor he is made comfortable, lying on a padded mat, and being provided with a cushion. He is then instructed in whatever exercises are suited to his condition.

Some useful exercises are as follows:

(a) Sitting up and lying down again.
(b) Rolling or turning from one side to the other.
(c) Moving backwards and forwards and across the mat.
(d) Turning right over to a prone lying position.
(e) Practising sitting balance.
(f) 'Propping' on either or both upper limbs. This involves sitting up for set periods, balancing on an extended arm.
(g) Moving into a crawling position.
(h) Coming to a kneeling position and practising balancing with the knees about 10 inches (25 cm) apart. (Throwing and catching a ball while kneeling can give variety to the exercise.)
(i) Sitting and balancing with crossed legs.

The Hand Class

Each patient is provided with a box or work bag containing a set of small common objects. Some suggestions are:

A match box containing 20 matches.
A handkerchief or piece of material of similar size.
A metre of thick string.
Three large beads threaded on to a length of 1 mm plastic tubing, knotted at each end.
A spring-type peg.
A small bean bag (3 inches × 2 inches/ 8 cm × 5 cm).
A ping pong ball.
A strip of material with a button on one end and a buttonhole on the other.

As well as these, the group as a whole should be provided with:

A length of cord to act as a clothesline.
A woolly ball about 5 inches (13 cm) in diameter.
A baton to pass from patient to patient. With two batons a 'relay' race may be included.

The exercises involve handling and manipulating these items. The list is not complete, and an interested leader will introduce ideas of her own. Some of the usual exercises are:

(a) Pass the woolly ball round the circle, in both directions.

(b) Throw the ball from patient to patient.

(c) Tip the matches out onto the table, and put them back in the box one at a time.

(d) Pick up the threaded beads, undo the knot and unthread the beads. Now thread them again and tie the knot.

(e) Take the length of thick string and tie a reef knot with the ends to make a circle. Put it over your head and round your neck like a string of beads. Take it off again and place it on the table to make a circle. Push the string with your finger so that it draws a face in profile.

(f) Ask every second patient to hold the clothesline steady. Those patients who are not holding the line, peg your handkerchief onto it. Now hold the line while the others peg their handkerchiefs. Repeat to unpeg the handkerchiefs.

(g) Place the handkerchief on the table and fold it neatly.

(h) Put the buttonhole strip on your knee and do up and undo the button.

(i) Place the bean bag on the back of your hand, and try to throw it up and catch it. Then transfer it to the back of the other hand and do the same.

(j) Put the string on the table and place the bean bag on the string. See if you can lift the bean bag with the string without it falling off.

APPENDIX D

TOOLS AND EQUIPMENT

Note. Every equipment list should be made with the needs of the individual institution in mind. A general list such as this can only serve as an indication of the type of equipment which might apply. The list given here is a general one, and many different activities could be introduced if such tools were available. Extra tools would be needed if more specialised crafts such as weaving, pottery or metal work were contemplated.

Tools needed for the making and adaptation of retraining equipment have been included so that they can serve a double purpose.

A Basic Tool List (Departmental Use and General Crafts)

Saws	Tenon saw — 12 inches (30 cm)
	Hand saw — 20 inches (50 cm)
Hammers	Claw hammer
	Tack hammer
Drill	Hand drill
	Set of bits for hand drill
	Rose counter sink
Plane	Smoothing plane — 8 inch × 1¾ in cutter (20 × 4.5 cm)
Screw drivers	Ratchet type — ⅜ inch (1 cm)
Pliers	Flat nosed with side cutter
	Round nose pliers·
	Diagonal nippers
Vice	Table vice
	Bench vice if a bench is available
	G clamps — 4 in (10 cm)
Rules and Squares	Folding rule — 3 foot (1 metre)
	Metal ruler — 12 in (30 cm)
	Metal straight edge — 24 in (60 cm)
	Metal set square — 15 in (38 cm)

444

	Perspex set squares — 45°, 8 in (20 cm)
	60°, 10 in (25 cm)
	Tape measure — 60 in (150 cm), metal ends
Knives	Stanley knife or equivalent with blades
	Bootmaker's knife — 4 in (10 cm) blade
Cutting Board	Cutting board or plate glass sheet — 18 in × 12 in (45 cm × 30 cm)
Punches	Revolving leather punch, six way
	Punch and eyelet pliers
	File punch (adjustable)
	Tools for inserting press studs
	Stapler, with long arm if possible
	Single hole punch — ⅛ in (3 mm)
	Nail punch
Awls etc.	Awl, long sharp point for piercing
	Awl, shorter blunt point for scoring
	Marlin spike
	Large straight bodkin, or refrigerator ice pick
Scissors	Cutting out shears — 8 in (20 cm)
	Scissors, blunt/sharp — 6 in (15 cm)
	Cutting out scissors — 7 in (18 cm)
Needles	Assorted sewing needles, particularly in larger sizes
	Darning
	Crewel
	Chenille
	Tapestry
	Packing needles
	Knitting needles, assorted metal types
	Crochet hooks, assorted metal types

Note. The following equipment can make a useful contribution to any programme for social stimulation, but being larger items it may not be possible to obtain them in the early stages of development. They do make suitable items to request if a donation is offered, or for the group as a whole to work for raffles, sales of work, and other fund raising activities.

Music	Record player with suitable records
	Piano
Household	Sewing machine
	Steam and dry iron
	Ironing board
	Electric fry pan
	Electric kettle
Games	Quoits
	Skittles or nine pins
	Indoor bowls
	Croquet mallets and hoops
	Mini golf

Equipment for Games

Note. The choice of games to be played, and therefore the equipment required, will depend upon the mental and physical abilities of the group concerned. No definitive list is possible but the following items have proved useful for a wide range of people.

Type of Game	Equipment
Blackboard	Blackboard and chalk, or
	Full sheets of 'butcher's paper' on a heavy sheet of cardboard. Writing in heavy black felt pen.
Table games	Boxed games to suit group. May include — Housie Housie, scrabble, checkers, draughts, ludo, dominoes, and others.
	Dice, dice box, score pads and pencils for beetle and other games.
	Cards, card holders for those who cannot hold a hand, and scorers.
	A tray holding small prizes such as combs, handkerchiefs, cakes of soap, sweets, fruit, plastic beakers or stamped envelopes.
Circle games	Bean bags to pass to music.
	Spring pegs to place on patients who are 'out' so that they can continue in the circle.

Quoits and pegs.

Soft balls and balloons for throwing between patients.

Floor games — Large cardboard sheets marked out to suit individual games and placed on the floor for play, e.g. waves for a fishing game, 'Hop Scotch' — throwing but not hopping, or a large 'dart board' for use with bean bags, waste paper baskets and balls for floor basket ball.

Quoits and a marked circle for modified deck quoits.

Outdoor games — Sunken jam tins, a golf ball and a putter for mini golf.

Hoops, ball and sticks for croquet.

Floor 'Darts'

The players take it in turns to throw small bean bags onto the board. They score when the bags fall wholly within the lines. The rules can be modified to suit the abilities of the group. More skill is required if the numbers must be taken in sequence.

Fishing

Rods are made of 8 mm handle cane, a length of string, and a toy magnet. The fish are cut out of fine cardboard, in assorted sizes and shapes. A paper clip is attached to the head of each fish. The fish are numbered for size, and placed on the board. The winner is the player who makes the highest catch.

Noughts and Crosses

Large cut out letters or bean bags of two different colours can be used to play this game. Players take turns to place their pieces. The aim is to get three in a row, across, down or diagonally, and to block the opponent from doing so. Pieces can be thrown into position, or moved by foot or with a stick.

Modified 'Hop Scotch'

Players throw a bean bag into each square in turn. When they reach home they place their team colours on any square they choose. The team which wins the most squares wins. In case of a tie the teams play off for 'home'.

Equipment made by Staff or Members of the Group

Waste paper baskets or bins. Covered or painted tins or cartons serve well.

Covered or painted boxes to place on shelves.

Work bags in various sizes. Both envelope and string pull varieties.

Labels for marking work. Tie on variety.

Knee rugs. Knitted or crochet squares, or patch work.

Cushions. Various sizes and shapes, including small 'bolsters' are useful.

Bean bags in various sizes.

Cut wool balls.

Skiffle band instruments.

Large Housie cards and counters.

Floor board games on large cardboard sheets (full Imperial).

GLOSSARY OF TERMS

Note. Technical terms are avoided in the retraining programme whenever possible because of the wide range of people who need to understand what is being discussed. For the same reason they have not been used in this book. There are, however, some ordinary terms which have come to have a more specific meaning in the retraining context, and these are defined in this glossary.

Word or Phrase	*Specific Meaning in Retraining*
Activity	Any occupation or function undertaken by the patient in the course of retraining.
• Nurse	A nurse who works in the retraining area as a full-time member of the retraining team.
• Sister	A Registered Nurse who is responsible for the retraining programme as it applies to nurses, and acts as a liaison officer between the nursing staff and the rest of the team.
• Nursing	The philosophy by which retraining activities and attitudes are incorporated into everyday nursing routines.
ADL	The activities of daily living.
• Assessment	An assessment of the patient's abilities and problems in caring for himself.
• Form	The form on which the details of the ADL Assessment are entered.
Back Slab	A splint placed behind the knee to support it in weight bearing.
Build Up	Any method used to raise the height of equipment such as beds, chairs, bathboards, boots, etc.
Day Centre	An organised group of patients who attend by day for activities and social contacts, but return home in the evening.
Day Hospital	As above, but also providing medical treatment.
Disability	A thing or a want that prevents one doing something.

449

• Residual	A disability which remains after treatment, and must be accepted as long-term or permanent.
Drill	A series of moves performed repetitively until they are perfected and become automatic.
• Bed Drill	The moves involved in getting in and out of bed, and in turning over, sitting up, etc.
• Chair Drill	The moves involved in standing up and sitting down, and in moving from one seat to another.
Elderly	Getting old. There is no fixed time of onset, and physiological rather than chronological ageing is inferred.
• Frail elderly	Elderly folk who need help in varying degrees for comfort and safety in everyday living.
Equipment	Articles used to help overcome disabilities.
• Basic Equipment	Those items which are used routinely in retraining and are stocked for immediate issue to patients for use after discharge.
• Personal	Equipment made or adapted to suit the
• Equipment	needs of an individual patient.
Gadget	Any small piece of equipment which helps a patient perform a task which would otherwise be difficult or impossible.
Geriatrics	The medical discipline which deals with the diseases of old age.
Gerontology	The study and science of the ageing process.
Goals	The aims which are set by the team in treating the patient, or which he sets himself.
• Intermediate	Small achievable goals, tackled one at a time, leading towards a larger, but more distant goal.
Helper	Any person assisting the patient with his retraining procedures.
Handicap	Any factor which makes it difficult for a patient to succeed in everyday tasks or to attain some specific goal. They may be physical, psychological, emotional or social in nature.

Job Breakdown	The analysis of a task so that its component parts can be tackled one by one in order to complete the whole by easy stages.
Lone Liver	A person who lives alone.
● 'Loner'	A person who enjoys his own company and dislikes group or co-operative activities.
Mock-up	A rough model of a new piece of equipment or adaptation in the development stage.
Night Care	The help needed by a disabled person during the night for toilet use, positioning in bed, or as a result of changed sleeping patterns.
Old Age	A time which varies in onset with different people, but in which physiological, mental and social deterioration tends to occur. The later stages of the ageing process.
Old Stroke	A previous stroke, the results of which are still evident and must be considered in current retraining plans.
Over Designed	Too complicated for its purpose, or made of too heavy a grade of material, and so unnecessarily expensive, or even unsuitable.
Placement	A euphemism for admission to permanent care in an institution.
Pylon	A wooden quadripod as used in the Newcastle retraining programme.
Quadripod	Any walking aid which is held in one hand and has four feet. Usually applied to the commercial metal varieties.
● Quad Stick	A colloquial term for quadripod.
Retraining	The process by which a patient who has disabilities as the result of disease or injury is brought back to as high a level of performance as he can attain.
Rehabilitation	Restoring a person to his place in the community. Used in the retraining unit to describe the end result rather than the process.
Relative	Used loosely of anyone who cares for the patient and takes responsibility during his illness. It may be used of a close friend or

neighbour as well as blood relations.

Rocking
Rhythmical swaying backwards and forwards or from side to side to help a patient initiate a required movement.

Social Neglect
The isolation of a person in the community, often leading to mental or physical deterioration or emotional problems.

Team
All those who work together in the retraining programme. This includes the relatives and the patient as well as all grades of staff.

Transfers
Movement from one situation to another, such as from bed to chair, or a chair onto the bathboard. The processes by which such moves are achieved.

Wall Bar
A bar placed on a wall, and preferably near a window, to be grasped by patients when practising standing and balancing.

Walking Frame
A metal walking aid with wheels at the front and rubbers at the back. Used for patients with problems of balance or weight bearing. bearing.

•Walker
The popular and more usual name for a walking frame.

INDEX

453